Supervised and Unsupervised Data Engineering for Multimedia Data

Scrivener Publishing
100 Cummings Center, Suite 541J
Beverly, MA 01915-6106

Advances in Data Engineering and Machine Learning

Series Editor: Niranjanamurthy M, PhD, Juanying XIE, PhD, and Ramiz Aliguliyev, PhD

Scope: Data engineering is the aspect of data science that focuses on practical applications of data collection and analysis. For all the work that data scientists do to answer questions using large sets of information, there have to be mechanisms for collecting and validating that information. Data engineers are responsible for finding trends in data sets and developing algorithms to help make raw data more useful to the enterprise.

It is important to have business goals in line when working with data, especially for companies that handle large and complex datasets and databases. Data Engineering Contains DevOps, Data Science, and Machine Learning Engineering. DevOps (development and operations) is an enterprise software development phrase used to mean a type of agile relationship between development and IT operations. The goal of DevOps is to change and improve the relationship by advocating better communication and collaboration between these two business units. Data science is the study of data. It involves developing methods of recording, storing, and analyzing data to effectively extract useful information. The goal of data science is to gain insights and knowledge from any type of data — both structured and unstructured.

Machine learning engineers are sophisticated programmers who develop machines and systems that can learn and apply knowledge without specific direction. Machine learning engineering is the process of using software engineering principles, and analytical and data science knowledge, and combining both of those in order to take an ML model that's created and making it available for use by the product or the consumers. "Advances in Data Engineering and Machine Learning Engineering" will reach a wide audience including data scientists, engineers, industry, researchers and students working in the field of Data Engineering and Machine Learning Engineering.

Publishers at Scrivener
Martin Scrivener (martin@scrivenerpublishing.com)
Phillip Carmical (pcarmical@scrivenerpublishing.com)

Supervised and Unsupervised Data Engineering for Multimedia Data

Edited by

Suman Kumar Swarnkar

J P Patra

Sapna Singh Kshatri

Yogesh Kumar Rathore

and

Tien Anh Tran

Scrivener Publishing

WILEY

This edition first published 2024 by John Wiley & Sons, Inc., 111 River Street, Hoboken, NJ 07030, USA and Scrivener Publishing LLC, 100 Cummings Center, Suite 541J, Beverly, MA 01915, USA

For more information about Scrivener publications please visit www.scrivenerpublishing.com.

Wiley Global Headquarters
111 River Street, Hoboken, NJ 07030, USA

For details of our global editorial offices, customer services, and more information about Wiley products visit us at www.wiley.com.

Library of Congress Cataloging-in-Publication Data

ISBN 978-1-119-78634-4

Front cover images created with Adobe Firefly
Cover design by Russell Richardson

Set in size of 11pt and Minion Pro by Manila Typesetting Company, Makati, Philippines

Printed in the USA

10 9 8 7 6 5 4 3 2 1

Dedication

To everyone who made this book possible, I recognize your efforts from the depth of my heart. My Parents, my Wife, my Son, Colleagues of the Computer Science and Engineering Department, the Institution head and the faculty members of Shri Shankaracharya Institute of Professional Management and Technology, Raipurwithout you people this book wouldn't have been possible. I dedicate this book to all of you.

Dr. Suman Kumar Swarnkar

To everyone who made this book possible, I recognize your efforts from the depth of my heart. My Parents, my Wife Sumitra, my Son Yuvraj, Colleagues of the Computer Science and Engineering Department, the Institution head and the faculty members of Shri Shankaracharya Institute of Professional Management and Technology, Raipurwithout you people this book wouldn't have been possible. I dedicate this book to all of you.

Dr. J P Patra

I would like to express our sincere gratitude to everyone who made this book possible. My Father Late S.L. Rathore, my Mother, my Wife Pooja, my Son Shivank, my Daughter Priyanshi, all my family members, Colleagues of the Department of Computer Science and Engineering and management of Shri Shankaracharya Institute of Professional Management and Technology, Raipur for their support and timely advice. I gladly dedicate this book to all of you.

Mr. Yogesh Kumar Rathore

Book Description

In the ever-evolving age of technology, Artificial Intelligence (AI) and Multimedia Data Engineering have become increasingly important tools for understanding and manipulating data. As AI and multimedia data engineering work together to create new technologies that can help us in our daily lives, it is essential to understand how these concepts interact with each other. This article will provide an overview of Artificial Intelligence and Multimedia Data Engineering, as well as their implications on modern society. Recent advances in AI have been aided by the development of multimedia data engineering techniques, which allow us to collect, store, analyze and visualize large amounts of information. By combining these two fields together we can gain a better understanding of how they interact with each other. The ability to extract meaningful insights from various types of datasets is becoming increasingly important in order to make decisions based on accurate data-driven analysis.

Contents

List of Figures

List of Tables

Preface

Artificial intelligence (AI) is a rapidly growing field of engineering that has the potential to revolutionize the way we interact with machines, process data, and even see our world. Multimedia Data Engineering (MDE) is an important branch of AI which focuses on how machine learning algorithms can be used to analyze and interpret large amounts of multimedia data. With this article, we will explore how AI technologies are utilized in MDE and the benefits they bring to professionals working in this domain.

At its core, MDE combines AI techniques with traditional computer science principles to make sense of vast amounts of multimedia data. By leveraging advances such as facial recognition technology, natural language processing tools, text-to-speech applications and more, engineers are able to transform unstructured data into valuable insights for businesses.

The research papers of this issue are broadly classified into current computing techniques, Artificial intelligence and Multimedia Data Engineering and implementation.

The editor thanks all the reviewers for their excellent contributions to this issue. I sincerely hope that you will enjoy reading these papers, and we expect them to play an important role in promoting advanced computing techniques and implementation research. I hope that this issue will prove a great success with the exchange of ideas, which will forester future research collaborations.

Dr. Suman Kumar Swarnkar
Department of Computer Science and Engineering Shri Shankaracharya Institute of Professional Management and Technology Raipur, Chhattisgarh, India
Dr. J P Patra
Department of Computer Science and Engineering Shri Shankaracharya Institute of Professional Management and Technology Raipur, Chhattisgarh, India

Dr. Sapna Singh Kshatri
Department of Computer Science and Engineering Shri Shankaracharya Institute of Professional Management and Technology Raipur, Chhattisgarh, India
Yogesh Kumar Rathore
Department of Computer Science and Engineering, Shri Shankaracharya Institute of Professional Management and Technology Raipur, Chhattisgarh, India
Dr. Tien Anh Tran
Vietnam Maritime University Haiphong, Vietnam

1

SLRRT: Sign Language Recognition in Real Time

Monika Lamba[1]* **and Geetika Munjal**[2]

[1]*Department of Computer Science and Engineering (CSE), The NorthCap University, Gurugram, India*
[2]*Amity School of Engineering and Technology, Amity University, Noida, Uttar Pradesh, India*

Abstract
An application called Sign Language Recognition (SLR) can recognise a variety of non-identical letter movements and translate them into text. In the area of science and technology, this application is extremely significant. It can be used in a variety of machine learning-based applications, including virtual reality. The purpose of the chapter is to develop a convolutional neural network that will recognise the signs captured or focused from the video capture and in turn provide us with correct or accurate output based on text and to improve the accuracy of the real-time sign language recognition via scanning and detecting that would aid other physically challenged individuals. For all individuals who want assistance in communicating with the rest of society, it offers an offline application. In order to produce quick, precise results and to ensure that the material isn't lost during the evaluation process, it tries to evaluate gestures more efficiently. Real-time sign language recognition involves first identifying images from a video feed that has been acquired using a machine learning model, then identifying edges and vertices, and then determining the desired result using a convolutional neural network. This method will be carried out at runtime to obtain results continuously while creating sign language with very little wait time utilising the CNN model. Character identification will be easier with this approach, and sentences can be constructed with high levels of accuracy using fewer letters.

***Keywords*:** Language recognition, real time, sign, convolutional neural network, machine learning

**Corresponding author*: missmonikalamba@gmail.com

Suman Kumar Swarnkar, J P Patra, Sapna Singh Kshatri, Yogesh Kumar Rathore and Tien Anh Tran (eds.) Supervised and Unsupervised Data Engineering for Multimedia Data, (1–26) © 2024 Scrivener Publishing LLC

1.1 Introduction

Nowadays, technology has taken an advanced leap forward in terms of improvement and efficiency. One of the many technologies that have taken such steps is Real Time Sign Language Recognition. Sign language recognition is an application to detect various gestures of different characters and convert them into text. This application has a huge importance in the field of science and technology. It has different applications based on machine learning and even in virtual reality. There are various types of sign languages such as ISL (Indian Sign Language) [1], BSL (British Sign Language) [2], ASL (American Sign Language) [3] and many more implemented differently at different parts of the world. Our aim is to apply American Sign language for sign to text recognition [3] [4] [5]. The American sign language is similar to other normal languages in that it can be expressed using gestures like hand or body movements. Although it shares many characteristics with other languages, it does not have English-like grammar. It is the most widely used sign language on earth. It is primarily used in nations like America, Africa, and much of southeast Asia. American sign language serves as a link between the deaf and hearing communities. They can textually describe their actions with the aid of this programme. This type of work has also been done in the past, with each instance producing unique outcomes and approaches, although few of them meet the standards for excellence.

The overall expansion of this language has been aided by its use in places like schools, hospitals, police stations, and other learning facilities. Since it is widely regarded as being simple to comprehend and fully independent of context, some people even choose to talk using this language. There are instances where newborn infants will receive this language from their mothers as their mother tongue. In fact, this is how sign language is meant to be understood. Figure 1.1 shows a visual representation of alphabets as signs.

Structure, grammar, and gestures are typically where sign languages diverge from one another. Unlike other sign languages, American Sign Language has a single-headed finger spelling alphabet. Compared to others, it is simpler to implement and interpret. The motions were also developed with consideration for various cultural traditions. Because people are accustomed to these gestures throughout their lives, this in turn draws a larger audience. The two-handed nature of BSL communication makes it difficult for non-BSL users to comprehend and interpret the language [5].

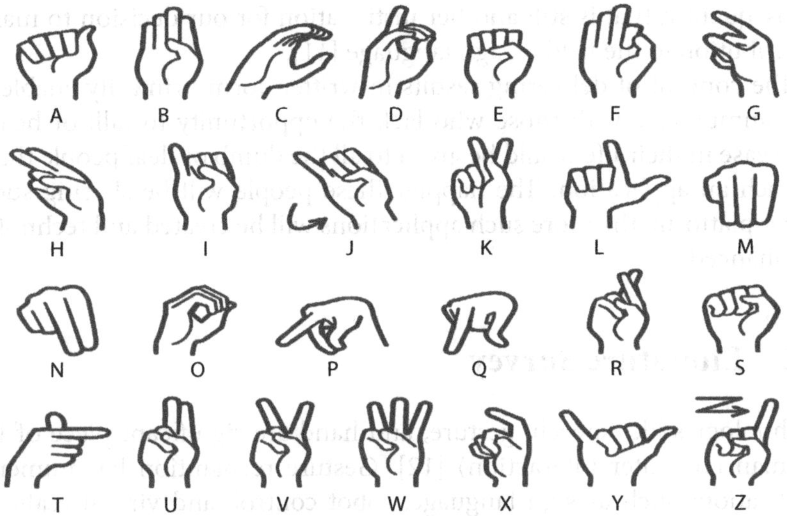

Figure 1.1 Basic sign language for each alphabet known characters.

The ISL is a well-known sign language in India; yet, because there are fewer studies and sources for accurate translations and because ASL has a larger audience, many individuals prefer ASL to other sign languages [6]. The ISL also has numerous identical motions with different meanings, which can be confusing when translated, even though all of these languages take roughly the same amount of time to translate letters and words. We needed ASL as the sign language converter because it is a more widely spoken language than English [7] [8].

The most fundamental need in society is for effective communication. Deaf and dumb people struggle greatly every day to communicate with regular people. Because those who are deaf or mute need to have their proper place in society, such an application was desperately needed. They experience secondary issues like loneliness and despair as a result of their basic weakness; thus it would be preferable if they could integrate more socially and forge more social ties [9] [10].

People also frequently offer alternative solutions, one of which is, "Instead of utilising another language to communicate, why don't deaf people just write it down and display it instead?" This explanation may appear reasonable and enticing from the perspective of a person without this disability, but the people who are experiencing these challenges require human solutions to their problems. These people need to express their feelings and activities, which cannot be done solely through writing.

Consequently, that is still another justification for our decision to make a contribution to the field of sign language [11].

The concept of delivering results in written form primarily enables us to communicate with those who lack the opportunity to talk or hear. A little ease in their life would be given to all the dumb or deaf people thanks to such an application. The happier these people will be sharing such a larger platform, the more such applications will be created and technology is enhanced.

1.2 Literature Survey

Technologies like speech, gesture, and hand are significant piece of HCI (human computer interaction) [12]. Gesture recognition has numerous applications such as sign language, robot control, and virtual reality. In the proposed method of Zhi-hua Chen [13], hand recognition is grounded on finger recognition and hence, it is more effective and uses a simpler rule classifier. The rule classifier used in real-time applications is highly efficient. The author used a simple camera to notice hand gesture rather than using data glove and special tape which are much more expensive. It includes fingers, hand detection, palm segmentation and hand gesture recognition. In the very first step, i.e., hand detection, the colour of the skin is measured using HSV model and the image is resized to 200 x 200. The output of this step generates a binary image in which white pixels represent the hand and black pixel represent the background. The next step is the segmentation of palm and fingers which is obtained with the help of palm point (center of pam), wrist line and wrist point. The labelling algorithm is applied to detect regions of fungus. Finally, hand gesture is recognized by counting fingers and identifying what figure. The dataset of 1,300 images is used to prove highly accurate results. The system takes 0.024 seconds to recognize a hand [13]. Zeenat [14] studied gesture as basically a form of non-verbal communication that involves gestures by which people communicate with each other. People can't communicate without gesture. They are the mode of communication which people use to communicate. Cooperation between people comes from various tactile modes like signal, discourse, facial and body articulations. The principle preferred position of utilizing hand signals is to connect with computer as an on-contact human computer input methodology. Hand gesture has eliminated the use of controlling of movement of virtual objects. One of the most broadly utilized examples for hand gesture recognition is data glove. Use of gesture recognition has also eliminated the use of data glove due to the expensive cost of gloves. There are three stages of gesture recognition: 1. Image pre-processing 2. Tracking 3. Recognition. The system developed was to capture the hand gesture in front of a web camera, which in turn would take a picture and then continue to recognize the reasonable motion through a specific algorithm. This paper fundamentally includes investigation and distinguishing proof of hand signals to perform suitable activities. Picture preparing is fundamentally an examination of digitized picture so as to improve its quality. EMGO-CV is fundamentally utilized for picture preparing. Emgu CV is a cross stage. Net wrapper to the Intel Open CV picture handling library. Permitting OpenCV capacities to be called from .NET perfect dialects, for example, C#, VB, VC++, Iron Python. The creator utilizes various procedures to discover number of fingers present close by signal.

Nayana presented a procedure for human computer communication exploiting open source like Python OpenCV. The proposed calculation comprises pre-handling, division and highlight extraction. Highlights include snapshots of the picture, centroid of the picture and Euclidean separation. The hand signal pictures are taken by a camera. The role of hand gestures is very important in day-to-day life. They basically convey expressive meanings by which people communicate with each other. This model presented a hand signal acknowledgment framework which utilizes just hand motions to speak. The calculation is partitioned into three sections: pre-handling, division and highlight extraction. The study utilizes forms, raised body and convexity deformities to discover the hand signal. In the course of the most recent couple of years a few explores are directed close by motion acknowledgment utilizing OpenCV and a few exhibitions correlations are led to improve the system. Picture changes are finished on the RGB picture to change over into YCBCR picture. The YCBCR picture changed into parallel picture. This computation needs uniform and plane establishment. OpenCV (Open-Source Computer Vision Library) is a library which mostly centres at continuous computer vision. OpenCV was structured for computational proficiency and with a solid spotlight on applications. It gives essential information structures for picture handling with productive improvements. Python is an object-oriented approach. For the implementation, Hand segmentation algorithm is used. In this calculation, hand division is utilized to extricate the hand picture from the foundation. There are a few strategies for division. The significant advance in division is change and thresholding. In this calculation, the BGR picture taken by a camera is considered as contribution to the calculation. The BGR picture is changed into a dark scale picture. The dark scale picture is obscured to get the definite limit. The obscured picture is edge to the specific worth. The creator introduced a procedure to locate the quantity of fingers present in the hand signal [15] [16].

Hand gesture recognition [17] is basically used for identifying the shapes or orientation depending on the feasibility of performing the task. Gestures are mainly used for conveying meaningful messages. They are the most important part of human life. Data gathering is the author's first action. The first step is to take a picture with the camera and identify a region of interest in the frame. This is important since the picture may contain a number of aspects that could lead to unfavourable outcomes and significantly reduce the amount of information that has to be prepared. A webcam is used to take the photo, which continuously records outline data and is used to gather basic planning information. Data pre-processing, which is done in two steps and comprises segmentation and morphological filtering, is the next phase. In order to have just two areas of interest in a photograph, segmentation is used to convert a dark-scale image into a two-fold image. In other words, one will be a hand, and the other a foundation. For this process, calculations known as "Otsu calculations" can be used. Dark-scale images are transformed into two-dimensional images with the area of interest serving as the hand and foundation. In order to ensure that there is no noise in the image, morphological filtering is used. Dilation, Erosion, Opening, and Closing are the basic filtering methods that can be used to assure that there is no noise. There is also a possibility of errors which can be termed as gesture noise [18].

Utilizing hand motions is one of the most regular ways of collaborating with the computer, and in particular right translation of moving hand signals progressively has numerous applications. In his paper, Nuwan Munasinghe [19] has planned and built up a framework which can perceive motions before a web camera ongoing utilizing movement history pictures (MHI) and feedforward neural systems. With the introduction of new technologies, new methods of interaction with computers have been introduced. Old methods were keyboards, mouse, joysticks and data gloves. Gesture recognition has been a commonly used method for interacting with computers and it also provides good interface for human computer interaction. It also has a lot of applications like sign language recognition, gameplay, etc. Gestures are non-verbal means of communication which are used to convey meaningful message. They can be static and dynamic. In this dynamic gesture recognition has been performed. Normally gesture recognition can be split into two parts: first, vision-based, and second, one that considers the use of keyboards, mouse, etc. The vision-based makes use of pattern recognition, image processing etc. In vision-based methodologies, a signal acknowledgment robot control framework has been created and hand presents and faces are distinguished utilizing various component-based layout coordinating systems, and to accomplish this, analysts have utilized skin shading–based division technique. Motions have perceived utilizing a standard-based framework where distinguished skin-like locales are coordinated with predefined motions. Feedforward neural network uses the concept of static hand gesture recognition to establish 10 different types of static gestures. There are a few algorithms which have been used for real-time gesture recognition using k-nearest neighbour and decision tree. The primary concern is how the computer vision-based methods and feed-forward neural systems-based grouping strategies have been utilized to build up an ongoing unique signal acknowledgment framework. In this paper, the author has basically made use of vision-based and neural network based real time-gesture recognition system.

In Ali [20] a steady vision-based structure is proposed to screen objects (hand fingers). It is built subject to the Raspberry Pi with camera module and changed with Python programming Language maintained by Open-Source PC Vision (OpenCV) library. The Raspberry Pi inserts with an image dealing with figuring called hand movement, which screens a thing (hand fingers) with its isolated features. The fundamental point of hand signal acknowledgment framework is to set up a correspondence between human and electronic frameworks for control. The perceived signals are utilized to control the movement of a portable robot progressively. The portable robot is constructed and tried to demonstrate the viability of the proposed calculation. The robot movement and route happy with various headings: Forward, Backward, Right, Left and Stop. Vision-based and picture handling frameworks have different applications in design acknowledgment and moving robots' route. Raspberry Pi is a little measured PC load up [20] reasonable for real-time ventures. The fundamental reason for the work exhibited in this paper is to make a framework equipped for distinguishing and checking a few highlights for objects that are predetermined by a picture handling calculation utilizing Raspberry Pi and camera module. The element extraction calculation is modified with Python upheld by OpenCV libraries, and executed with the Raspberry Pi connected with an outer camera. In this paper, it is displayed convenient robot using Raspberry Pi, where its advancement is constrained by methods for the camera related with Raspberry Pi that forward headings direct to the driver of a two-wheel drive portable meanderer. It used hand signal computation to recognize the article (hand) and control the improvement of the robot. Moreover, it made this robot work with living circumstance poor brightening condition. Software used for the implementation of the system is Raspbian OS which is developed for Raspberry Pi. Python and OpenCV are used also. Python, as we already know, is a very high-level programming language with fewer lines of code. It is simple and easy to execute. It has an extensive number of libraries. OpenCV is a free library that joins a few APIs for PC dreams used in picture taking care of to propel an authentic time application. There are a couple of features in OpenCV which support data dealing with, including: object area, camera arrangement, 3D multiplication and interface to video planning. Python programming language was utilized to manufacture the hand motion acknowledgment framework.

David [21] proposed a method that detected two hands simultaneously using techniques like border detection and filters. The application is divided into two parts: Robot and GPS use. In the Robot, the hand gestures are used to control the robot and in GPS, the GPS is controlled using gestures. The data of 600 gestures is used which is performed by 60 users. The application gave 93.1% accuracy and successively detected hand gesture. The least detected hand gestures are showing one figure but still is 75% accurate.

VivekBhed [22] displays the Sign language which is a kind of correspondence that regularly goes on understudied. Where the interpretation procedure among signs and communicated in or composed language is officially called understanding it assumes the job which is equivalent to the interpretation for the communicated in language. Nowadays, the usage of depth-sensing technology is growing in popularity; the Custom Designed Colour Gloves makes the feature extraction much more efficient. Though the depth-sensing technology is not used for automatic sign language recognition, there have also been successful attempts at using CNNs to handle task of classifying images of ASL letter gesture. The general design was a reasonably CNN engineering; it has various convolutional and thick layers. The information incorporates an assortment of 25 pictures from 5 individuals for every letter set and digits 1-9, a pipeline was built up that can be utilized so individuals can add pictures to this dataset. The performances will be improved and observed in the Data Augmentation process. A Deep Learning approach for a classification of ASL, the method used here shows potential in solving the problem using a simple camera which is easy to access, also bringing out the huge difference in performance of algorithms.

Hand gestures are also known as sign language; it is a language basically used by deaf people and by people who are unable to speak. There is a process known as the hand gesture recognition process focused on the recognition of meaningful expression of form and motion by the involvement of only the hands. Hand gestures recognition is applied in plenty of the applications for the purpose of accessibility, communication and learning.

This paper includes information about different experiments conducted on different types of the convolutional neural network, and it is evaluated on marcel dataset. Gjorgji [23] presented an approach, i.e., mainly divided into Data-glove-based approach which collects the information from the sensor attached to the glove and mounted on the hand of the user. The approach describes the artificially visual field to complement biological human vision. Hand motions are a basic part in human-to-human correspondence. The effectiveness of data move utilizing this procedure of correspondence is remarkable; thusly it has started thoughts for usage in the region of human-PC collaboration. For this to be conceivable the PC needs to perceive the motion appeared to it by the individual controlling it.

Various individuals and background were utilized so as to build assorted variety and data contained inside the dataset. Since the profound models that we prepared in our analyses require an enormous mass of information to prepare appropriately, we utilized information expansion on the pictures in the dataset. This was done so as to pick up amount while as yet presenting some curiosity as far as data to our dataset. GoogLeNet is a profound convolutional neural system structured by Google highlighting their prevalent Inception engineering [24].

Gesture-based communications, which comprise a blend of hand developments and outward appearances, are utilized by hard-of-hearing people the world over to communicate. Be that as it may, hearing people once in a while know gesture-based communications, making obstructions to consideration.

The expanding progress of portable innovation, alongside new types of client collaboration, opens up potential outcomes for overcoming such obstructions, especially using signal acknowledgment through cell phones. This literature review discusses works from 2009 to 2017 that present answers for motion acknowledgment in a versatile setting just as facial acknowledgment in gesture-based communications. Among an assorted variety of equipment and methods, sensor-based gloves were the most utilized extraordinary equipment, alongside animal power correlation with order motions.

1.3 Model for Sign Recognition Language

The main ideas of the content up to this point have been what sign language is and why American sign language was chosen above other sign languages.

What compelled us to research this topic even more? Now the question is, how are we going to accomplish such a task? To answer that, we must be able to comprehend the idea that this research is trying to portray as well as the procedures or strategies that will be employed to carry out this research sequentially.

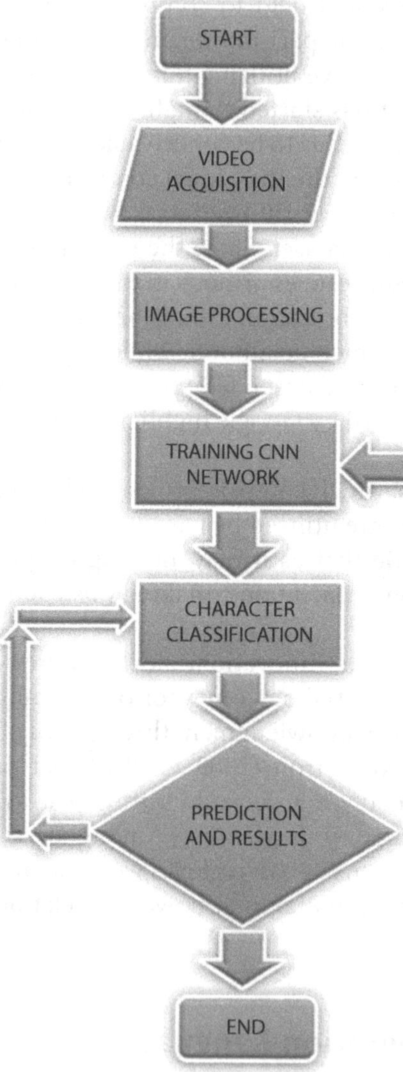

Figure 1.2 Block diagram of phases of sign language recognition.

The fundamental assumption of this chapter is that whenever people need to communicate with each other, especially the deaf or dumb, they cannot comprehend each other, even persons with no physical issues with deaf or dumb people. By bridging that communication gap, this application will help.

Consequently, how do these sign languages function? Unlike commonly spoken languages, signs occasionally express their meaning by hand, facial, or body motions. Given that grammar is different from spoken language, this also applies to the way it is presented. Non-manual action is the term used to describe the act of communicating with sign languages.

The process shown in Figure 1.2 shows how to guarantee accurate and correct input recognition. Each phase is broken down into numerous substeps, all of which will be covered in detail in this chapter.

1.4 Experimentation

Real-time sign language recognition is a challenging application; therefore, system requirements must be kept in mind. Such research can typically be implemented using both low- and high-resolution cameras as well as more advanced systems. In order to ensure that neural network implementation is still effective even with low-resolution photos, this research will capture the primary input from the webcam of the laptop.

Python will be needed for this research's programming language, and it will also need tools like PyCharm or Jupiter Notebook [25] for the research's internal operations. For the training dataset, there will be at least 200 data sets for each character. Additionally, this research will apply effective machine language algorithms and aim to raise the baseline accuracy level.

The research will make use of well-known platforms and libraries to compute data and present results in a certain format, such as:

1. TensorFlow – It is an open-source platform for developing and building applications based on machine learning. It contains all the tools and libraries for the development of machine learning–powered applications.
2. Keras – It was founded to provide ease in deep neural network applications. It is mainly an application programming interface which can be performed using Python programming language. It is mostly helpful in back-end working.

3. OpenCV – It is a library which contains the material to operate real-time applications. It can be used with Python language. It is mainly for front end purposes.
4. Libraries such as NumPy or Os are also used to calculate mathematical procedures as well as file reading and writing executions.

Dataset

Humans have been accustomed to using two dimensions, yet occasionally three dimensions are employed as well, much like throughout evolution. What if, however, there are n dimensions to consider? When seemingly straightforward situations become completely unmanageable for human interactions, machine learning becomes useful.

We have a really helpful dataset that is directly related to computer vision and is used for sign language recognition. This data collection was created by MNIST:

M-Modified
N-National
I -Institute
S-Standards
T-Technology

The MNIST dataset was produced using Sign language in all of its possible manifestations [26]. A few samples of MNIST are mentioned in Figure 1.3. The data set's signs have size of 200*200 pixels on both the horizontal and vertical axes. The sequences and each element of the dataset have been numerically labelled according to the class to which they belong.

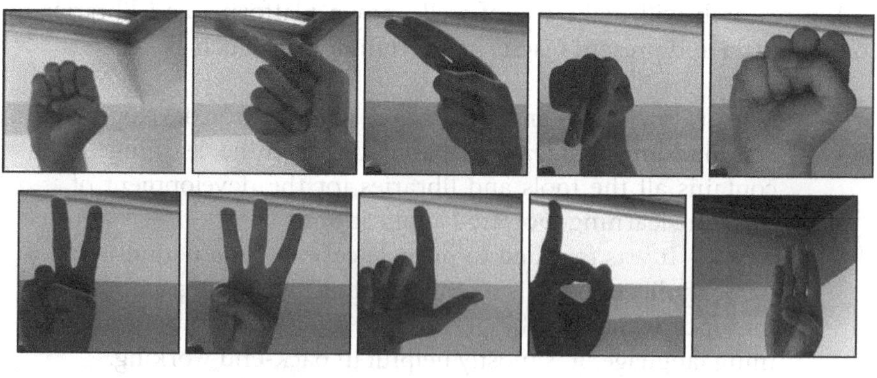

Figure 1.3 A few samples of MNIST sign language dataset.

Data Vectorization

Prior to data pre-processing, data vectorization is the first and most crucial stage. The produced code is vectorized to alter the linear reading of the vectorized data. In turn, this modifies the data in matrix form. These vectors use numerous samples at once to produce a vector array for logistic regression, which may then be used for image processing. The procedure will be split into two phases to accomplish vectorization. It will be created in pixelated form in the first portion, and data will be stored in much more exact form in the second. Figure 1.4 discusses the specific actions in detail.

Each array will contain values ranging from 0 to 255 when the matrix has been formed, which corresponds to the RGB values. In linear format, the system will read these data. Even though the user may not see this procedure as you do, the system need this data flow for binary thresholding.

The second stage of vectorization, which involves storing and resizing the raw data for the system to read, follows the initial vectorization. Before the validation split shown in Figure 1.5 is implemented, the saved data will serve as the training repository.

Binary Class Matrix

The binary version of the stored pixelated values must be used after data vectorization is finished. Why, then, must the array values be converted into binary?

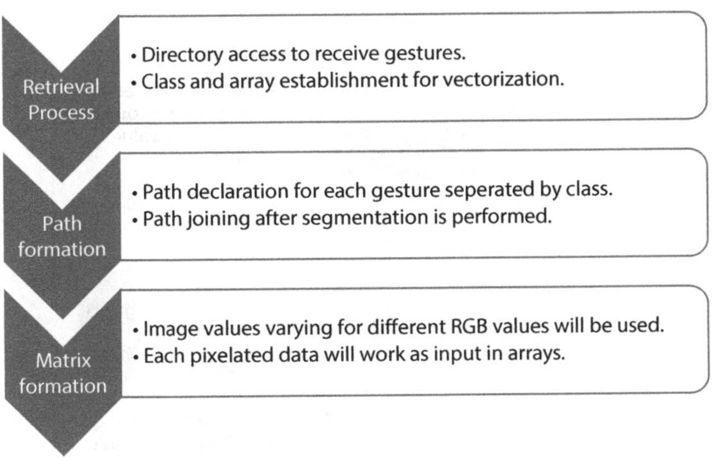

Figure 1.4 Initial vectorization of data.

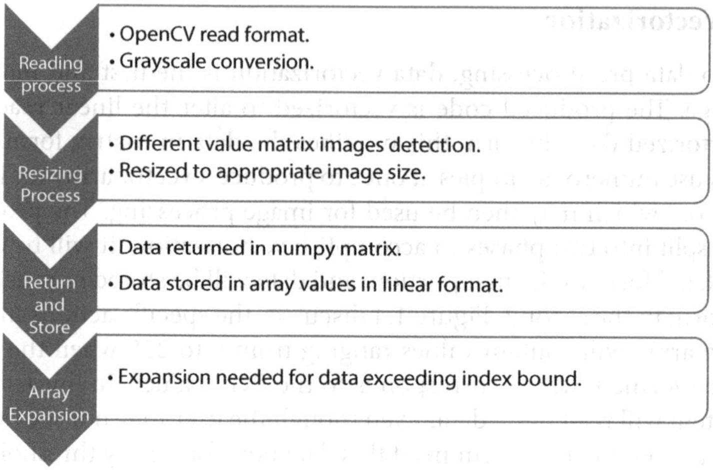

Figure 1.5 Final vectorization of data.

The values collected will be split into the training set and the testing set, or two states. A dictionary representing characters from each class will have each of these values. The required values should be in binary when

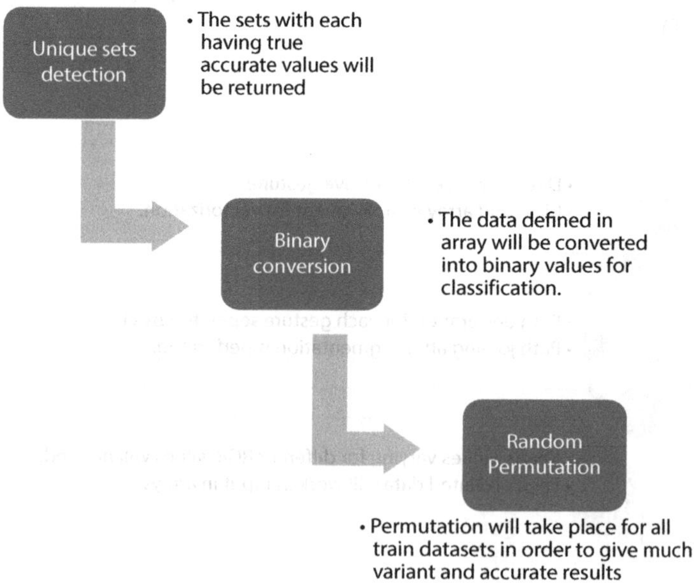

Figure 1.6 Phases of binary class conversion.

compiling these values to train so that shuffling is possible. A detailed description of the binary class conversion is described in Figure 1.6.

Thus, all of the distinct values required for training will be found using NumPy, and they will all be returned.

Learning Model

To further improve the validity and accuracy of our forecast, the learning model on which we trained our data generates results based on accuracy, loss, or time. Because this is a supervised learning topic, we need supervised learning for this research. We can classify this issue on the basis of which we can predict class labels.

Basic convolutional neural models will be the focus of this study. It will have several layers of convolutions, followed by pooling and a few fully linked layers. Rectified Linear Unit, or ReLu, will be required as the activation function. It is superior to a sigmoid function in a number of respects, which will be discussed later. Additionally, the pooling type will be maximum pooling in a single layer. The only size available for the kernel or filter is 3*3.

A simple model with the capacity to stack layers specified by users is a sequential model. In Figure 1.7, a sequential model with more layers is explored. A model object is started to add another layer in order to enable this model. Additional layers that will make the research process easier will be defined after the model's basic structure. We have previously discussed

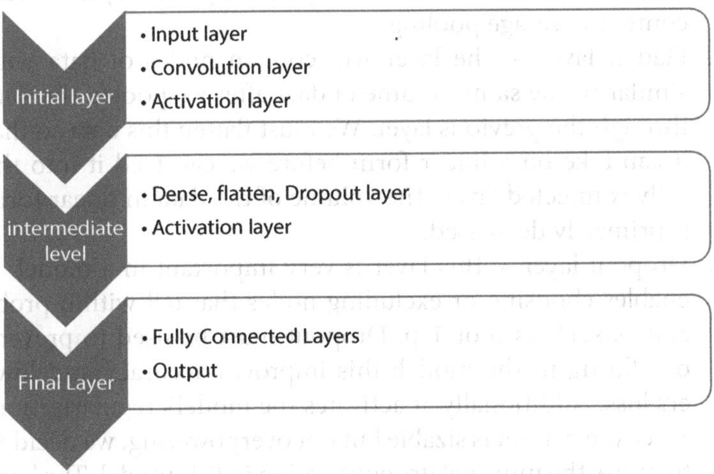

Figure 1.7 Sequential model with added layers.

the usage of layers in this research, but each layer serves a different purpose. Some of the layers with various functions and their purposes in this research are described below.

1. Convolution Layer – Using kernels or filters, this layer will convolve the supplied input matrix into customizable data. The kernel is the component that creates universal data that can be used during training by using the dot product of its matrix with the input picture matrix.
2. Another question that comes up before convolutions is why the convolution network is superior to the feed-forward network when implementation is simple.
3. The necessity for this is that even if we flatten the data and input it into the network, the result will not produce accuracy since the picture complexity would not drop and will modify the output significantly.
4. Pooling Layer – The convolution layer and this layer are very similar. The data that is received from the convolution layer is altered or made smaller. By doing this, the image's resolution is shrunk, and the amount of computer power required to finish the procedure is also reduced. The pooling is done in two different ways: the maximum value present in the chosen matrix region is returned by the max pooling method, and average data is produced by the average pooling method. The noise in the photos is also decreased by the maximum pooling. Maximum pooling yields superior outcomes to average pooling.
5. Flatten layer – The layer will contain nodes of data with similar or the same volume of data after we pooled the data through the previous layer. We must flatten this data so that it can take on a linear form before we can feed it into the fully connected layer. The volume of the data in linear form is primarily decreased.
6. Dropout layer – This layer is very important in a model. It enables choosing or excluding nodes that fall within probability, such as p or 1-p. Dropout must be used to prevent overfitting in the model; this improves accuracy and lowers loss. Additionally, it activates the model's regularisation. Since the dataset is sizable but not overpowering, we decided to utilise the minimal dropout option in this model. The level of dropout suggested by this model is more than sufficient.

Model Compilation and Loss Calculation

The model is assembled using the machine learning techniques after the layers have been formed or added. SGD (stochastic gradient descent) has been employed as the optimizer in this research [27]. In order to produce outcomes that are added as input to another node, the neurons serve as functions and the weights serve as the parameters of the functions. The equation, which has a fixed learning rate and parameters including both ground truth and hypothetical tests, is provided in eq 1:

$$\theta_j = \theta_j - \alpha(\hat{y}^i - y^i)x_j^i \tag{1.1}$$

Categorical cross entropy computations are used in the next step. The data that was compiled for these calculations contains binary classes of data for testing and training validation. This allows for a comparison between the binary class matrix and the true distribution of all forecasts, or the set of all data. This therefore provides us with an output that will have minimal loss and the highest likelihood of the expected result. Simply said, this algorithm will determine or forecast one particular result from all other potential outcomes. Classification can be accomplished in this manner. The following formula can be used to determine cross entropy loss:

$$L(y,\hat{y}) = -\sum_{j=0}^{M}\sum_{i=0}^{N}(y_{ij} * \log(\hat{y}_{ij})) \tag{1.2}$$

Image Processing

This technique for improving images will be utilised with OpenCV [28]. These methods enable picture modification based on accurate computer vision identification and the removal of any impediments prior to image analysis. There will be a variety of image processing methods employed, including:

1. Picture Enhancement – The dataset will be enhanced in varying degrees for contrast, sharpness, colour, and brightness. The ability to distinguish contours on each image depends on the degree of contrast changes. The borders of each image's specific details will be more heavily emphasised, which is more crucial.
2. Line Enhancement – This method enables us to precisely determine those edges that are challenging to improve. The

grayscale effect is used to identify the outlines of each fingertip. Additionally, it much more clearly identifies the hand-to-border ratio. This will significantly improve the neural network's ability to recognise the outcome.

3. Image Whitening – In this method, values representing a particular colour were dissolved using the pixel matrix. Additionally, it eliminates unnecessary data to free up storage space and simplify the system. It enables a neural network to discover intricate patterns that can produce better outcomes. During convolutions, we can employ the identity or zero matrix for this purpose. To create a distinction between low-intensity pixels and high-intensity pixels, we employed the threshold function.
4. Colour Model – The HSV colour model, RGB colour model, and YCbCr colour model are only a few of the various colour models that will interact in this research. With the HSV colour model, colour information can be distinguished from image brightness. When displaying colour in a picture, HSV should be used. As a result, skin edges will be used to detect contours. Other colour models employ various techniques to enable image pre-processing, and those processes are shown in the figure below. We will use the RGB colour model and convert it to grayscale for this research.

Figure 1.8 shows the order of the image processing steps.

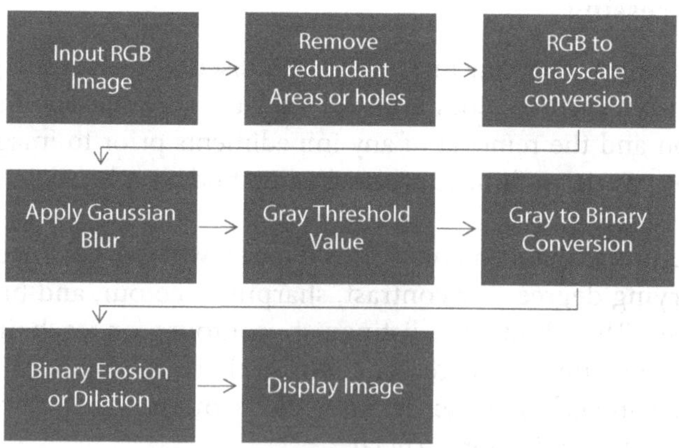

Figure 1.8 Image processing techniques and steps.

1.5 Methodology

The Convolutional Neural Network (CNN) serves as the manuscript's main structural component; nevertheless, it differs from Artificial Neural Networks in that it proposes using images as input, both in their raw and non-raw forms, rather than a linear data array [29]. In order to predict the required output in the form of an image or video presentation, images are essentially needed as a learning set. Convolutions are necessary because they can capture the spatial and temporal requirements or dependencies in the images. The network may generate a result that can comprehend the matrix form of an image as a result of changes in weights and complicated parameter forms. These layers need filters to show how photographs function in their raw state and convert through pre-processing procedures to provide results that are significantly more accurate. The structure of CNN is given in Figure 1.9.

CNN (Convolutional neural network) Layers:

These layers appearing repeatedly suggest the formation of a deep neural network. These layers are distinguished in the following format:

1. Input layer – The input is provided as images.
2. Convolutions – A matching channel must be provided by the layers in order to get the desired outcome. These matches are made using the kernel, and the outcome also shows edge detection and high-value features.
3. Activation layer – The Activation function primarily transforms the input data from every node into output, which

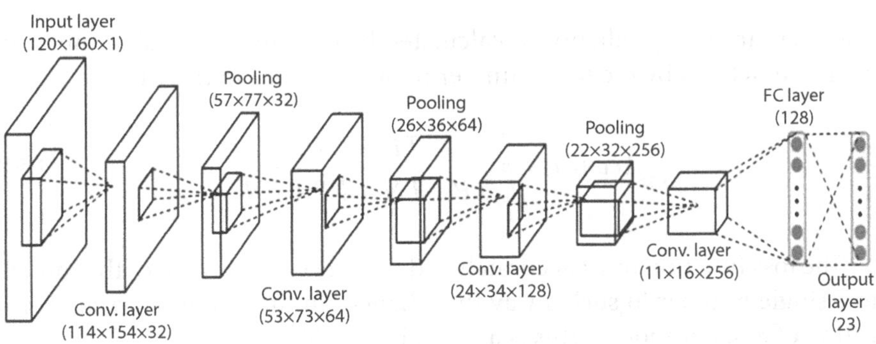

Figure 1.9 A basic convolution for feature learning and classification.

is made up of data generated using modified weights and parameters and is then fed to another layer's node.
4. Pooling layer – It plays with the data volume and selects the pixel that best captures the image data.
5. Fully connected layer – The output from this layer is based on distinct high-level and low-level properties. To generate the desired results, it learns non-linear functions.

Activation Function (AF)

To map the input to the output, AF is used. The main applications of AF are to integrate nonlinear functionality in data and to support output that is precise and range-limited. ReLu and Softmax are two of the AFs used. Rectified linear unit is referred to as ReLu. ReLu has an advantage over other AF in that it never activates all of the neurons at once, as specified in eq. 1.3. Numerous sigmoids make up Softmax, which treats probabilities of data linking to the class used for the multiclass problem mentioned in equation 4 and returns values between 0 and 1 [14].

$$L_i = -\log\left(\frac{e^{f_{y_i}}}{\Sigma_j e^{f_j}}\right) \tag{1.3}$$

$$R = \max(0, z) \tag{1.4}$$

Performance Measure

The accuracy of a prediction is calculated by dividing the total number of right predictions by the total number of observations in the dataset.

$$Accuracy = \frac{TP + TN}{TP + TN + FP + FN} \tag{1.5}$$

The loss function must accurately reduce every component of the model to a single number in such a way that changes in that number are an indication of a better model. This is a crucial task [30].

```
x_train = np.expand_dims(x_train, axis=-1)
x_train.shape
Out[40]: (4823, 100, 100, 1)
```

Figure 1.10 Vectorized data outcome.

1.6 Experimentation Results

Each epoch's running repository comprised 200 photos with 200 pixels of resolution. As a result, each epoch took close to three minutes, but the data was accurately trained. The validation split and dropout were required to prevent overfitting, which led to a decrease in val_loss and an increase in val_accuracy shown in Table 1.1.

The array size after resizing and reading each variable's output during vectorization, as well as the axis at which it is defined, are all clearly determined by the output form mentioned in Figure 1.10.

The model training result is shown in Table 1.2. This displays accuracy, and loss generated after each epoch. Given that our system could handle such huge computations, we performed a total of 30 epochs. On 30th Epoch, promising results are obtained in terms of accuracy and loss with training and testing data, highlighted in bold text.

Table 1.1 Accuracy and loss values per epochs.

Top highest accuracy	Top lowest loss
97.88	5.97
97.60	5.63
97.51	6.42
97.33	7.35
96.71	8.30
95.60	8.78
95.35	8.05

Table 1.2 Experimental results of training and testing data for accuracy and loss.

Number of epochs	Highest training accuracies (First two) (%)	Lowest training loss (Last two) (%)	Highest testing accuracies (First two) (%)	Lowest testing loss (Last two) (%)
2	70.2	55.1	72.2	60.5
	61.1	67.4	67.9	68.1
5	89.9	35.7	87.1	58.5
	86.6	43.6	86.2	61.2
10	96.7	11.1	93.5	21.5
	95.8	13.5	91.3	34.8
20	97.2	6.57	95.4	24.5
	97	7.14	95.2	26.6
30	**97.8**	5.97	**96.7**	**10.5**
	97.6	**5.63**	96.6	10.9

1.7 Conclusion

This study shows that CNN can accurately identify various signs used in sign languages even when users and their surroundings are not part of the training set. RTSL (Real Time Location Systems) entails first utilising an ML model to identify images from a video feed that has been collected, then further identifying the edges and vertices, and then using CNN to assess the desired result. This paradigm aids in creating software that enables communication between deaf and mute persons. With a 97% accuracy rate, the suggested sequential approach has been successful in understanding sign language.

The first step in the process is to extract the video's frames. A single frame is not taken into account to create the final prediction in order to give the machine a sense of the sequence. Instead of using a single frame for classification, a group of frames from a certain segment of the video are employed. For each epoch, various optimizers are employed to produce outcomes depending on accuracy, loss, and time complexity. Using 10-fold validation, each optimizer enhanced the model's performance, with accuracy reaching more than 95%.

Additionally, these stage components ought to provide the minimal administration qualities (QoS) that the programme requires (processor speeds, memory limits, correspondence transmission capacities, and so forth).

Future Scope

There is potential for the suggested system to be improved and its application in daily life expanded by a number of other improvements. Its use in some domains is restricted by the current dynamics of its capabilities. The training model's repository enhancement may be increased in the future, and the system's accuracy might be increased.

This research concentrated on a sequential model with extra layers, such as dropout layers and additional activation layers. In the future, a more optimised model, like Google Neural Network, may be employed. If more extensive processing is done on the photos, such as contrast modification, background removal, and possibly cropping on a more sophisticated and deeper level, the classification task could be made much simpler. Building a bigram and trigram language model would enable us to handle sentences rather than individual characters, leading to improved letter segmentation.

References

1. U. Zeshan, M. N. Vasishta, and M. Sethna, "Implementation of Indian Sign Language in educational settings," *Asia Pacific Disabil. Rehabil. J.*, vol. 16, no. 1, pp. 16–40, 2005.
2. R. L. Thompson, D. P. Vinson, B. Woll, and G. Vigliocco, "The Road to Language Learning Is Iconic," https://doi.org/10.1177/0956797612459763, vol. 23, no. 12, pp. 1443–1448, Nov. 2012, doi: 10.1177/0956797612459763.
3. E. L. Newport and R. P. Meier, "The Acquisition of American Sign Language," *Crosslinguistic Study Lang. Acquis.*, pp. 881–938, Jul. 2017, doi: 10.4324/9781315802541-12.
4. S. K. Liddell and R. E. Johnson, "American Sign Language: The Phonological Base," *Sign Lang. Stud.*, vol. 64, no. 1, pp. 195–277, 1989, doi: 10.1353/SLS.1989.0027.
5. M. Strong *et al.*, "A Study of the Relationship Between American Sign Language and English Literacy," *J. Deaf Stud. Deaf Educ.*, vol. 2, no. 1, pp. 37–46, Jan. 1997, doi: 10.1093/OXFORDJOURNALS.DEAFED.A014308.

6. A. S. Ghotkar, R. Khatal, S. Khupase, S. Asati, and M. Hadap, "Hand gesture recognition for Indian Sign Language," *2012 Int. Conf. Comput. Commun. Informatics, ICCCI 2012*, 2012, doi: 10.1109/ICCCI.2012.6158807.
7. D. Deora and N. Bajaj, "Indian sign language recognition," *Proc. 2012 1st Int. Conf. Emerg. Technol. Trends Electron. Commun. Networking, ET2ECN 2012*, 2012, doi: 10.1109/ET2ECN.2012.6470093.
8. H. Muthu Mariappan and V. Gomathi, "Real-time recognition of Indian sign language," *ICCIDS 2019 - 2nd Int. Conf. Comput. Intell. Data Sci. Proc., Feb. 2019*, doi: 10.1109/ICCIDS.2019.8862125.
9. R. T. Barker and K. Gower, "Strategic Application of Storytelling in Organizations," http://dx.doi.org/10.1177/0021943610369782, vol. 47, no. 3, pp. 295–312, Jun. 2010, doi: 10.1177/0021943610369782.
10. E. Suter, J. Arndt, N. Arthur, J. Parboosingh, E. Taylor, and S. Deutschlander, "Role understanding and effective communication as core competencies for collaborative practice," https://doi.org/10.1080/13561820802338579, vol. 23, no. 1, pp. 41–51, 2009, doi: 10.1080/13561820802338579.
11. R. B. Wilbur and E. Malaia, "Contributions of Sign Language Research to Gesture Understanding: What can Multimodal Computational Systems Learn from Sign Language Research," *Int. J. Semant. Comput.*, vol. 2, no. 1, p. 5, Mar. 2008, doi: 10.1142/S1793351X08000324.
12. I. S. MacKenzie, "Human-computer interaction.," p. 370, 2012.
13. Z. H. Chen, J. T. Kim, J. Liang, J. Zhang, and Y. B. Yuan, "Real-time hand gesture recognition using finger segmentation," *Sci. World J.*, vol. 2014, 2014, doi: 10.1155/2014/267872.
14. Z. Afroze, S. U. Rahman, and M. Tareq, "Hand Gesture Recognition Techniques For Human Computer Interaction Using OpenCv," *Int. J. Sci. Res. Publ.*, vol. 4, no. 12, 2014, Accessed: Nov. 25, 2022. [Online]. Available: www.ijsrp.org
15. S. Nayana, P. B., & Kubakaddi, "Implentation of hand gesture recognition technique for HCI using open CV," *Int. J. Recent Dev. Eng. Technol.*, vol. 2, no. 5, pp. 17–21, 2014.
16. Y. Luo, G. Cui, and D. Li, "An Improved Gesture Segmentation Method for Gesture Recognition Based on CNN and YCbCr," *J. Electr. Comput. Eng.*, vol. 2021, 2021, doi: 10.1155/2021/1783246.
17. A. P. Ismail, F. A. A. Aziz, N. M. Kasim, and K. Daud, "Hand gesture recognition on python and opencv," IOP *Conf. Ser. Mater. Sci. Eng.*, vol. 1045, no. 1, p. 012043, Feb. 2021, doi: 10.1088/1757-899X/1045/1/012043.
18. F. Zaklouta and B. Stanciulescu, "Real-time traffic sign recognition in three stages," *Rob. Auton. Syst.*, vol. 62, no. 1, pp. 16–24, Jan. 2014, doi: 10.1016/J.ROBOT.2012.07.019.
19. M. I. N. P. Munasinghe, "Dynamic Hand Gesture Recognition Using Computer Vision and Neural Networks," 2018 *3rd Int. Conf. Converg. Technol. I2CT 2018*, no. January, 2018, doi: 10.1109/I2CT.2018.8529335.

20. A. A. and S. A., "Python-based Raspberry Pi for Hand Gesture Recognition," *Int. J. Comput. Appl.*, vol. 173, no. 4, pp. 18–24, 2017, doi: 10.5120/ijca2017915285.
21. D. J. Rios-Soria, S. E. Schaeffer, and S. E. Garza-Villarreal, "Hand-gesture recognition using computer-vision techniques," *21st Int. Conf. Cent. Eur. Comput. Graph. Vis. Comput. Vision, WSCG 2013 - Commun. Pap. Proc.*, pp. 1–8, 2013.
22. S. Lan, Z. He, W. Chen, and L. Chen, "Hand Gesture Recognition Using Convolutional Neural Networks," *2018 Usn. Radio Sci. Meet. (Joint with AP-S Symp. Usn. 2018 - Proc.*, no. September, pp. 147–148, 2019, doi: 10.1109/USNC-URSI.2018.8602809.
23. M. Al-Hammadi, G. Muhammad, W. Abdul, M. Alsulaiman, M. A. Bencherif, and M. A. Mekhtiche, "Hand Gesture Recognition for Sign Language Using 3DCNN," *IEEE Access*, vol. 8, pp. 79491–79509, 2020, doi: 10.1109/ACCESS.2020.2990434.
24. P. Ballester and R. M. Araujo, "On the performance of googlenet and alexnet applied to sketches," *30th AAAI Conf. Artif. Intell.* AAAI 2016, pp. 1124–1128, 2016, doi: 10.1609/aaai.v30i1.10171.
25. Q. Hu, L. Ma, and J. Zhao, "DeepGraph: A PyCharm Tool for Visualizing and Understanding Deep Learning Models," *Proc. - Asia-Pacific Softw. Eng. Conf. APSEC*, vol. 2018-December, pp. 628–632, Jul. 2018, doi: 10.1109/APSEC.2018.00079.
26. L. Fernandes, P. Dalvi, A. Junnarkar, and M. Bansode, "Convolutional neural network based bidirectional sign language translation system," *Proc. 3rd Int. Conf. Smart Syst. Inven. Technol. ICSSIT 2020*, pp. 769–775, Aug. 2020, doi: 10.1109/ICSSIT48917.2020.9214272.
27. L. Bottou, "Stochastic gradient descent tricks," *Lect. Notes Comput. Sci.* (including *Subser. Lect. Notes Artif. Intell. Lect. Notes Bioinformatics*), vol. 7700 LECTURE NO, pp. 421–436, 2012, doi: 10.1007/978-3-642-35289-8_25/COVER.
28. G. R. Bradski and A. Kaehler, "Learning OpenCV : computer vision with the OpenCV library," p. 555, 2008.
29. K. O'Shea and R. Nash, "An Introduction to Convolutional Neural Networks," Nov. 2015, doi: 10.48550/arxiv.1511.08458.
30. X. Lei, H. Pan, and X. Huang, "A dilated CNN model for image classification," *IEEE Access*, vol. 7, pp. 124087–124095, 2019, doi: 10.1109/ACCESS.2019.2927169.

2

Unsupervised/Supervised Feature Extraction and Feature Selection for Multimedia Data (Feature extraction with feature selection for Image Forgery Detection)

Arun Anoop M.[1*], Karthikeyan P.[2] and S. Poonkuntran[3]

[1]*Alva's Institute of Engineering & Technology, Mijar, Moodbidri, Karnataka, India*
[2]*Velammal College of Engineering and Technology, Viraganoor, Madurai, Tamilnadu, India*
[3]*VIT Bhopal University, Sehore, Bhopal, Madhya Pradesh, India*

Abstract

Multimedia data needs to be protected from unauthorized duplication, otherwise, data may lead to tampering which may not be identified by the naked eye. Features and feature vector are collections of local and global features of digital images. Features can determine the image level classification accurately nowadays. So, the importance of feature extraction is high. Some redundant and irrelevant data may be many in the case of feature extraction. To avoid it, feature scaling and feature selection approaches are mandatory to get an accurate prediction. Multimedia data are mostly image, video and audio technologies. In this paper, we demonstrate different supervised and unsupervised feature extraction algorithms and forgery classification technique of 42 features to check the accuracy of detection and supervised image classification based on GLCM(24), GLDM(4) and GLRLM(7) feature extraction combination with LBP(7) variants. Later the same method will process, based on a different correlation map, a threshold-based feature selection approach with different cross-validation methods. After that, the same system will process based on different feature selection approaches, especially bio-inspired methods. Finally, it will check based on some pre-trained CNN

**Corresponding author*: arunanoopm@gmail.com

Suman Kumar Swarnkar, J P Patra, Sapna Singh Kshatri, Yogesh Kumar Rathore and Tien Anh Tran (eds.) Supervised and Unsupervised Data Engineering for Multimedia Data, (27–62) © 2024 Scrivener Publishing LLC

models to conclude which is the best approach based on classification accuracy. Finally, significant journal comparisons have also been done to show the novelty of our research work.

***Keywords*:** Image forgery and its detection, pre-trained CNN models, feature selection approaches, bio-inspired methods, feature extraction algorithms

2.1 Introduction

Digital image authenticity is one of the challenging tasks in this digital era especially in digital camera-based or format-based or camera still lens based. The advancement of digital cameras and the Internet have made it simple for anybody to catch forged regions from digital images. Digital image manipulation tools are there to modify and circulate the images around the world. For marketing strategies there are huge reasons for the creation of manipulated images. Some prefer manipulation for improving brightness, some fake people use brightness and they hide some important portions or they add new regions with original ones to spread false data in order to make a false image. A lot of research has now been done on the detection and localization or recognition of image manipulations, but proving authenticity and integrity are the real issues still, even if all tools or methods are available. As the main forgeries are copying and moving in a desired object or background or foreground regions, combining of two or more images in one, merging of digital images, resizing of digital images and its regions, therefore, multimedia manipulation detection is a very big task.

Types of Image forgery attacks with Image (Related works):

1. Figure 2.1 shows copy-move forgery prevention and detection. Attacks often use forensic analysis and advanced picture processing. Image forensics programs scan images for duplicated patterns to reveal interference or fabrication. The identification process may examine statistical traits or incongruities within duplicated areas to reveal suspected manipulation and preserve digital material authenticity.
2. Figure 2.2 may show a photomontage attack. These assaults involve malicious actors mixing photos to create scenarios or change the context. Photomontage assaults can spread false information, create images, or change public perception. Advanced picture forensics is often needed to identify

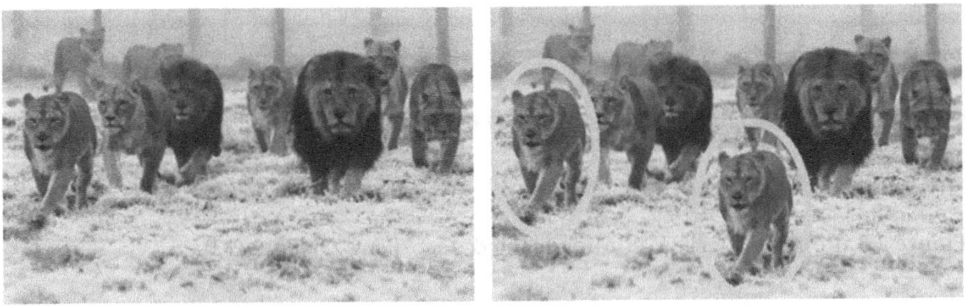

Figure 2.1 Copy move forgery attack (Rahul Dixit & Ruchira Naskar 2017).

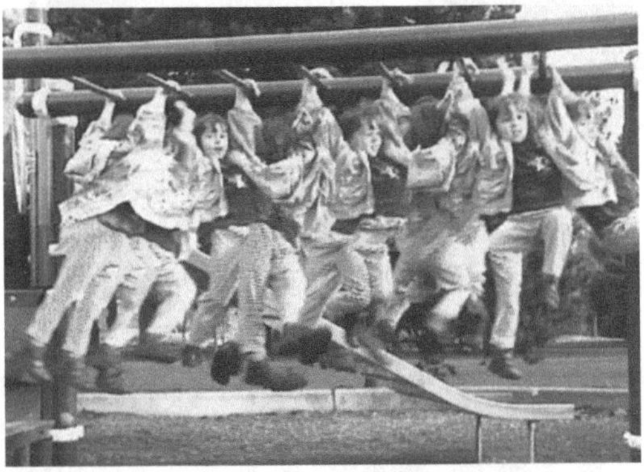

Figure 2.2 Photomontage attack (Aseem Agarwala *et al.*, 2004).

and prevent photomontage assaults. These approaches detect manipulation in pixel-level details, shadows, and lighting to protect digital photos.

3. Figure 2.3 likely depicts a resizing attack. With malicious intent, this attack can alter how people see a photograph.

   Enlarging an image, often called "upscaling," may lower image quality and pixels, impacting its appearance. Shrinking a photograph reduces transparency and blurs details.
4. In Figure 2.4, an image splicing attack combines elements of multiple photos into one. Creating a false world to fool or dominate others is widespread.
5. The hues in Figure 2.5 have probably been altered or manipulated with potentially malicious intentions. This type of attack may involve altering the color distribution, saturating or desaturating specific regions, or introducing synthetic hues to deceive or manipulate the viewer.

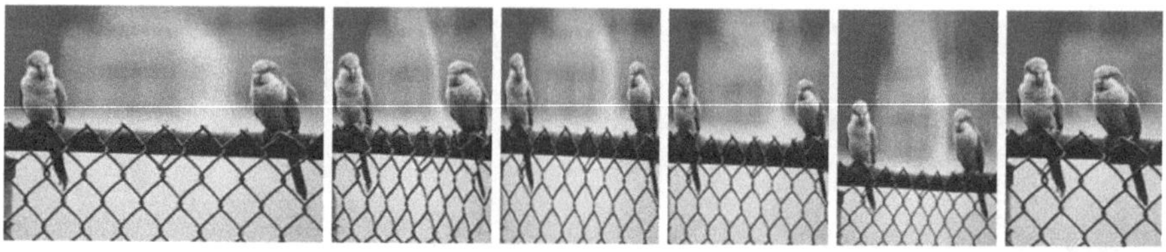

Figure 2.3 Resizing attack (Wei-Ming Dong & Xiao-Peng Zhang, 2012).

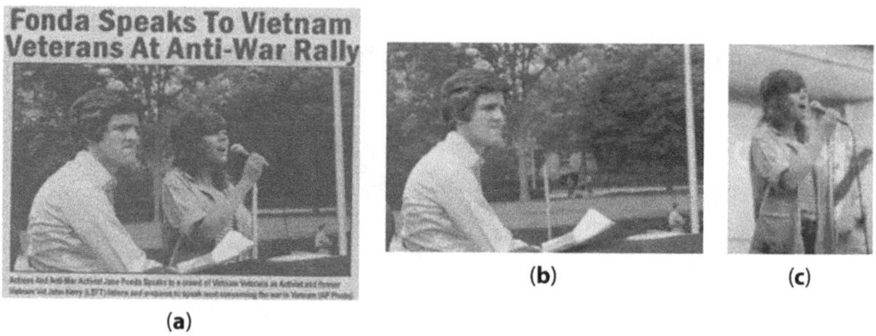

Figure 2.4 Image splicing attack (Yun Q. Shi *et al.*, 2007).

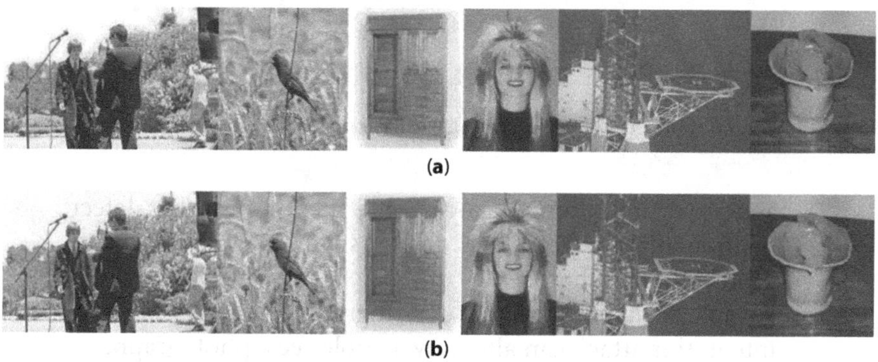

Figure 2.5 Colorized image attack (Yuanfang Guo *et al.*, 2018).

6. Figure 2.6 shows camera-based image assaults, including blurring, lens distortions, or other alterations during picture acquisition. These attacks may violate privacy, propagate misinformation, or create fake visual content.

   Understanding manipulation artifacts and properties is often necessary to identify camera-based picture attacks. Forensic analysis may include metadata analysis, image quality analysis, and manipulation pattern identification.

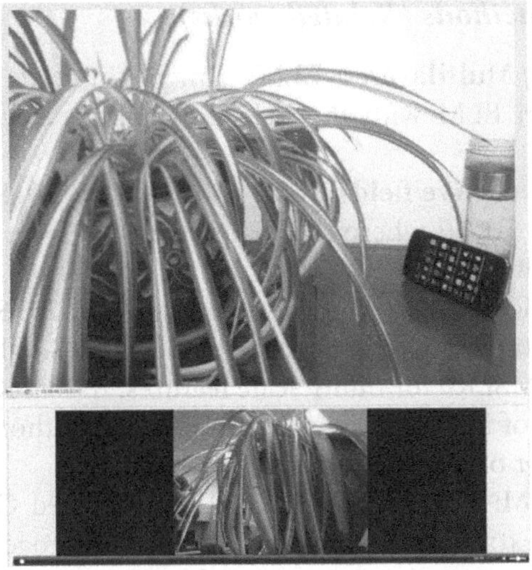

Figure 2.6 Camera-based image attack (Longfei Wu *et al.*, 2014).

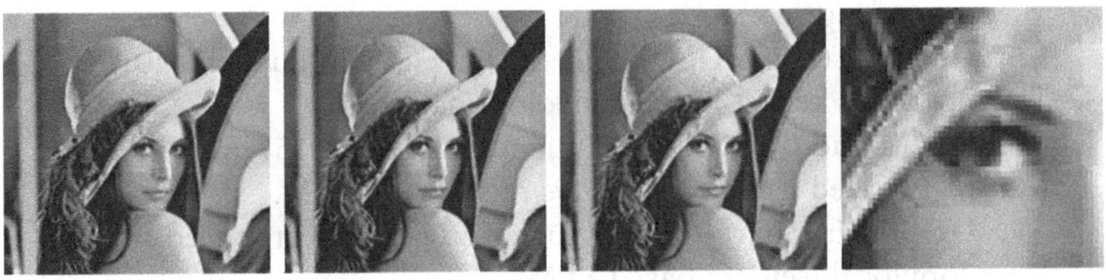

Figure 2.7 Format-based images (LK Tan, 2006).

Legal and investigative settings require the capacity to identify and understand camera-based picture assaults to maintain image integrity and reliability.

7. “Format-based images” do not describe Figure 2.7’s features or contents. However, it refers to a group of graphics that may be associated with a file format. Images can be stored in JPEG, PNG, or GIF, each with its characteristics.

   Understanding format-based images in forensics or security may require examining image file format vulnerabilities or features. Different formats’ compression, color representations, and metadata structures may affect image authentication and analysis.

Types of ELM methods (Related works):

1. **Pruning Multilayered ELM**: (Jingyi Liu *et al.*, 2021) proposed an ELM with the help of Cholesky decomposition method.
2. **Local Receptive fields ELM**: (Bo He *et al.*, 2018) proposed LRF and HLRF, where HLRF is the hybrid form of LRF and Gabor filter.
3. **SS/MSLRF ELM**: (Jinghong Huang *et al.*, 2016) proposed local features-based approaches SSLRF, for single-scale features & MSLRF for multi-scale features. In that K is the total number of feature maps. Based on K, the authors evaluated texture or object classification process.
4. **ARF ELM**: (Chao Wu *et al.*, 2019) proposed Convolution feature extraction and feature coding approach and it is called Autoencoder receptive fields ELM, which consist of local and global receptive fields. Feature coding consists of feature dimension reduction and two hidden layers for ELM processing.
5. **CKELM**: (Shifei Ding *et al.*, 2016) (Huijuan Lu *et al.*, 2016) proposed kernel-based convolutional ELM.
6. **RELM and CS-RELM**: (Huijuan Lu *et al.*, 2015) proposed a regularized and cost sensitive regularized ELM.
7. **DC-ELM**: (Shan Ping & Xinyi Yang, 2016) proposed random local weights-based ELM.
8. **CAE-ELM**: (Yueqing Wang *et al.*, 2015) proposed a method which consists of voxel data and it is processed based on feature maps, pooling maps with different auto encoders outputs inputted to ELM classifier.
9. **Multilayer ELM**: (Yimin Yang & Q.M. Jonathan Wu, 2015) proposed a machine learning with subnetwork nodes.
10. **Hierarchical Ensemble ELM**: (Yaoming Cai *et al.*, 2018) proposed an ELM for reducing overfitting training data issues.
11. **EK-based multilayer ELM**: (Chi-Man Vong *et al.*, 2018) proposed empirical kernel map–based multilayer stacked auto encoder ELM.
12. **Ensemble ELM**: (Sen Hui Wang *et al.*, 2019) proposed EELM for predicting iron ore sintering characters. It is the improved version of Ada-boost-rt algorithm.
13. **Voting-based ELM**: (Jiuwen Cao *et al.*, 2012) proposed a voting-based ELM and measured performance based on 19 datasets.

14. **GEELM**: (Chao Wang *et al.*, 2022) proposed global extended ELM for tea gas information prediction and e-nose gas feature recognition.
15. **Sae-ELM**: (Jiuwen Cao *et al.*, 2012) proposed SVM and Levenberg-Marquardt algorithm for Self-adaptive evolutionary ELM.
16. **FC-ELM**: (Ming-Bin Li *et al.*, 2005) proposed fully complex ELM.
17. **I-ELM**: (Guang-Bin Huang *et al.*, 2008) proposed Incremental ELM based on fully complex hidden nodes.
18. **2-stage ELM**: (Yuan Lan *et al.*, 2010) proposed two-stage ELM.
19. **O-ELM**: (Wan-Yu Deng *et al.*, 2010) proposed Ordinal ELM for SLFNs.
20. **EELM**: (Qin-Yu Zhu *et al.*, 2005) proposed Evolutionary ELM.
21. **SELM**: (Xueyi Liu *et al.*, 2013) proposed Symmetric ELM.
22. **OS-ELM**: (Guang-Bin Huang *et al.*, 2005) proposed Online-Sequential ELM and they compared method based on Fuzzy-ELM. OS-ELM produced better generalization performance at very fast learning speed.
23. **EM-ELM**: (Guorui Feng *et al.*, 2009) proposed Error Minimzed ELM.
24. **DBELM**: (Arun Anoop M & Poonkuntran S) proposed BAT optimized ELM for Image Forgery detection. Four kernels Tribas, Sigmoidal, Radian, Sinusoidal considered for their work in the case of ELM. Combination of Tribas achieved better results than others. And also random hidden neurons (0-30) processed for their work.

A comprehensive compilation of a wide range of machine learning classifiers that are commonly employed in a variety of contexts is displayed in Table 2.1. The subsequent classifiers are machine learning algorithms employed to make decisions and identify patterns.

The proposed diagram is shown in Figure 2.10, and digital forgery detection proposed flow is shown in Figure 2.11, algorithm pseudo code added after Figure 2.12. In today's digital world, there are many different image look and feel changing tools; most of them are used for the quality changing of images for people who are interested to place their images in front of the public. In most cases, the improved image may not show any clues regarding the original, especially if the original image is not readily available.

Table 2.1 Different ML classifiers.

<table>
<tr><td>1</td><td>Naïve Bayes</td><td>Here picked Forged image, need to find the probability of that image being Genuine.
Probability of finding Genuine in total images, P(Genuine). Then probability of finding Forged in total images, P(Forged).
Probability of finding Forged in Genuine images, that's $P\ (Forged/Genuine)$.
Naïve Bayes equation of the work will be,

$$P\left(\frac{Genuine}{Forged}\right)=\frac{P(Forged/Genuine)*P(Forged)}{P(Genuine)} \tag{2.1}$$
</td></tr>
<tr><td>2</td><td>Decision Trees</td><td>Tuning parameters mainly are Information gain, Gini Index, Chi Square.
"Entropy" is a metric for impurity measuring. Entropy's reduction measured by "Information Gain". "Gini Index" is the measure of both purity and impurity. It is always used in CART of decision trees.

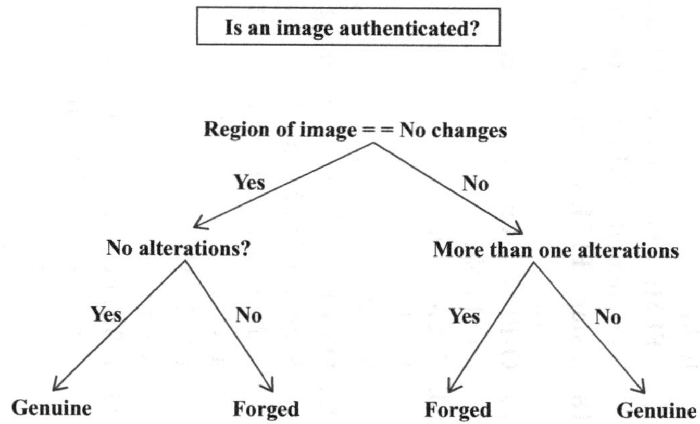

Figure 2.8 Decision tree working scenario.</td></tr>
</table>

(*Continued*)

Table 2.1 Different ML classifiers. (*Continued*)

3	Support Vector Machine	Can call "sklearn.svm" and process the code based on LinearSVC() function.
4	Random Forest Classifier	It is in ensemble and it can process by using Random Forest Classifier() function.
5	Extreme Learning Machine	It is Single Hidden layer feed forward Neural Network. ELM support single/different layers of hidden nodes. Hidden nodes are arbitrarily doled out and never refreshed.

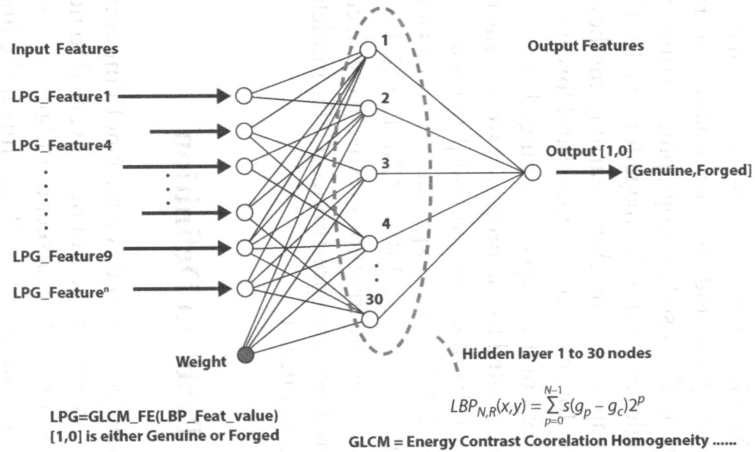

Figure 2.9 Modified ELM-LPG working mechanism (Zaher Yaseen *et al.* 2017).

Due to these readily available image editing windows or android tools, the authenticity of a given image is always a big security task in the research field.

This article presents mainly about forgery detection method that is applicable in the case of different image forgery cases. The proposed transform domain technique relies on both the second-order statistical method, GLRLM, GLCM, GLDM and Local Binary Pattern's variants. It used feature scaling methods for redundant and irrelevant features from feature dataset. It also used lexicographic sorting and Euclidian distance method for single and multiple image forgery localization. And finally it applied some supervised machine learning methods, model stacking and voting method for predicting genuine and forgery images.

The rest of the chapter is arranged as follows. Section 2 presents a survey of work related to the proposed work. This is followed by the presentation of the problem definition and proposed method in Sections 2.2 and 2.3. Section 2.4 discusses experimental results and gives a performance evaluation of LBPGLRLM, LBPGLCM, LBPGLDM with ELM based on different machine learning methods respectively. Section 2.5 presents Feature selection methods and pre-trained CNN models. Finally, a conclusion to the chapter is offered.

2.2 Problem Definition

The main issue noted is a false noticing image region inside the original image. As any image can be converted to normal or abnormal, this leads to crime rates always keeping high. Dangerous situations like this type of forgery may happen all the time if the image is with the wrong person. A person who has expert knowledge to manage image editing decreases the visual nature of the digital image and that can lead a court to make a false determination. It might affect good person to become culprit without correct prediction or wrong person can escape also in case of his or her fake document's forgery nature not noticed while evaluation. So, this problem might be noticed before processing for final decision, so that genuine people will not suffer for fake prediction and based on the issues.

We developed a fused approach. Advanced Local Patterns of Graylevel (LBPSOSA) is the combination of LBP-variants and second-order statistical feature extraction algorithm. And this algorithm will not have the capacity to identify the features for predicting medical image forgeries.

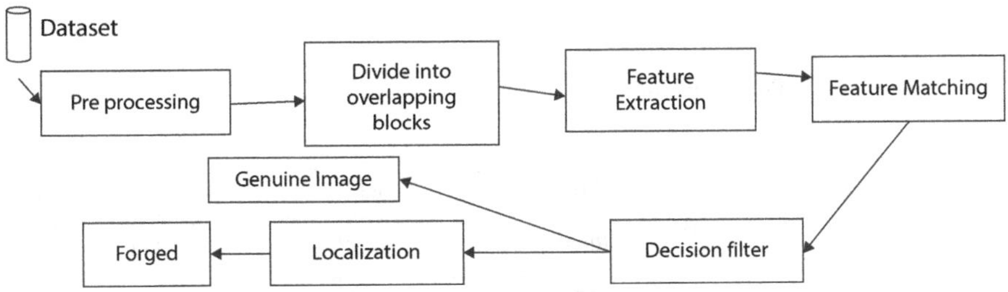

Figure 2.10 General diagram.

For that, ***ALBPVG(ML and CNN)*** have been developed previously. It outperforms previous accuracy rates, mentioned in the experimental evaluation section.

2.3 Proposed Methodology

The block diagram of the proposed system (shown in Figures 2.11, 2.12) demonstrates the detection of digital image manipulations in digital image forensics research area.

The digital image can be processed based on second-order statistical feature extraction algorithm and LBP variants. In LBPSOSA, different machine learning methods have been processed. Also feature scaling results used to remove noises and redundant features. Supervised learning algorithms processed are Extreme learning Machine, Naïve Bayes, Decision Trees, Support Vector Machine, and Random Forest Classifier.

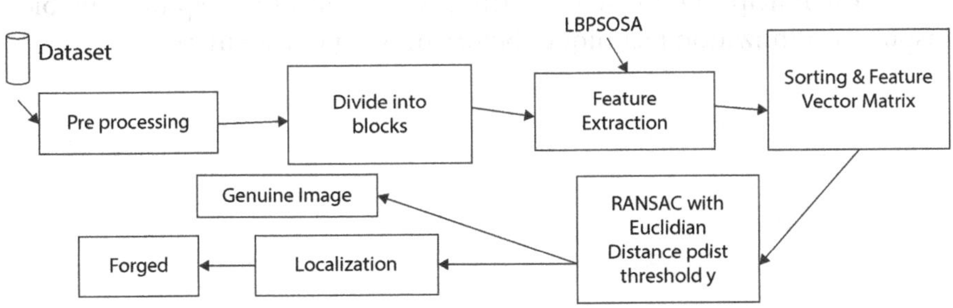

Figure 2.11 Proposed advanced LBPSOSA for image forgery detection.

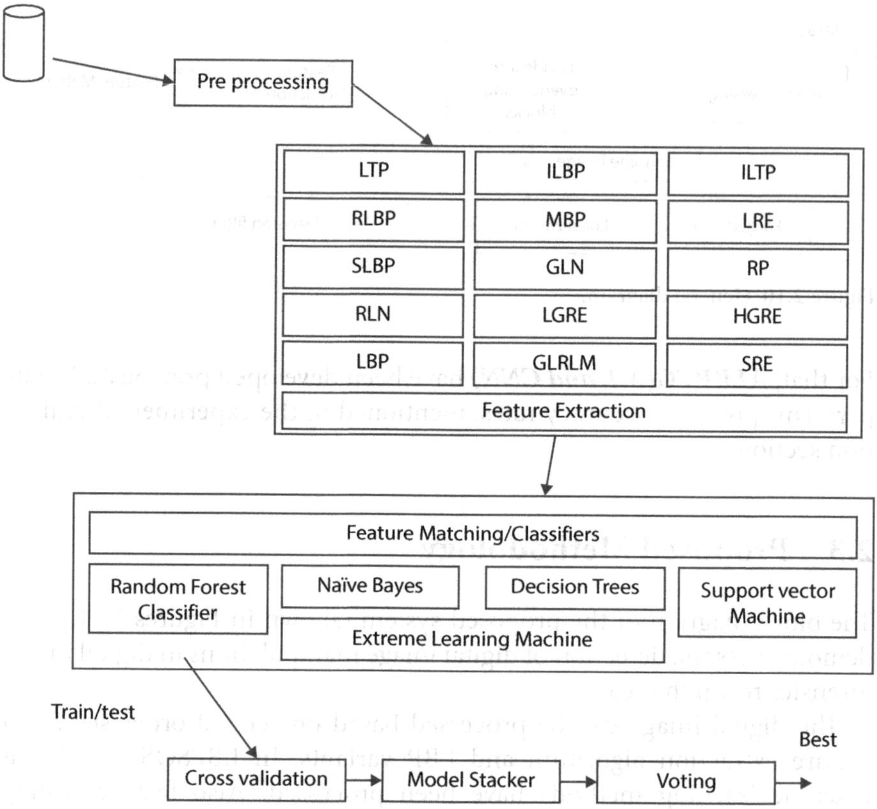

Figure 2.12 Proposed flow of Local Binary Pattern Second-Order Statistics Algorithm (LBPSOSA) for Image Forgery Detection.

In future Advanced Efficient Local LBP variants of Gray level (LBPSOSA) method will help to remove overfitting issues, with the help of some bio-inspired optimization techniques before moving to classifiers.

```
Data: N_dimensional Feature Vector of LBPSOSA
Result: Final Prediction either Genuine or Forged
Initialize data_file ← [featurevalues..];
data_file ← f1, f2, ....f42;
Base_Estimators ← [
if Classifier Accuracy is Higher then
    NaiveBayes()
    DecisionTree()
    SupportVectorM()
    RandomForest()
    ExtremeLearningM()
    ];
    Choose Best Classifer
end
if FV is processed for Matching then
    Total Features: f1, f2, ....f42
    X ← f1, f2, ....f42
    Modified LBP That is Seven wonders of LBP
    LBP_{N1,R1}(x, y)
    S/RLBP_{N1,R1}(x, y, k)
    MBP_{N1,R1}(x, y)
    LTP_{N1,R1}(x, y)
    ILB/TP_{N1,R1}(x, y)
    LBP + GLCM
    LBP + GLDM
    LBP + GLRLM
    Y ← f43
    YisforLabelling
    Example:ELM only mentioned here to show Classification
      Accuracy
    from sklearn.model_selection import train_test_split
    from sklearn.preprocessing import StandardScaler
    from sklearn.base import BaseEstimator
    from sklearn.base import TransformerMixin
    from sklearn.pipeline import make_pipeline
    from sklearn.linear_model import LogisticRegression
    class MyOwnTransformer(BaseEstimator, TransformerMixin)
    elm ←
      make_pipeline(MyOwnTransformer(), LogisticRegression(random_state =
      10, solver =' lbfgs', multi_class =' auto'))
    elm.fit(X_test, y_test)
    elm_pred ← elm.predict(X_test)
    elm_score ← elm.score(X_test, y_test)
    elm_score
end
if Final_Prediction: then
    scores ← [model_A, model_B, .....model_n]
    algorithms ← ["Algorithm_1, Algorithm_2, ....Algorithm_n]
    for i ← range(len(Algorithms)) :
      print(algorithms_i + str(scores_i) + "%")
      sns.barplot(algorithms, scores)
end
```

Algorithm 1: LBPSOSA-A NOVEL APPROACH FOR FORGERY DETECTION

Hybrid Feature Extraction Approach is the combination of LBP-variants (Seven wonders of LBP) and second-order statistical feature extraction method, GLRLM. Working with LBPSOSA to detect Image forgery detection:

1. **In preprocessing,** color image was converted to grayscale image for processing images. In the case of LBP, seven variants were considered with small modifications. LBPs variants generated 16X205 features, among those maximum values calculated in that 16X205, and its average value considered as final feature value for every LBP-variants. Feature vector consists of features and they formed a matrix for carrying those extracted features. People can represent these matrices based on Jacobian or hessian matrix if they required.
2. **In feature extraction,** extraction based on LBP variants and GLRLM-algorithms. **Types of LBP-variants method:** The following are the different inventions of LBPs.

Table 2.2 Modified LBP variants (Seven wonders of LBP) and second-order statistical feature extraction, GLRLM algorithm.

1	$(x_{p1}, y_{p1}) = (x_{c1} + R\,cos(2\pi p/N), y_{c1} - R\,sin(2\pi p1/N))$ (2.2) $LBP_{N1,R1}(x,y) = \sum_{p1=0}^{N1-1} s(g_{p1} - g_{c1})2^{p1}$ (2.3) $s(x) = \begin{cases} 1, x \geq 0 \\ 0, otherwise \end{cases}$ Based on the above equation, updated equation for LBP is the following, $BV \leftarrow Vector\ of\ 2^0, 2^1, 2^2, \ldots, 2^7$ $BI \leftarrow zeros(253,253)$ $BI_{j-1}^{i-1} \leftarrow \sum BV$ (2.3) $RI_{j\pm1}^{i\pm1} X_k, Y_k \geq RI_{j\pm1}^{i\pm1} 2,2$ (2.4) $b_p \leftarrow 1$ $else$ $b_p \leftarrow 0$ $LBP \leftarrow (205\ columns, 16\ rows)$ $205cols\ 0s\ of\ two\ rows + 14Images = 16rows$ $LBP_{feature}\ of\ 1cell = Each\ cell/MAX_{value}$

(Continued)

Table 2.2 Modified LBP variants (Seven wonders of LBP) and second-order statistical feature extraction, GLRLM algorithm. (*Continued*)

2,3	$SLBP_{N1,R1}(x,y,k)=\sum_{p1=0}^{N1-1} s(g_{p1}-g_{c1}-k)2^{p1}$ (2.5) (Gustaf Kylberg *et al.*2013), (Gustaf Kylberg *et al.*2016). $RLBP_{N1,R1}(x,y,t_1)=\sum_{p1=0}^{N1-1} s(g_{p1}-g_{c1}-t_1)2^{p1}$ (2.6) For SLBP and RLBP, features modified is almost same, some positive negative notations only used to differentiate both methods for our work. Modified feature calculation steps are the following, $LBI_{j-1}^{i-1} \leftarrow \sum BV_{lbp}$ (2.7) $UBI_{j-1}^{i-1} \leftarrow \sum BV_{ubp}$ (2.8) $SLBP_{N1,R1}(x,y,k)=\left\{\begin{matrix} RI_{j\pm1}^{i\pm1}X_k, Y_k - RI_{j\pm1}^{i\pm1}2,2-t<0 \\ lbp \leftarrow 1 \\ RI_{j\pm1}^{i\pm1}X_k, Y_k - RI_{j\pm1}^{i\pm1}2,2-t>0 \\ ubp \leftarrow 1 \end{matrix}\right\}$ (2.9) $RLBP_{N1,R1}(x,y,t_1)=\left\{\begin{matrix} RI_{j\pm1}^{i\pm1}X_k, Y_k - RI_{j\pm1}^{i\pm1}2,2+t_1<0 \\ lbp \leftarrow 1 \\ RI_{j\pm1}^{i\pm1}X_k, Y_k - RI_{j\pm1}^{i\pm1}2,2+t_1>0 \\ ubp \leftarrow 1 \end{matrix}\right\}$ (2.10) $(S\ or\ R)LBP \leftarrow (205\ columns,\ 16\ rows)$ *205cols 0s of two rows + 14Images = 16rows* $(S/R)LBP_{feature} = Each\ cell/MAX_{value}$

(*Continued*)

Table 2.2 Modified LBP variants (Seven wonders of LBP) and second-order statistical feature extraction, GLRLM algorithm. (*Continued*)

4	$MBP_{N1,R1}(x,y)=\sum_{p1=0}^{N1-1} s(g_{p1}-g_{med})2^{p1}+s(g_{c1}-g_{med})2^{N1}$ (2.11) $g_{med}=median(\{g_0, g_1, \ldots, g_{N1-1}, g_{c1}\})$ (Girisha *et al.* 2013) (Zaher *et al.* 2017). $DN \leftarrow Directory$ $GI \leftarrow rgb\ to\ gray$ $RI \leftarrow Image\ Resizing$ $X \leftarrow Vector\ of\ 1-3$ $Y \leftarrow Vectore\ of\ 1-3$ $BV \leftarrow Vector\ of\ 2^0, 2^1, \ldots \ldots, 2^7$ $BI \leftarrow zeros(RI)$ $MBP_{N1,R1}(x,y)=RI_{j\pm1}^{i\pm1}X_k, Y_k - RI_{j\pm1}^{i\pm1}2,2$ (2.12) $MBP_{N1,R1}(x,y)=BI_{j-1}^{i-1} \leftarrow \sum BV$ (2.13) $MBP \leftarrow (205\ columns,\ 16\ rows)$ $205cols\ 0s\ of\ two\ rows + 14Images = 16rows$ $MBP_{feature} = Each\ cell/MAX_{value}$
5	$LTP_{N1,R1}(x,y)=\sum_{p1=0}^{N1-1} s_3(g_{p1}, g_{c1}, t_1)2^{p1}$ (2.6) (X Tan *et al.*2007) (Zaher *et al.* 2017) (Dijana Tralic *et al.* 2014). $s_3(g_{p1}, g_{c1}, t_1)=\begin{cases}1, g_{p1} \geq g_{c1}+t_1\\ 0, g_{c1}-t_1 \leq g_{p1} < g_{c1}+t_1\\ -1, otherwise\end{cases}$ (2.13) $LTP_{N1,R1}(x,y)=LBI_{j-1}^{i-1} \leftarrow \sum BV_{lbp}$ (2.14) $LTP_{N1,R1}(x,y)=UBI_{j-1}^{i-1} \leftarrow \sum BV_{ubp}$ (2.15) $LTP_{N1,R1}(x,y)=\begin{Bmatrix} RI_{j\pm1}^{i\pm1}X_k, Y_k < RI_{j\pm1}^{i\pm1}2,2-t\\ lbp \leftarrow 1\\ RI_{j\pm1}^{i\pm1}X_k, Y_k > RI_{j\pm1}^{i\pm1}2,2+t\\ ubp \leftarrow 1\end{Bmatrix}$ (2.16) $LTP \leftarrow (205\ columns,\ 16\ rows)$ $205cols\ 0s\ of\ two\ rows + 14Images = 16rows$ $LTP_{feature} = Each\ cell/MAX_{value}$

(*Continued*)

Table 2.2 Modified LBP variants (Seven wonders of LBP) and second-order statistical feature extraction, GLRLM algorithm. (*Continued*)

6,7	$ILBP_{N1,R1}(x,y)=\sum_{p1=0}^{N1-1} s(g_{p1}-g_{mean})2^{p1}+s(g_{c1}-g_{mean})2^{N1}$ (2.17) $g_{mean}=\frac{1}{N1+1}(\sum_{p1=0}^{N1-1} g_{p1}+g_{c1})$ (Gustaf Kylberg *et al.* 2013). (2.18) $ILTP_{N1,R1}(x,y)=\sum_{p1=0}^{N1-1} s_3(g_{p1}-g_{mean})2^{p1}+s_3(g_{c1}-g_{mean})2^{N1}$ (2.19) (7) (L Nanni *et al.* 2010). For ILBP and ILTP, features modified is almost same, some positive negative notations only used to differentiate both methods for our work. Modified feature calculation steps are the following: $ILB/TP_{N1,R1}(x,y)=RI_{j\pm1}^{i\pm1}X_k,Y_k \pm Mean\big(Mean(RI_{j\pm1}^{i\pm1}X_k,Y_k)\big) + RI_{j\pm1}^{i\pm1}2,2 \pm Mean(Mean(RI_{j\pm1}^{i\pm1}X_k,Y_k)$ (2.20) $ILBP_{N1,R1}(x,y)=BI_{j-1}^{i-1} \leftarrow \sum BV$ (2.21) $(ILB/TP) \leftarrow (205\ columns,\ 16\ rows)$ $205cols\ 0s\ of\ two\ rows + 14Images = 16rows$ $ILB/TP_{feature} = Each\ cell/MAX_{value}$
8-14	LBPSOSA$_{\{\text{SHORT RUN EMPHASIS (SRE), LONG RUN EMPHASIS (LRE), GRAY LEVEL NON-UNIFORMITY (GLN), RUN PERCENTAGE (RP), RUN LENGTH NON-UNIFORMITY (RLN), LOW GRAY LEVEL RUN EMPHASIS (LGRE), HIGH GRAY LEVEL RUN EMPHASIS (HGRE)}\}}$ (Wout Oude Elferink, 2015,University of Twente, The Netherlands) $image_{location} \leftarrow imreadfunction$ $masking \leftarrow ones\big(size(image_{location})\big)$ $quantizing \leftarrow 8\ to\ 16$ $[SRE, \dots\dots, HGRE] = glrlm(image_{location}, quantitzing, masking)$ (2.22)

3. **In feature matching,** some different feature matching methods are mentioned.
4. **Second-order statistical feature extraction and Feature vector collection stages are mentioned below (In case of LBPGLRLM),**

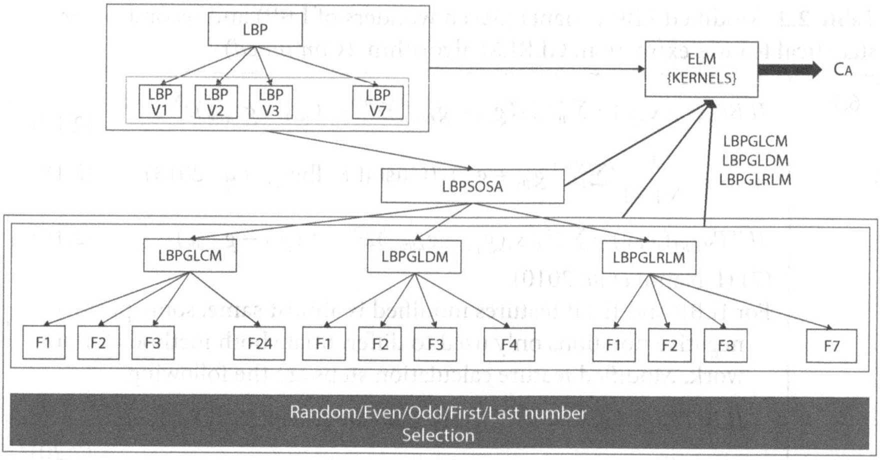

Figure 2.13 LBPSOSA different features for ELM classification accuracy prediction.

$$Feature\_Vector(FV)_{ALPvG2}$$

$$= \{LBP_{N1,R1}(x, y), ILBP_{N1,R1}(x, y), MBP_{N1,R1}(x, y),$$

$$LTP_{N1,R1}(x, y), ILTP_{N1,R1}(x, y), RLBP_{N1,R1}(x, y, t_1),$$

$$SLBP_{N1,R1}(x, y, k), SRE_{GLRLM}$$

$$LRE_{GLRLM}, GLN_{GLRLM}, RP_{GLRLM}, LGRE_{GLRLM},$$

$$HGRE_{GLRLM}, RLN_{GLRLM}\} = 14 \text{ features} \tag{2.23}$$

In order to obtain precise information regarding the influence of LBPSOSA on the prediction of classification accuracy for Extreme Learning Machines (ELM), it is necessary to consult the primary source material, which may consist of a research paper, thesis, or document containing the depicted figure. The figure caption and the accompanying text in the primary source are expected to explain the results and approach illustrated in Figure 2.13 comprehensively.

5. **Features processed by different ML methods:** For evaluation, selected supervised machine learning algorithms are Extreme Learning Machine, Naïve Bayes, Decision Trees, Support Vector Machine, and Random Forest Classifier. Model stacking identifies the best accuracy generating

Table 2.3 Schema of 1-5 database.

F1	F2	F3	F4	F5	F6	F7	F8	F9	F10	.....	F42

classifier combination based on voting process. Euclidian distance with threshold method processed for image forgery prediction in natural digital images.

2.4 Experimentation and Results

The proposed method is processed based on five datasets (Arun Anoop M & Poonkuntran S, 2020). Following datasets are used,

1. CASIA: 100 original & 100 tampered.
2. CoMoFoD: 3GB small images considered for this work. 10402 original images. Out of that 300 original and 300 forged images considered.
3. MICC-F220: 150 original and 150 tampered.
4. HiFoD: 1,216 original & 1,216 forged.
5. Kodak: Aerials (36,36); Misc (37,37). Out of four, two categories considered.

Schema is overall design of dataset. Declaration of variables is in the form of a table, which here consists of different features or attributes namely F1, F2, ..., F42. Based on the image count values must be added in this database schema. Database schema is the collection of database objects and it is associated with database username. Here database username is the name of the database. Seven wonders of LBP generate seven feature algorithms and its values and its collection are already mentioned in Table 2.2. In addition to that GLRLM features are generated. LBP seven wonders is not new but have modified that deriving steps for this work. Many researchers have already used LBP variants in the field of face recognition and facial feature extraction. It results in high accuracy, so the motivation behind this work is for getting better accuracy. Utilized LBP variants for work that helped to get better features and better accuracy rates. These utilized LBP variants, modified based on this work, helped to get high accuracy for image forgery detection.

The presentation of proposed technique LBPSOSA-based duplicate move falsification identification is assessed by specific execution measures. LBPSOSA is the hybridization of LBP and second-order statistical feature extraction algorithm, GLRLM. Furthermore, done execution in view of ELM AI approach. LBP-variations produces seven elements, GLRLM creates seven different component pixel values. GLRLM+LBP variants => 14 features. Utilized AI approaches considering Neural Network, Naive Bayes, SVM and ELM utilized for LBPSOSA Copy Move Forgery Detection, CMFD. ELM performed high effectiveness contrasted with other three calculations. ELM is the best one for our examination work in view of execution assessment. Our calculation will work in all datasets which have unique and manufactured pair. Original pictures isolated by '1' and produced '0' separately. Exactness determined considering 'rad','sig' and 'tribas' actuation capabilities or portions of ELM. The boundaries like Precision(p), Recall(r), F1-score and exactness % are used. The p and r are assessed and tried with different clinical pictures. Execution estimates utilized here are depicted as Tp1 is Valid Positive, TN1 is Valid Negative, Fp1 is Misleading Positive and FN1 is Bogus Negative. **Calculated_Precision(p):** It connotes the right and exact discovery of phony is evaluated as a falsification picture. It connotes the accuracy of the strategy. **Calculated_Recall(r):** It is a negligible portion of the pertinent phony picture that is really recuperated and it demonstrates the fortitude of the procedure. **Calculated_F1-score:** F1-score or F-measure is the proportion of test exactness. Exactness % is the extents of the classifier to make an exact fabrication picture grouping.

$$Calculated\_Precision, Cp = \frac{T_{p1}}{T_{p1} + F_{p1}} = \frac{Fdetected_{Image} \cap Manipulated_{Image}}{FDetected_{Image}} \tag{2.17}$$

$$Calculated\_Recall, Cr = \frac{T_{p1}}{T_{p1} + F_{N1}} = \frac{FDetected_{Image} \cap Manipulated_{Image}}{Manipulated_{Image}} \tag{2.18}$$

$$Calculated\_F1-score = \frac{2 * p1 * r}{Calculated\_Precision + Calculated\_Recall} \tag{2.19}$$

Table 2.4 Image forgery detection & recognition (**original & forged**).

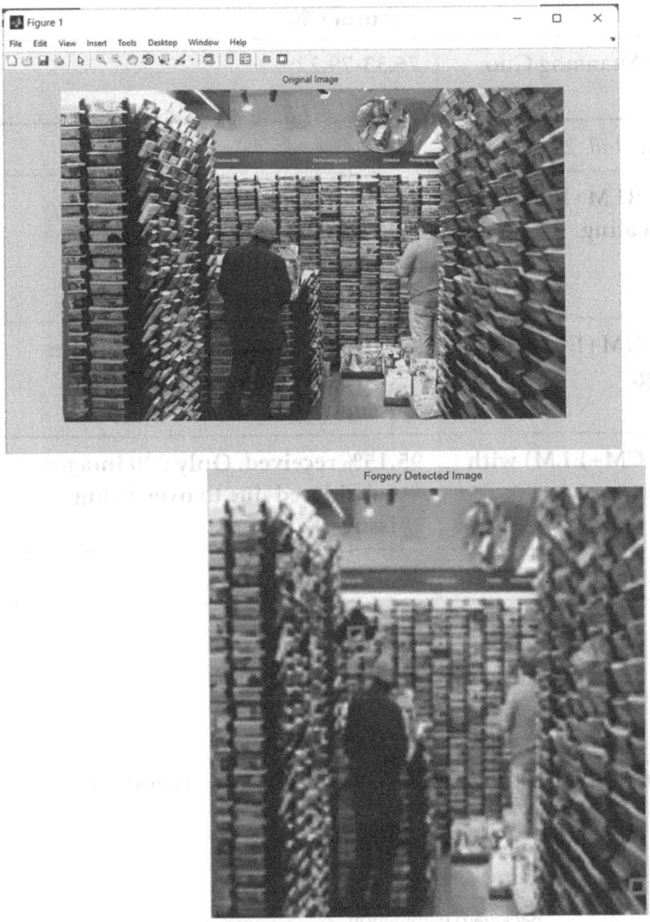

Figure 2.14 Forgery localization.

In Table 2.5 is the classification accuracy of the proposed approaches. Initially 1,839 original and forged images were considered. There were overfitting issues, so only 50% of upper bound 1,839 were considered. That is 920 images considered for the work. Seven wonders of modified ELM and hybrid of LBP and second-order statistical measures like GLRLM, GLDM and GLCM were used. CNN and bio-inspired algorithms were introduced next for avoiding overfitting issues.

Table 2.5 Accuracy for different methods.

Methods	Accuracy %
FCID-HIST & FE (Yuanfang Guo *et al.* 2018)	76.33-79.22%
BusterNet (Yue Wu *et al.* 2018)	78.0%
Proposed (LBPGLRLM+ELM) with standard scaling.	**96.05% received 50% of 1,839 original & forged. Only 920 images considered due to overfitting issues.**
Proposed (LBPGLDM+ELM) with standard scaling.	**94.31% received. Only 920 images considered due to overfitting issues.**
Proposed (LBPGLCM+ELM) with standard scaling.	**95.15% received. Only 920 images considered due to overfitting issues.**
Overall LBPSOSA+ELM	**96.01%**

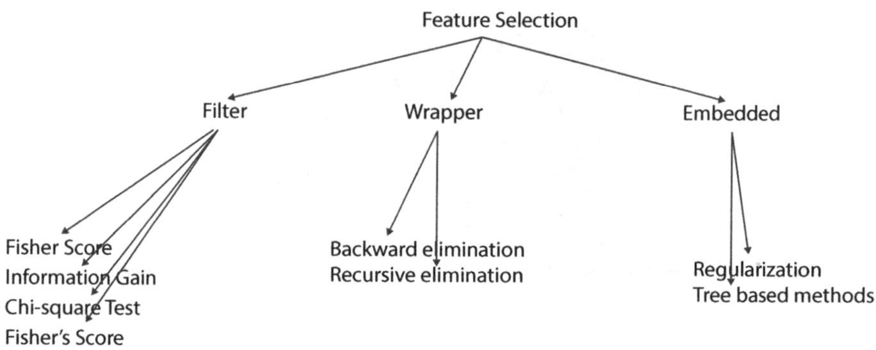

Figure 2.15 Feature selection methods.

2.5 Feature Selection & Pre-Trained CNN Models Description

Below are the details of feature selection methods like Information gain, Fisher score, Laplacian score, PCA, ADAM optimizer, Elephant herding algorithm, Genetic algorithm, BAT algorithm, etc.

Sl. no	Feature selection method name	Details with equation
1	Information gain	It is characterized as how much information was given by the feature to distinguish the objective worth and measures decrease in the entropy values. The biggest information gain is identical to the smallest entropy.
2	Fisher Score	Fisher's Score selects each feature freely as indicated by their scores under Fisher basis, prompting a suboptimal set of features. The bigger the Fisher's score is, the better is the selected feature.
3	Laplacian score	For each element, its Laplacian score is processed to mirror its territory saving power.
4	PCA	PCA lessens the dimensionality without losing data from any features. Principal Component Analysis (PCA) is an element reduction strategy frequently utilized in clustering undertakings.
5	ADAM optimizer	Adaptive Moment Estimation (ADAM) works with the calculation of learning rates for every boundary utilizing the first and second moment of the gradient.
6	SGD	Beginning from an underlying worth, Gradient Descent is run iteratively to track down the optimal upsides of the boundaries to track down the base conceivable worth of the given cost function.

(Continued)

(*Continued*)

7	Elephant herding algorithm	This algorithm is roused by the herding behavior of the elephant bunch. Elephants are gathered as far as clans and their leader is a Matriarch. The adult male elephants get away from their family bunch. Hence, these two behaviors of the elephant bunch lead to two operators, i.e., tribe refreshing operator and isolating operator.
8	Genetic Algorithm	Genetic algorithms depend on the thoughts of natural selection and genetics.
9	BAT algorithm	All bats use echolocation to detect distance, and they moreover "know" the bearing of the food/prey.

Below are the details of pre-trained CNN models, which are LeNet, ResNet, AlexNet, etc.

Sl. no	Pre-trained CNN models	Details with equation
1	LeNet	LeNet is a convolutional neural network structure proposed by LeCun *et al.* in 1998. In general, LeNet alludes to LeNet-5 and is a basic convolutional neural network.
2	ResNet	ResNet, which was proposed in 2015 by specialists at Microsoft Research presented another design called Residual Network.
3	VGG	VGG represents Visual Geometry Group and it is a standard profound Convolutional Neural Network (CNN) engineering with different layers. Ordinary forms are VGG 16 and 19.
4	GoogleNet	GoogLeNet is a kind of convolutional neural network in light of the Inception engineering.

(*Continued*)

(Continued)

5	AlexNet and ImageNet	AlexNet, named after Alex Krizhevsky, is a changed rendition of ImageNet which train on 15 million pictures having a place with 20,000 classes.
6	Mask R-CNN	Mask R-CNN is an adaptable framework created for the purpose of object instance segmentation.
7	Inception	Inception is a CNN model which is a network trained on more than 1,000,000 pictures from the ImageNet data set.
8	YOLO	YOLO is an ultra-popular item recognition framework for deep learning applications.
9	MobileNet	MobileNet is an architecture intended for mobile gadgets.

Below are different learning types with examples.

Sl. no	Unsupervised/Supervised learning methods
1	Regression models, Clustering methods, Support Vector Machine, Decision Tree, Random Forest, Boosting algorithms, Artificial Neural network, Convolutional Neural Network, Extreme Learning Machine classifiers.

BAT Algorithm

The BAT algorithm (BA) is a bio-inspired algorithm developed by Xin-She Yang in 2010.

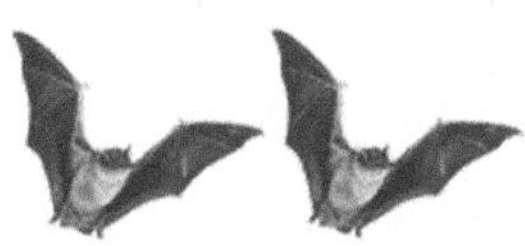

emit high-frequency sound waves, which hit and return from the objects around them; they find their direction, generate sounds and escape from obstacles, and find prey for food. They emit waves for identifying obstacles and they generate waves for food. They choose food based on best value. The term "best" means they select very nearest one while flying for prey. Bats ecolocation is like "sonar system". Bats use sonar characteristics for movement or hunting. Bats use these characteristics, so at least they can hunt or move anything and anywhere without hitting any obstacles. Bats mainly use wavelength, loudness and velocity. Bats can hear frequencies up to 120KHz.

Xin-She Yang's Rules

1. All bats use echolocation to identify distance for food, prey, or obstacles recognition.
2. Bats randomly fly at constant frequency (f_{min}), speed (v_i), position (x_i), with wavelength (λ), and loudness (A_0) to find their prey. They can automatically adjust emitting pulse frequency, and adjust the emitting pulse rate of r in [0, 1].
3. The loudness varies from a large value A_0 to a minimum value A_{min}.

In general the frequency f in a range [f_{min}, f_{max}] range of [20kHz, 500kHz] and $f \in [0, f_{max}]$ corresponds to a range of wavelengths [λ_{min},λ_{max}] range of wavelengths from 0.7mm to 17mm.

The rate of pulse in the range of [0,1] where 0 for no pulses notation, and 1 for maximum rate of pulse emission notation.

Equations mainly are,

$$f_i = f_{min} + (f_{max} - f_{min})\beta$$

$$v_i{}^t = v_i{}^{(t\text{-}1)} + (x_i{}^t - x_*)f_i$$

$$x_i{}^t = x_i{}^{t-1} + v_i{}^t$$

Xin-She Yang's BAT algorithm is described below:

Data: Total Features
Result: Best values

Optimization function f(x), wherein x = $(x_1, ..., x_d)^T$
For each bat of the population x_i.
let there be a corresponding velocity v_i and pulse frequency f_i.
Let the pulse rates be r_i.
Having loudness A_i
while (time < max) do
Obtain new solutions by continuously altering frequency, and changing velocity and location
if rand > r_i then
Optimize the given solutions
Select from the given set of optimized solution, a locally acceptable solution
One random solution to be generated
end if
if random < A_i
and
$f(x_i) < f(x)$ then
Where, x is the current best solution
Accept this newly generated solution Increment and Decrement loudness A_i
end if
Rank bats in order of r_i and rank the current best solution
end while

Algorithm 2: BAT optimization Algorithm

Data: N_dimensional Feature Vector of ALBPVG
Result: Final Prediction either Genuine or Forged
Initialize $i \leftarrow 1, 2, \ldots., N$ *training samples*
$\beta \leftarrow [\beta_1, \beta_2, \ldots..\beta_L]^T$ *output of matrix between hidden and output neurons*
$h(x) = [\alpha_1, \alpha_2, \ldots.\alpha_n]$ *hidden neuron outputs*
x_i *Randomized hidden feature*
$h_i(x)$ i^th *hidden neuron*
$h_i(x) = G(a_i, b_i, x), a_i \in R^d, b_i \in R$ $G(a_i, b_i, x)$ *using hidden neuron parameters* (a, b), *is a non − linear piecewise continuous function*
Log Sigmoid $\leftarrow G(a, b, x) \leftarrow \frac{1}{1+\exp(-ax+b)}$
$||H\beta - T||$ *where, Hiddenlayer(H), T,* β^* *is the procedure step of ELM and 'H' is the randomized hidden layer output then it is notated below*
$[g(x_1), g(x_2), ...g(x_n)]$
$[t_1^1, t_2^2, ...t_n^T)]$
$\beta^* = H^+T$
where, H^+T *is Moore Penrose generalized inverse function+*

ALBPVG based on ELM Algorithm

2.6 BAT ELM Optimization Results

Feature Selection is dimensionality reduction method to identify best features in order to get good classification accuracy. Nature inspired and bio-inspired feature selection approaches normally using for Machine Learning and Deep Learning (ML or DL) based predictions. Feature selection methods are Information gain, Fisher score, Laplacian score, PCA, ADAM optimizer, Elephant herding algorithm, Genetic algorithm, BAT algorithm, etc.

CNN is enough for feature extraction and classification process. In CNN, we need not worry about feature extraction and scaling process. We just need to process images and reshaping or resizing of images for further CNN algorithmic process. Managing a huge number of images is a big task; in the case of CNN, it may lead to training and testing errors. Sometimes testing accuracy will be higher than training accuracy, training accuracy may be higher than testing, testing loss may be higher than training loss, and testing loss may be lower than training loss. Sometimes while processing large dataset, Google Colab may get stuck and it may stop processing for classification. As CNN is slow in case of large dataset

Figure 2.16 BAT optimized CNN-ELM image forgery localizer.

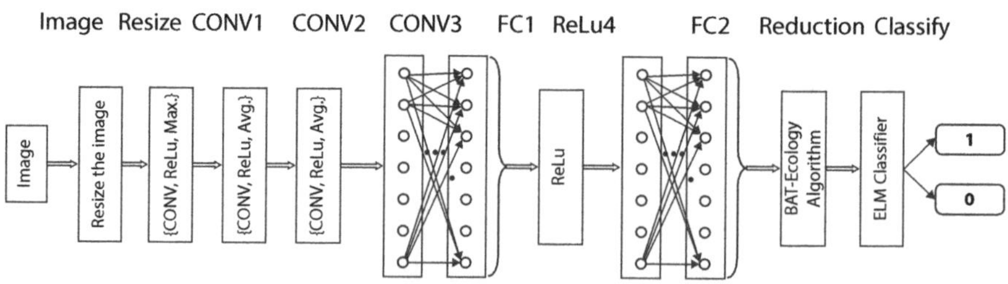

Figure 2.17 BAT optimized CNN-ELM for image forgery predictor.

managing, there should be a bio-inspired algorithm framework after the last fully connected layer.

Data: Dataset of Test and train Images
Result: Final Prediction either Genuine or Forged

//PredictionModelDetails//
Images
Resize = 64,64,3 of Data_images
Conv2D_2
Conv2D_2
Conv2D_2
FullyConnectedlayer1
ReLu
FullyConnectedlayer2
Alexnet CNN for feature extraction feature maps
BAT ecology
ELM Classifier

//BAT Optimized ELM-CNN Prediction
Intialize the neurons
Initialise Loudness, frequency, Pulse rate, velocity
Evaluate the fitness function
Calculate the best value
Calculate the classification accuracy(Ac)
Stop Criterion
If Ac < At
Select best features
Update the loudness, Frequency,Pulse rate, velocity
else
goto step 2 and repeat it until to reach best match results.
Created a BAT ecology framework for data collection
Population size
Number of generations
Minimum frequency
Maximum frequency
Initial loudness
Loudness Adaptation measure(below 1)
Initial pulse rate
Pulse rate Adaptation measure(below 1)
Activation function
Number of Epochs
ELM processed
Classification Accuracy Received

Algorithm 3: BAT optimized CNN-ELM for Image Forgery Predictor

Table 2.6 Accuracy for different methods.

Methods	Accuracy %
AlexNet+ELM	97.47%
AlexNet+BAT+ELM	99.24%

Conclusion

Proving authenticity is a difficult task nowadays due to freely available image editing software. Metadata retrieval or extraction is an easy task but if anyone modified or deleted data about data, then it will be a difficult task to identify the genuine information regarding images or other multimedia resources. The proposed approach demonstrated authenticity in view of various forgery datasets. Among supervised machine learning classifiers ELM with various activation functions demonstrated and also checked AlexNet-based pre-trained CNN model with BAT-ELM framework. The proposed system outperforms previous results and mainly features extracted based on second-order statistical algorithms like GLCM, GLDM, GLRLM, and Seven wonders of LBP variants-based features. The performance was evaluated and concluded using tables. Based on ALEXNET-CNN with BAT-ELM strategies, highest classification accuracy achieved was in between 97-99.24%. The next work will be based on BAT-ecology-bio-inspired algorithm with Benchmark functions like Ackley-function, Rastrigin-function testing and it will identify mean-standard-deviation measures and compare different bio-inspired algorithms.

Declarations

Availability of data and materials: Data sharing is not applicable to this article as the dataset used here is Suckling's dataset, which is already cited in our article.

Competing interests: The authors declare that they have no competing interests.

Funding: This work has no funding source. This paper's work implementation was completed from Research Laboratory, Department of Computer Science & Engineering, Velammal College of Engineering & Technology, Viraganoor, Madurai, Tamilnadu, India. This chapter is a part of "LPG: a novel approach for medical forgery detection in image transmission," *Journal of Ambient Intelligence and Humanized Computing*, Springer.

Consent for Publication

No informed consent was required for us, as the study does not involve any human participant. This article does not contain any studies or analysis with animals or humans performed by any of the authors.

Conflict of Interest

Dr. Arun Anoop M, Dr. P. Karthikeyan & Dr. S. Poonkuntran declare that they have no conflict of interest.

Acknowledgement

The authors would like to thank Velammal College of Engineering & Technology for the completion of the work. No funding was involved in the present work. Also, we thank the anonymous reviewers for their suggestions.

References

1. Suckling, J., Parker, J., Dance, D., Astley, S., Hutt, I., Boggis, C., Ricketts, I., Stamatakis, E., Cerneaz, N., Kok, S-L., Taylor, P., Betal, D., Savage, J., Mammographic Image Analysis Society Digital Mammogram Database, Elsevier, 375-378, 1994.
2. H. Farid, "Image forgery detection," in *IEEE Signal Processing Magazine*, vol. 26, no. 2, pp. 16-25, March 2009, doi: 10.1109/MSP.2008.931079.
3. Jingyi Liu, Xinxin Liu, Chongmin Liu, Ba Tuan Le, and Dong Xiao,"Pruning Multilayered ELM Using Cholesky Factorization and Givens Rotation Transformation," *Hindawi Mathematical Problems in Engineering*, Volume 2021, Article ID 5588426, pp. 1-11.
4. Bo He, Yan Song,Yuemei Zhu, Qixin Sha, Yue Shen, Tianhong Yan, Rui Nian, Amaury Lendasse, "Local receptive fields based extreme learning machine with hybrid filter kernels for image classification," Springer, *Multidim Syst Sign Process*, June 2018.
5. Jinghong Huang, Zhu Liang Yu, Zhaoquan Cai, Zhenghui Gu, Zhiyin Cai, Wei Gao, Shengfeng Yu, Qianyun Du,"Extreme learning machine with multi-scale local receptive fields for texture classification," Springer *Multidim Syst Sign Process*, April 2016.
6. Chao Wu, Yaqian Li, Zhibiao Zhao, Bin Liu,"Extreme learning machine with autoencoding receptive fields for image classification," Springer *Neural Computing and Applications*, June 2019.
7. Shifei Ding, Lili Guo,Yanlu Hou,"Extreme learning machine with kernel model based on deep learning," Springer *Neural Comput & Applic*, Dec 2015.
8. Huijuan Lu, Bangjun Du, Jinyong Liu, Haixia Xia, Wai K. Yeap,"A kernel extreme learning machine algorithm based on improved particle swam optimization," Springer Memetic Comp., Amrch 2016.

9. Huijuan Lu, Shasha Wei, Zili Zhou, Yanzi Miao, Yi Lu, "Regularised extreme learning machine with misclassification cost and rejection cost for gene expression data classification," *Int. J. Data Mining and Bioinformatics*, Vol. 12, No. 3, pp. 294-312, 2015.
10. Yueqing Wang, Zhige Xie, Kai Xu, Yong Dou, Yuanwu Lei, "An Efficient and Effective Convolutional Auto-Encoder Extreme Learning Machine Network for 3D Feature Learning," Elsevier *Neurocomputing*, Oct 2015.
11. Yimin Yang, Q. M. Jonathan Wu, "Multilayer Extreme Learning Machine with Subnetwork Nodes for Representation Learning," IEEE Transactions on Cybernetics, pp. 2168-2267, 2015.
12. Yaoming Cai, Xiaobo Liu, Yongshan Zhang, Zhihua Cai, "Hierarchical Ensemble of Extreme Learning Machine, Pattern Recognition Letters," Elsevier *Pattern Recognition Letters*, 2018.
13. Chi-Man Vong, Chuangquan Chen, Pak-Kin Wong, "Empirical Kernel Map-Based Multilayer Extreme Learning Machines for Representation Learning," Elsevier *Neurocomputing*, 2018.
14. Sen-Hui Wang, Hai-Feng Li, Yong-Jie Zhang, and Zong-Shu Zou, "A Hybrid Ensemble Model Based on ELM and Improved AdaBoost.RT *Algorithm for Predicting the Iron Ore Sintering Characters*, Jan 2019.
15. Jiuwen Cao, Zhiping Lin, Guang-Bin Huang, Nan Liu, "Voting based extreme learning machine," Elsevier *Information Sciences*, pp. 66-71, 2012.
16. Chao Wang, Jizheng Yang, and Qing Wu, "A global extended extreme learning machine combined with electronic nose for identifying tea gas information," *Measurement and Control* 2022, Vol. 55(7-8) 746–756.
17. Jiuwen Cao, Zhiping Lin, Guang-Bin Huang, "Self-Adaptive Evolutionary Extreme Learning Machine," Springer Science & Business Media *Neural Process Lett* 36:285–305, 2012.
18. Ming-Bin Li, Guang-Bin Huang, P. Saratchandran, N. Sundararajan, "Fully complex extreme learning machine," Elsevier *Neurocomputing* 68, 306–314, 2005.
19. Guang-Bin Huang, Ming-Bin Li, Lei Chen, Chee-Kheong Siew, "Incremental extreme learning machine with fully complex hidden nodes," Elsevier *Neurocomputing* 71, 576–583, 2008.
20. Yuan Lan, Yeng Chai Soh, Guang-Bin Huang, "Two-stage extreme learning machine for regression," Elsevier *Neurocomputing* 73, 3028–3038,2010.
21. Wan-Yu Deng, Qing-Hua Zheng, Shiguo Lian, Lin Chen, Xin Wang, "Ordinal extreme learning machine," Elsevier *Neurocomputing* 74, 447–456, 2010.
22. Qin-Yu Zhu, A.K. Qin, P.N. Suganthan, Guang-Bin Huang, "Rapid and brief communication: Evolutionary extreme learning machine," *Pattern Recognition* 38(10):1759-1763,2005.
23. Xueyi Liu, Ping Li, Chuanhou Gao, "Symmetric extreme learning machine," Springer-Verlag London Limited, *Neural Comput & Applic* 22:551–558, 2013.

24. Guang-Bin Huang, Nan-Ying Liang, Hai-Jun Rong, P. Saratchandran, and N. Sundararajan, "On-Line Sequential Extreme Learning Machine," *The IASTED International Conference on Computational Intelligence (CI 2005), Calgary, Canada, July 4-6, 2005.*
25. Xin-She Yang, "Bat Algorithm for Multi-objective Optimization," *Int. J. Bio-Inspired Computation*, Vol. 3, No. 5, pp. 267-274, 2011.
26. Xin-She Yang and Amir H. Gandomi, "Bat Algorithm: A Novel Approach for Global Engineering Optimization," *Engineering Computations*, Vol. 29, Issue 5, pp. 464–483, 2012.
27. Xin-She Yang, "A New Metaheuristic Bat-Inspired Algorithm," Springer NICSO 2010, SCI 284, pp. 65–74, 2010.
28. Yang, X.-S., and Xingshi He, "Bat Algorithm: Literature review and applications," *Int. J. Bio-Inspired Computation*, Vol. 5, No. 3, pp. 141–149, 2013.
29. Longfei Wu and Xiaojiang Du, "Security Threats to Mobile Multimedia Applications: Camera-Based Attacks on Mobile Phones," *IEEE Communication Magazine, Security in Wireless Multimedia Communications*, pp 80-87, March 2014.
30. Yuanfang Guo, Xiaochun Cao, Wei Zhang and Rui Wang, "Fake Colorized Image Detection," Arxiv, 2018.
31. Wang, Gai-Ge & Deb, Suash & Coelho, Leandro, "Elephant Herding Optimization," *3rd International Symposium on Computational and Business Intelligence*, 2015.
32. Li, Juan & Lei, Hong & Alavi, Amir & Wang, Gai-Ge., "Elephant Herding Optimization: Variants, Hybrids, and Applications", MDPI Mathematics. 8. 1415, pp. 1-25, 2020.
33. LK Tan, MBiomedEng, "Image file formats," *Biomedical Imaging and Intervention Journal Technology in Imaging Tutorial* 2(1), 2006.
34. Rahul Dixit, Ruchira Naskar, "Review, analysis and parameterisation of techniques for copy–move forgery detection in digital images," *Institution of Engineering and Technology* 2017.
35. Seyedali Mirjalili, Seyed Mohammad Mirjalili, Xin-She Yang, "Binary bat algorithm," Springer *Neural Comput & Applic*, 2013.
36. Monalisa Nayak, Soumya Das, Urmila Bhanja, Manas Ranjan Senapati, "Elephant herding optimization technique based neural network for cancer prediction," Elsevier *Informatics in Medicine Unlocked* 21 100445, 2020.
37. Xiaofei He, Deng Cai, Partha Niyogi, "Laplacian Score for Feature Selection," *NIPS'05: Proceedings of the 18th International Conference on Neural Information Processing Systems*, pp 507–514, 2005.
38. Aseem Agarwala, Mira Dontcheva, Maneesh Agrawala, Steven Drucker, Alex Colburn, Brian Curless, David Salesin, Michael Cohen, "Interactive Digital Photomontage," *ACM SIGGRAPH conference Proceedings*, 2004.
39. Dong WM, Bao GB, Zhang XP, and Jean-Claude Paul "Fast multi-operator image resizing and evaluation," *Journal of Computer Science and Technology* 27(1): 121–134, 2012.

40. Yun Q. Shi, Chunhua Chen, Wen Chen, "A natural image model approach to splicing detection," MM&Sec '07: *Proceedings of the 9th Workshop on Multimedia & Security*, pp 51–62, 2007.
41. Cristina Malegori, Laura Franzetti, Riccardo Guidetti, Ernestina Casiraghi, "GLCM, an image analysis technique for early detection of biofilm," Elsevier *Journal of Food Engineering*, 2016.
42. Neda Ahmadi, Gholamreza Akbarizadeh, "Iris tissue recognition based on GLDM feature extraction and hybrid MLPNN-ICA classifier," Springer *Neural Computing and Applications*, 2018.
43. Sonali Mishra, Banshidhar Majhi and Pankaj Kumar Sa, "GLRLM-Based Feature Extraction for Acute Lymphoblastic Leukemia (ALL) Detection," Springer *Recent Findings in Intelligent Computing Techniques, Advances in Intelligent Systems and Computing* 708, 2018.
44. Abu Sayeed Md. Sohail, Prabir Bhattacharya, Sudhir P. Mudur, and Srinivasan Krishnamurthy, "Local Relative Glrlm-Based Texture Feature Extraction for Classifying Ultrasound Medical Images," IEEE CCECE 2011.
45. Wei Yu, Lin Gan, Sha Yang, Yonggang Ding, Pan Jiang, Jun Wang, Shijun Li, "An improved LBP algorithm for texture and face classification," Springer-Verlag London 2014.
46. Thomas Raths, Jens Otten and Christoph Kreitz, "The ILTP Problem Library for Intuitionistic Logic Release v1.1," Kluwer Academic Publishers, 2006.
47. Guangjian Tian, Hong Fu, David Dagan Feng, "Automatic Medical Image Categorization and Annotation Using LBP and MPEG-7 Edge Histograms," *Proceedings of the 5th International Conference on Information Technology and Application in Biomedicine*, in conjunction with *The 2nd International Symposium & Summer School on Biomedical and Health Engineering*, 2008.
48. Mingyi Liu, Zhiying Tu, Tong Zhang, Tonghua Su, Zhongjie Wang, "LTP: A New Active Learning Strategy for CRF-Based Named Entity Recognition," *Neural Processing Letters* volume 54, pp. 2433–2454. 2022.
49. Meng Yang, Lei Zhang, Lin Zhang and David Zhang, "Monogenic Binary Pattern (MBP): A Novel Feature Extraction and Representation Model for Face Recognition," *IEEE International Conference on Pattern Recognition*, 2010.
50. J. Chen, V. Kellokumpu, G. Zhao, M. Pietikäinen, "Rlbp: Robust Local Binary Pattern," *British Machine Vision Conference*, 2013.
51. Jeonghyun Baek, Jisu Kim and Euntai Kim, "Part-based Face Detection using SLBP," *14th International Conference on Control, Automation and Systems*, 2014.
52. Mingxing Jia, Zhixian Zhang, Pengfei Song, and Junqiang Du, "Research of Improved Algorimth Based on LBP for Face Recognition," *CCBR* 2014, LNCS 8833, pp. 111–119, 2014.
53. Arun Anoop M, Poonkuntran S, "Dbelm for Image Forgery Detection," *International Journal of Computing and Technology*, Volume 7, Issue 10, 2020.

54. Dr. Arun Anoop M, Dr. Karthikeyan P, Dr. Poonkuntran S, "Medical Image Detection and Recognition using Machine learning and Deep learning (ALBPVG-A NOVEL APPROACH FOR MEDICAL FORGERY DETECTION IN IMAGE TRANSMISSION)," Machine learning and Deep Learning techniques for Medical Image Recognition, CRC T & F Book Chapter (Major Revision process).
55. Yang, X. S., & He, X. (2013). Bat algorithm: literature review and applications. International Journal of Bio-inspired computation, 5(3), 141-149.
56. Chaitra, B., and PV Bhaskar Reddy. "An approach for copy-move image multiple forgery detection based on an optimized pre-trained deep learning model." Knowledge-Based Systems 269 (2023): 110508

3

Multimedia Data in Healthcare System

Sarita Gulia[1], Pallavi Pandey[2] and Yogita Yashveer Raghav[3]*

[1]*Department of Computer Science and Engineering, K. R. Mangalam University, Gurugram, Haryana, India*
[2]*School of Engineering & Technology, K. R. Mangalam University, Gurugram Haryana, India*
[3]*Computer Science Department at K. R. Mangalam University, Gurugram, Haryana, India*

Abstract

Data that combines many media is multimedia. Types of data include text, numbers, images, audio, and video. Multimedia is crucial for presenting information. It has diverse applications in education, training, business, advertising, and entertainment. Multimedia data can feed neural network models for disease diagnosis and prediction, benefiting the healthcare business. Feature identification, extraction, and analysis can use several machine learning methods. Multimedia technology allows subjects to view diagnosis images such as X-rays, CT scans, and MRI scans to grasp the issue better. Detection and staging of illness are possible. Combining multimedia techniques and technology can improve doctor-patient communication. With multimedia technology, patients may easily recall offered information, promoting therapeutic progress. New algorithms in a cloud system can improve multimedia data management, including patient, specialized doctor, and nursing details. Multimedia components include text, images, sounds, videos, and graphics. Video representation of data improves understanding of diseases and therapy, according to the survey. Using multimedia technology in diagnostic methods such as CT scans, X-rays, and MRI has enhanced patients' quality of life. It also enhances the quality of life for those with disabilities. Digital media data can be quickly adjusted and comprehended by patients, improving therapy satisfaction. The surgical process can be enhanced with multimedia tools and methods. This chapter covers multimedia tools and strategies for smart healthcare systems. Interactive multimedia tools and machine learning will be introduced to healthcare. Critical applications include

**Corresponding author:* Yogita.raghav@krmangalam.edu.in

Suman Kumar Swarnkar, J P Patra, Sapna Singh Kshatri, Yogesh Kumar Rathore and Tien Anh Tran (eds.) Supervised and Unsupervised Data Engineering for Multimedia Data, (63–92) © 2024 Scrivener Publishing LLC

Multimedia data visualization, Computer vision for healthcare monitoring, and Machine learning for brain dysfunction, and cancer detection. This article will cover machine learning methods for disease diagnosis and prediction using diagnostic tools. The use of multimedia tools can improve patient care compared to traditional methods. Deep learning algorithms can be utilized for image and video analysis. This chapter will also address the security of multimedia data in healthcare. We will also focus on neural networks for diagnosing multimedia-based data.

Keywords: Multimedia data, healthcare, K-prototype clustering, emerging trends, robotics in E-healthcare

3.1 Introduction

In this rapidly growing world, everything has been made easy with the assistance of new technology. Similarly, in the field of medical management evolution of applied sciences has paved a way for better health analysis. Data-driven decision-making solutions are more in demand in the healthcare industry for research, testing, and trials; they are meant to be used in both homes and hospitals. This chapter offers researchers and engineers insightful viewpoints on creating powerful multimedia medical data analytics systems and enhancing remote patient care. Using multimedia in the medical industry provides an elaborate and clear understanding of a particular condition, which helps to explore more accurate and robust solutions.

What is Multimedia?
Multimedia is a combination of two words, "multi," meaning many, and "media," meaning means of communication. Multimedia can be described in two ways. First, the technological perspective [1]. It can be defined with the common technical traits that multimedia possesses such as Multidimensional presentation techniques, the combination of text, pictures, sound, etc., Multimodal Interactions, the use of modalities such as voice, gesture, etc., or Hypermedia Techniques, non-linear data structure consisting of nodes and links. Secondly, the user-centered perspective. It would describe multimedia as systems which allow multiple modalities to be used at the same time and a single modality to be used by many users. This would allow the user to use multiple modalities such as voice, gestures simultaneously and multiple users to use the same modality at the same time. This would allow multi-tasking from both the user's end and the system's side as well [2].

Forms of Multimedia
Diverse forms of multimedia are depicted visually in Figure 3.1. The use of multiple forms of content within a singular presentation or application,

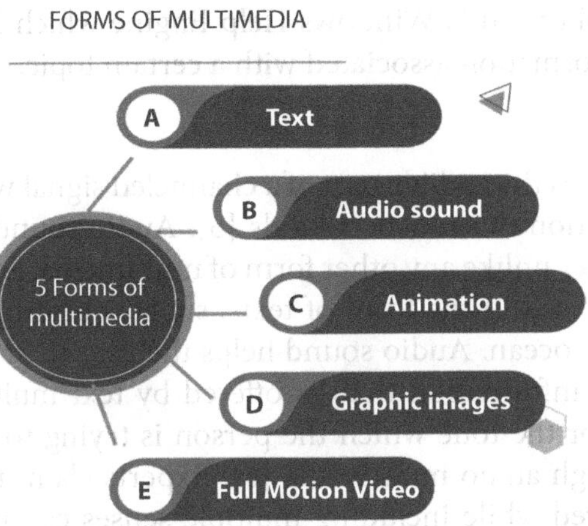

Figure 3.1 Different forms of multimedia.

including text, images, audio, video, and interactive components, is called multimedia. The figure exhibits many multimedia content examples, showcasing the multifunctionality and abundance of media integration. This may consist of visual and aural elements, videos, audio snippets, and interactive components such as simulations or animations. The purpose of the illustration is to underscore the wide range of multimedia components, emphasizing their synergistic influence in generating captivating and ever-changing user encounters across various platforms and applications.

Text

Text is the most basic and common form of communication. It consists of alphanumeric characters combined to create information [3]. Text multimedia is often overlooked but it serves as an effective way to convey information in multimedia. It can be used as headlines, slogans, subtitles, etc. It can be used to pass information or to fortify conveyed information. It can also be used as a substitute in case of unavailability of other forms of multimedia. Text is the foundation of various word processors and multimedia applications. Multimedia applications are used to display text information related to a certain topic which is most viewed by the users. This computerized information provides convenience to the user and helps in finding appropriate information to the user in the minimum amount of time [4]. As a multimedia programmer, you can display the information which you want to convey in the most attractive manner with the help of formatting; you can select desired font style, font size and various other options to make your document look appealing. One such example of text multimedia application is Windows Help Engine which helps the user to easily access information associated with a certain topic.

Audio Sound

Audio in general is the audible part of a channeled signal which is a recording or reproduction of acoustic sounds [5]. Audio sound provides information to the user unlike any other form of multimedia. Some information cannot be expressed in the form of texts, such as beating of the heart or the sound of the ocean. Audio sound helps the user to get a better understanding of the information than is offered by text multimedia, such as the expression or the tone which the person is trying to convey is better expressed through audio multimedia [6]. Experts claim that information which is delivered while including multiple senses can help the receiver to get a finer understanding of the topic; it also makes the information more interesting for the recipient. Audio can be categorized into two parts, namely sound and music.

Sound can be used in multimedia to provide essential sound effects. These are used to highlight certain aspects. These are referred to as "Sound FX" intending "effects". This vernacular is not based on dictionary definitions; rather, it evolved through everyday discourse and widespread common application. However, it is frequently employed in this sector [7].

The denotation of the expression music is more widely used in multimedia compared to other common areas. It may also contain sound. The music track, however, is anything which is audible in a multimedia production except for the incorporated Sound FX which are synchronized to the key events.

Animation

The human eye can perceive up to 60 frames per second. It means that if multiple related images are simultaneously shown at high speed, then the images appear to be moving. The same application is used in Animation multimedia. It provides the user with an apparition that the graphic image is moving. Animation refers to a series of images put together to give it an effect of motion. Multimedia includes both 2D as well as 3D animation. Animation is used to add visual appeal or to highlight certain information or links. It can explain the mechanism or can convey useful details in interesting ways [8]. Animation is a dynamic, media-rich form of information that remains contained in one area on a page and is a particularly effective form of communication. Animation focuses on amplifying the details that affect movement.

For example, if CPR (Cardiopulmonary resuscitation) must be explained to the user, then conveying the information in the form of text may not be effective. Though providing images for the same can be helpful, providing an animation of CPR may prove to be the best course of action as it provides a detailed explanation and involves multiple senses, which makes it easy to gain the attention of the receiver [9].

Graphic Images

Graphic images are one of the most integral parts of multimedia. Humans prefer to receive information in the form which is visually appealing as it makes it easy to grasp the facts which are being conveyed. There is no movement in these pictures. Static or still pictures are used alongside text, which further strengthens the understanding of the details. While applying multimedia photos are more than just showpieces. These are used to catch the user's attention. They are used in various websites or on social media as slideshows or galleries to highlight facts which may benefit the user or to narrate/describe something. These can also consist of clickability, which will direct the patron to the location or another element such as audio or video as decided by the keeper of the page [10]. Various multimedia applications include graphics, which provide the viewer the ability to communicate through interactive visual effects. Creation of graphics consists of certain formats and can be created by following numerous courses of action. There are an unlimited number of static graphics available describing or related to various topics. There is a limitless archive of graphics which can be used to create a wide variety of multimedia applications. Graphics on a website or in social media include pictures such as photos, illustrations, sketches, clip art, icons, or any other non-text elements [11].

Full-Motion Video

Full-motion videos are a kind of visual multimedia application which integrates multiple images to configure into moving pictures and sound. Videos can be elaborate explanations about some topic. The effect of videos on various social media platforms, websites, etc., is unique and can impact it in a powerful way [12]. You can notify the world about the existence of your company, you can advertise about your company, you can grab the attention of the target audience and let them know about the benefits which you can provide. One can also spread information about a procedure to achieve a certain goal or finish a task, introduce a new product into the market, etc. As more and more visitors expect it, videos on websites, and particularly on social media platforms, already have a strong presence and will only continue to grow in popularity [13]. Marketing professionals can post pertinent videos on social media platforms like Facebook, Twitter, and LinkedIn thanks to the inclusion of videos on these networks' platforms. Short movies may be an effective marketing tool and a great way to set yourself apart from your rivals.

3.2 Recent Trends in Multimedia Marketing

The user interface of video and audio programmes as well as the architecture of multimedia computer hardware are now being improved continuously. Particularly by implementing the plan that is software, architecture design and algorithm, the power of the computer may be boosted. Therefore, in order to meet the requirements of a multimedia network environment, to make multimedia software smarter, we wish to create and research it. Users can use multimedia systems for industrial control, commercial administration, medical electronic devices, multimedia mobile phones, PDAs, hand navigators, and other purposes [14].

More Short-Form Videos

There is no denying TikTok's growth. The number of monthly active us ers increased from 11 million in 2018 to over 700 million in 2020, making it the media platform with the highest growth. The first part of its secret is, of course, its brief, 60-second videos.

Only in that they have a limited amount of time to impart information, TikTok's shorter videos are similar to old-school TV commercials. Modern short-form videos must be lively, fast-paced, visually engaging, and most importantly, relatable.

More User-Generated Content

The collection of user-generated material, which enables the public to participate in the creation process and inspire other users, is the second aspect of TikTok's success story (just as it was for YouTube). Traditional TV commercials and infomercials talk down to the audience, pushing as much information about the good or service as they can into a small amount of time.

A discourse and connection between a brand and its target audience are the goals of contemporary corporate video advertisements (see the Geico and Progressive commercials, for instance). It's more important to cultivate enduring brand loyalty than to make a single transaction.

More Online Training and Educational Videos

The e-learning market was expanding even before COVID-19 mandated all institutions in the country to go online (think Kahn Academy or TEDTalks). Students can pause and replay instructions as many times as they wish, unlike in a typical classroom. Additionally, anyone in the world can access the movies at any time. The fact that the instructors and tutors do not have to be actual people is another advantage of online training and educational videos. Videos that are animated often have significantly more movement and fascinating visuals. Furthermore, animated diagrams or explanations can be considerably simpler to comprehend. It truly is a personalised learning process that respects each student's schedule and learning preferences.

These films can be used in the business world to promote new products, inform current clients on usage, welcome new staff members, and instruct cooperating organisations. Explainer videos aid in product uptake and persuade potential customers to buy in the marketing sector.

More AR Content

You might want to consider ways to incorporate augmented reality (AR) and virtual reality (VR) aspects into your video marketing plan given the expanding popularity of these technologies.

Retail giants like IKEA and Warby Parker have already adopted augmented reality apps that let customers try new furniture and clothing before making a purchase. Additionally, *Forbes* believes that 40% of customers are willing to pay more for a product if they can see it first through AR/VR. This proves that the AR system is effective. That was before the pandemic forced the temporary closure of the great majority of brick-and-mortar shopping malls.

Include augmented reality (AR) components in your multimedia marketing to help potential buyers engage more quickly and directly with your product or service while also demonstrating the best ways to use it.

More Virtual Events

Given the widespread use of Zoom (or Microsoft Teams) in businesses, this shouldn't be shocking. Even when limitations and mask requirements are abolished, many activities will probably still take place virtually.

Virtual conferences save costs associated with travel and lodging while also making it simpler for attendees from other countries to join and gain knowledge. Importantly, they also offer a brand-new platform for chances in multimedia marketing where users may interact directly with the material.

Companies are escaping the webinar mentality and developing truly engaging experiences thanks to new tools and platforms. Virtual events could be your next major marketing platform and your key to reaching a completely new audience when used in conjunction with innovative content and value-driven message.

3.3 Challenges in Multimedia

Cost

Despite falling technological costs, daily increases in development expenditures are occurring. The price reflects the complexity of the technology and the requirement for acquiring the rights to utilise a significant amount of content, before others. Due to the usage of numerous media, multimedia production is more expensive than other methods of production. It requires expensive electronic equipment, which is required. The cost of using it is increased by the fact that it needs electricity to operate.

Equipment Failure

In comparison to more conventional media, multimedia frequently requires more technology to deliver a message. There is always a danger of equipment failure when it is used.

Technical Barriers

Organizations that use multimedia applications need to be aware of the latest hardware and software developments. The most recent multimedia features include:

a. personal computers or workstations that can accommodate multimedia data must be provided by this upgrade.
b. Modern files servers that can manage the data volumes.
c. New software tools that can regulate the information quality of various forms.

In commercial buildings, it is occasionally necessary to transfer excessively large multimedia data in the form of continuous streams via local and wide area networks. The incompatibility between the user's equipment and the information sender's equipment can occasionally be attributed to a lack of standards.

Social and Psychological Barriers

Multimedia technology development has led to an increase in teleworking that is happening every day. Loneliness, isolation, lack of emotion, and a lack of interaction with clients and other professionals ensue as a result.

Due to the ambient noise, the typical workplace setting does not facilitate multimedia engagement. The background movements can occasionally cause videoconferencing participants to get disengaged, which results in a poor-quality image.

Legal Problems

"Ownership of content" is one of the main issues with the development of multimedia applications. If someone copies a piece of work protected by a copyright without the owner's consent, it will be illegal. The copyright holder may file a lawsuit for damages in such a situation.

Copyright is the exclusive and transferable legal right granted to the creator for a specific period of time to print, publish, perform, screen, or record works of literature, art, or music. When networks are utilised to encourage teamwork, there could be issues with intellectual property rights. Data integrity must be protected, and access to information must be restricted.

3.4 Opportunities in Multimedia

Journalism

[Earns an Average of $35,495 per Year]

News articles must be produced and presented to an audience in a variety of ways by a journalist. They might produce broadcasts and movies, write essays, offer pictures, or take part in radio shows. Journalists conduct the necessary background research on a story or issue, conduct expert interviews, and produce objective, truthful work.

Video Production Editor

[Earns an Average of $43,424 per Year]

A video editor is in charge of combining and editing videos to create a finished work that can be presented to an audience. Depending on the purpose of the video, the audience it is intended for, the industry or group it is for, and the location where it will air, a video editor may employ special effects and graphics, music, camera angles, text, and other aspects. Video producers who create narratives may need to edit an existing video to fix mistakes or add material that was omitted.

Animator

[Earns an Average of $44,673 per Year]
Motion picture products are made by animators. They use their production to tell tales, educate an audience, or motivate viewers to take action. Storyboards are made by animators, who also consult with clients and stick to a production budget. It's typical for animators to use specialised computer programmes to create drawings, stop-frame animations, or 2D or 3D animation.

Technical Writer

[Earns an Average of $57,513 per Year]
A technical writer creates writing that explains to a user how a product works. To explain the features, advantages, and applications of the product, they might produce articles, manuals, paperwork, diagrams, and guidelines. Technical writers aim to simplify too technical language and make their writing easy to grasp for both their readers and the product's consumers.

Video Game Designer

[Earns an Average of $58,096 per Year]
A storyline and created characters are used in the creation of video games by a video game creator. They create unique gaming elements to keep them entertaining and difficult for players. To ensure that the video game is developed in accordance with specifications and the needs of the video game end user, video game designers regularly update design documents and collaborate with production.

Multimedia Designer

[Earns an Average of $61,392 per Year]
Using photos, written text, graphics, and videos, a multimedia designer makes presentations, similar to marketing campaigns, for a target audience. Multimedia designers may produce work for websites, television, video games, or motion pictures. They employ a variety of design tools, animate characters, collaborate with a project team to ensure they stay within budget and adhere to a deadline, and more to finish their work.

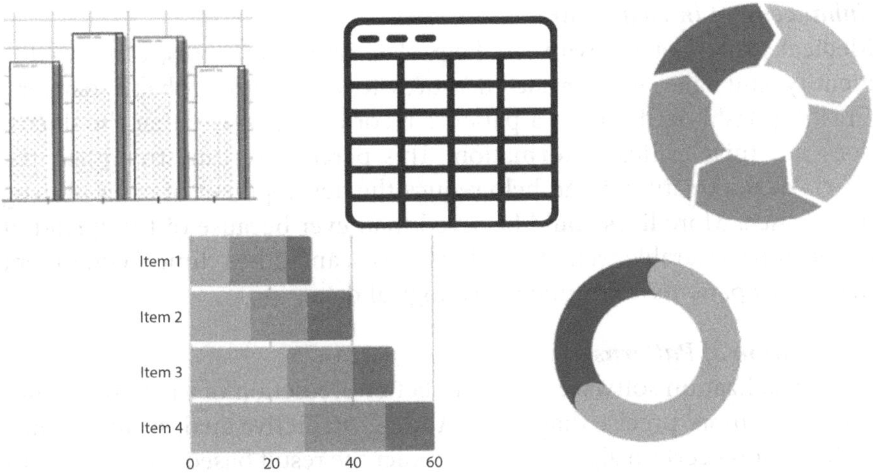

Figure 3.2 Data visualization method.

3.5 Data Visualization in Healthcare

Various charts, diagrams, and visualization tools are illustrated in Figure 3.2 to illustrate data patterns, trends, and relationships. Potential methods for representing data may encompass a variety of graphical representations, such as line graphs, scatter plots, pie charts, heat maps, or network diagrams. The figure is presumed to illustrate the wide range of visualization techniques that can effectively convey the information obtained from data analysis.

Data visualization in the healthcare industry refers to a combination of data from a variety of sources into a graphical format for easy understanding and quick access of the information. Data visualization can be of great advantage to healthcare professionals as it may help them to accelerate the understanding of the problem, interpret data, recognize trends, and boost the quality of decision making [15]. Charts are a means to depict a large amount of information in an abstract and easily understandable form. Multimedia healthcare data comprises Electronic health records (EHR), home monitoring equipment, disease registers, and much more. The availability of wearable devices and various other Internet of Things' devices provides with the healthcare data.

The following are some effects of data visualization on healthcare.

Enhancement in Healthcare

Medical professionals, with the help of visualization tools, can speedily identify and take appropriate measures to deal with probable dangers. Creating dashboards about a patient's records can ensure that the doctor does not miss critical information. This perception can strengthen the effects of the treatment and help reduce the development of cases of drug intolerance. More lives could be saved than ever because of the spread of fitness apps, wearable technology, biosensors, and other clinical equipment that tracks patients' real-time physiological data.

Recognition of Patterns

Data visualization software can aid in better prediction of a patient's health and create more precise diagnoses. Adding predictive analysis in the mix, which follows certain algorithms to predict the result based on the patterns in data, will further help in providing better health facilities to patients. Furthermore, the data collected through fitness apps and wearable devices will assist the doctors in detecting and treating illnesses at an early stage.

Increased Efficiency

Real-time data visualization significantly speeds up the understanding of information, compared to labor-intensive manual reporting, enabling healthcare firms to decrease inefficiencies, make decisions more rapidly, and save money. Visualizing factors relating to a patient's experience at the hospital can also assist the hospital in improving the facilities provided to patients.

Determining Mistakes and Identifying Frauds

The yearly cost of Medicare fraud and abuse is estimated to be between \$58.5– \$83.9 billion. In the healthcare field, fraud is practiced by both professionals and patients. Examples include double or ghost billing, several bills for a single service, counterfeit prescriptions, insurance fraud, and other schemes. The relation between patients, doctors, insurance companies and hospitals can be better understood by the relevant professionals through the assistance of data visualization, which will help in minimizing such fraudulent activities [16].

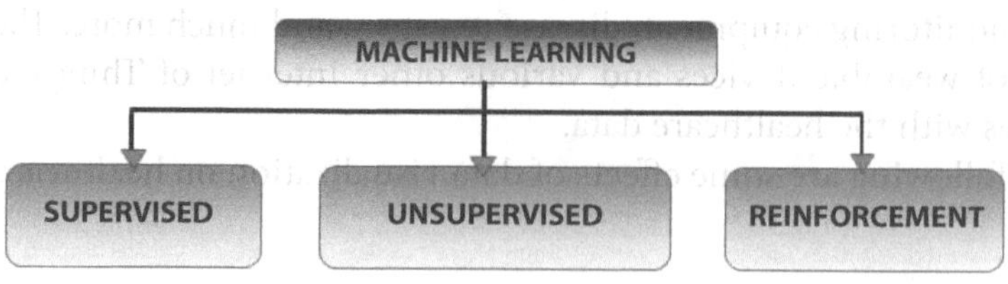

Figure 3.3 Types of machine learning.

3.6 Machine Learning and its Types

A subfield of Artificial Intelligence (AI) and computer science called Machine Learning uses data and algorithms to gradually improve the accuracy of its output in an effort to mimic human learning processes. In the new big data era, they are regarded as the workhorses. Machine learning techniques are successfully used in a wide range of fields, including pattern recognition, computer vision, aerospace engineering, finance, entertainment, and computational biology, as well as biomedical and medical applications [17].

Machine learning is the practise of programming computers to maximise a performance criterion using test data or past knowledge. Learning is the application of a computer programme to optimise the model's parameters using training data or past knowledge. A model has been defined up to a particular point. The model may be descriptive to draw conclusions from the data, predictive to foretell the future, or both [18].

Types of Machine Learning

Supervised Machine Learning

Supervised learning is a type of machine learning where a model is trained on labeled data, meaning that the correct output is provided for each example in the training data. The model is then able to make predictions on new, unseen examples by using the patterns it learned from the training data. The goal of supervised learning is to build a model that can make predictions that are as accurate as possible [19].

By integrating the features and finding patterns shared by each class in the training data, the class of each testing instance is determined. The classifying process involves two steps. A classification technique is first used to the training data set to assess the model's performance and accuracy, and the extracted model is then validated against a labelled test data set [20].

Unsupervised Machine Learning

Unsupervised learning is a type of machine learning where a model is trained on unlabelled data, meaning that the correct output is not provided for each example in the training data. Instead, the model is expected to discover the underlying structure of the data through the use of various algorithms and techniques. The goal of unsupervised learning is to find hidden patterns or relationships in the data that can be used for various purposes, such as data compression, anomaly detection, and density estimation. Some examples of unsupervised learning algorithms include clustering, dimensionality reduction, and auto encoders. Unsupervised learning techniques are gaining popularity in networking due to their favourable outcomes in other fields such as computer vision, natural language processing, speech recognition, and optimal control. Furthermore, unsupervised learning roughly calculates the requirement for labelled data and manual feature engineering, allowing for more flexible, general, and automated machine learning methods [21].

Hierarchical Learning
A visual representation of hierarchical learning can be found in Figure 3.4. Hierarchical learning is an approach to machine learning or artificial intelligence in which models are hierarchically arranged, frequently exhibiting a tree-like configuration. In the learning procedure, distinct degrees of abstraction or complexity are represented at each tier of the hierarchy.

Learning fundamental and complex features from a hierarchy of several linear and nonlinear activations is referred to as hierarchical learning. A computable feature of the input data is a feature in learning models. Independent, discriminative, and informative are the ideal desirable attributes. In statistics, features are commonly referred to as independent or explanatory variables. A group of methods known as feature learning, sometimes known as data representation learning, can be used to learn one or more features from input data. Unprocessed data must be transformed into a calculable and comparable representation that is particular to the input's property while being sufficiently inclusive to allow comparison to inputs with related qualities. Functionalities are typically developed especially for the current application. The reliance on domain expertise leads to the automated learning of generalised features from the underlying structure of the input data, but even then they do not generalise effectively to the variety of real-world data. Like other learning approaches, feature learning is divided into supervised and unsupervised learning domains depending

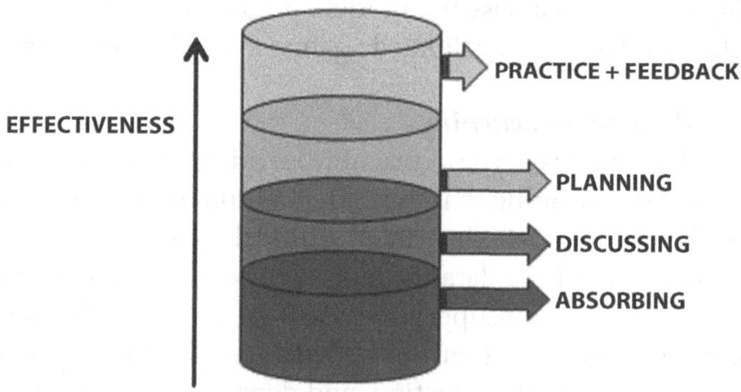

Figure 3.4 Hierarchical learning.

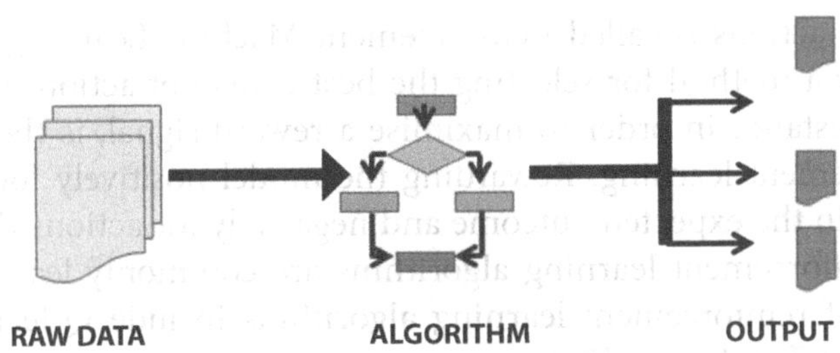

Figure 3.5 Data clustering.

on the type of data that is available. Nearly all unsupervised learning algorithms undergo a stage known as feature extraction in order to learn data representation from unlabelled data and build a feature vector on which to base subsequent tasks.

Data Clustering

Finding latent patterns in unlabelled input data in the form of clusters is the aim of the unsupervised learning task of the cluster. It entails grouping the data into meaningful natural groupings based on the similarity of various attributes in order to comprehend the structure of the data. A high level of intra-cluster and a low level of inter-cluster similarity must be achieved when organising data for clustering. "Data" is the concept used to describe the final structured data. Machine learning, data mining, network analysis, pattern recognition, and computer vision all use clustering in a variety of ways. Clustering algorithms are widely utilised in networking for tasks like traffic monitoring and anomaly detection in many types of networks.

Latent Variable Models

The relation between the observed variables and the underlying, hidden variable is described by the assistance of latent variable models which are a grade of statistical model. These hidden variables are called "latent" because they cannot be directly observed, but they are assumed to affect the observed variables in some way. Latent variable models are used in many fields, such as, natural language processing, computer vision, and social sciences. Latent Dirichlet allocation, factor analysis, and probabilistic latent semantic analysis are some examples of latent variable models. These models are typically trained using maximum likelihood estimation or variational inference [22].

Reinforcement Machine Learning

The type of machine learning where a model learns to make decisions by carrying our actions and observing the rewards or consequences that result from those actions is called Reinforcement Machine Learning. Learning a policy, or a method for selecting the best course of action in a particular circumstance in order to maximise a reward signal, is the objective of reinforcement learning. Rewarding the model positively for activities that result in the expected outcome and negatively for actions that do not is how reinforcement learning algorithms are commonly learned. Some examples of reinforcement learning algorithms include Q-learning and Monte Carlo Tree Search [23].

3.7 Health Monitoring and Management System Using Machine Learning Techniques

There are several uses for machine learning in the healthcare industry. Machine learning can be used in everything from administration to healthcare treatment. Data mining techniques like classification, clustering, regression, etc., are frequently employed in the healthcare industry. Heart disease is the leading cause of death in the modern world due to stressful lifestyles. Machine learning algorithms is the most effective and cost-effective technique to identify the risk for this disease. According to data analysis from the Centers for Disease Control, heart attacks caused close to 80% of deaths in the previous ten years. In medical terminology, heart diseases are sometimes referred to as cardiovascular diseases. Cardiovascular disease is particularly prevalent in people 40 years and older, and it needs to be identified and treated as soon as possible. It has been determined that the conventional approach to treating cardiac disease is ineffective [24].

The security of the country is crucial in the modern world. Soldiers in the army play one of the most significant and crucial roles. There are numerous elements that affect the soldiers' safety. Therefore, numerous systems are put on soldiers for security purposes that allow others to see their health status and current whereabouts [25]. The modern health monitoring system for soldiers must therefore be integrated with the command centre for data communications and real-time GPS (global positioning system) transmission and reception. To connect with the control unit and other military personnel stationed side by side, the soldier needs wireless communication networks. The soldier will then need to be safe to defend himself with modern weapons. Then, for security purposes, we combine the soldier with the bio-medical monitoring sensors and processes in this study. The integrated components must be compact and power efficient. The fundamental problem is that soldiers cannot communicate with the control unit during military operations. Then, between the soldiers' positions and the control unit, proper navigation is crucial. It is therefore more beneficial for the control unit room station to be able to pinpoint the precise positions of the soldiers and guide them accordingly when the job is concentrated on the routing system location of the soldier using GPS.

The pulse sensor, ECG module, moisture and heat sensor, bomb detector, etc., are all combined in smart bio-medical sensors. The LoraWAN (long-range wide area network) is used to connect all of these sensors. These sensors are connected via the WBAN and protected by the low-cost, low-power LoraWAN module (wireless body area network). The procedures for creating two effective monitoring methods for the Intensive Care Unit (ICU). We describe two innovative methods that contract with massive amounts of information and make clear the key issues with the current monitoring setup. The current control process in the ICU has numerous problems dealing with critical and non-critical patient situations [26]. ICU frequently develops a collection of false alarms that have an adverse impact on working conditions and can endanger patient lives while deceiving medical staff.

To combat these false alerts in the ICU, we employ machine learning methods that have been effective in resolving the problem of the high volume of false signals. By using the K-prototypes clustering techniques with the SVM (support vector machine) approaches KP-ISVM [27] and KP-LASVM[5], the K-means clustering technique can be applied to regulate the statistics gathered at the base station for better prediction. The WBAN sensor mechanisms are proven to be less reliable, have more complex nodes, and have fewer nodes overall than the WSNs. In addition, the WSNs do not allow precise specifications or connectivity between the network and the human body.

Machine Learning Method

K-Means Clustering will be used to create sensor observations from the sensor data collected during darkness, such as temperature, moisture, and heartbeat. It offers any statements or conclusions regarding the connections between the many factors that we are accumulating are irrelevant particularly when it comes to the problem of individual training. Each cluster classifies these remarkable behaviours based on the data acquired from the observation data of numerous sensors for unique circumstances or things like going, running, resting, experiencing an air attack, and suffering. The K-Means Classification treads include:

Data Assignment

One of the flocks is represented by each centroid. Centred upon the rectangular Euclidean gap, each data situation is given to its nearest centroid in this step. To put it more accurately, if is the number of centroids in set C, then each numbers location x is given to a flock depending upon:

$$\arg_{ci \in c} \min \text{dist}\ (Ci, x)^2$$

here optimal Euclidean gap is dist (ci, x). Let Si be the data collection appointment limit for each ith bundle centroid.

Centroid Update

The centroids are recalculated at this step. The least desirable of all data places assigned to that centroid's flock is used to determine this.

$$C_i = 1/S_i \, \Sigma_{xi \in Si}\, x^i$$

3.8 Health Monitoring Using K-Prototype Clustering Methods

The most important responsibility in the intensive care unit (ICU) is to control the patients. In the emergency room, a unique procedure known as the control approach is used to keep track of patients who are in danger and to measure various treatment frameworks in the intensive care unit. Then, each acted structure includes a certain threshold denoting the patient's condition. A signal is triggered if the amount of the specification exceeds its limits. The therapy team in the clinics recognises the sounding of sirens as a sign of a perilous situation. Therefore, this patient requires instant medication as a result. However, not all panic attacks that are triggered resemble a serious condition; there are several mistaken fears, and the observe operation can reflect the clinic's medicinal personnel inaccurately.

Clustering Methods

The K-Prototypes Method

Huang proposed the partitional clustering method known as "k-models" for mixture data, which includes absolute and numerical data. This chart shows how the k-factors method has changed throughout time. The k-models method makes use of two copies of the trace-to-trace distances. The basic matching dissimilarity measure and the Euclidean distance for numerical traces were used between specific properties. Pretend we have two items, X and Y, with characteristics that have standards that are a

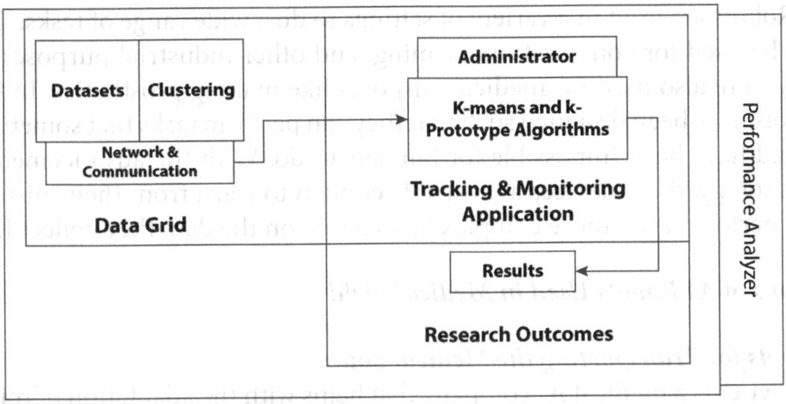

Figure 3.6 K-Prototype method.

combination of definite and numeric. The following formula can be used to determine the difference d (X, Y) between these phenomena:

$$d(X,y)=\sum_{j=1}^{p}(X_j-y_j)^2+Y\sum_{j=P+1}^{m}\delta(X_j,y_j)$$

The number of numerical and absolute qualities is appropriately represented by p and m, and is a substance required to avoid accepting any kind of associates. In our practise, we devised a way to use the k-prototypes technique to collect examples that had measurable costs that were both numerical and categorical in relation to preventive frameworks. Patients with the same diseases will be grouped together as the clustering.

3.9 AI-Based Robotics in E-Healthcare Applications Based on Multimedia Data

AI-based robotics in e-healthcare applications based on multimedia data is an innovative approach to explore deep understanding of human disease and to develop novel prognostic and predictive models, which will contribute to improving patient care through the customization of treatment.

Robotics in Healthcare has opened new opportunities and uses for robotic devices by developing AI solutions that can assist in improving human health. This technology is widely used in hospitals and clinics, but it can also be used to automate processes across multiple industries, allowing the use of big data and efficient solutions to benefit all sides involved.

Robots are used in a variety of settings to do a wide range of tasks. They can be used for construction, farming, and other industrial purposes but they were also used for medical purposes like making prosthetics. In fact, robots have been designed such that they can perform tasks that sometimes would have been impossible for humans to do. With the advancement in technology, these devices are capable enough to learn from their mistakes and perform even more complex tasks based on the data they collect [28].

Forms of AI Robots Used in Medical Field

Robots for Transporting the Medical Sources

Anolytics is a medical AI company that helps with the adaptation of robots to the medical industry. The company states, "We work with a number of hospitals, clinics and healthcare organisations to provide them with highly adaptable robots that are trained using large sets of data. This ensures that our robots can learn to navigate their way around a hospital or clinic both within and without crowds. They can also perform well in poorly lit environments and when they are not supervised by humans. The sensor fusion technology in Anolytics means that we can create self-navigated robot solutions for many different situations".

Robots Used for Disinfection and Hygiene

Robots have been used to clean and disinfect infected areas, which is especially important because they can clean huge areas with extreme speed and efficiency. This can drastically reduce human contacts in the cleaning process and protect against highly infectious diseases like COVID-19 and more viruses.

AI robots in several areas can be used for cleanliness and sanitation, where they are exposed to the infection of a diseased area. In contrast, human beings exposed to such sick areas may become ill. So AI machines or robots can be applied for neatness or cleansing at various locations.

Robots to Work as Surgical Assistants

AI is being used to develop robot assistants that can assist surgeons in performing complex surgeries. The robots are designed with a wide range of sensors and neural infrastructure, with the aim of generating great results in challenging environments.

These robots have enhanced natural stereo vision capabilities and augmented reality capabilities. Through computer vision, these robots are also trained with various forms of training data so they can comprehend circumstances and respond appropriately.

Robotics for Prescription Dispensing Systems

AI robots can move faster and more accurately. This is an essential phase for the healthcare industry to offer accurate features and medicines, work faster and treat patients faster and treat them in time.

Similarly, automated dosing systems with advanced capabilities are being developed, demonstrating that robots can now manage powders, solutions, and highly sticky materials faster and more accurately. Such robots can distribute many other items when fitted in hospitals and medical centres.

3.10 Future of AI in Health Care

Given the rate at which AI is becoming more prevalent in healthcare, we can expect AI to assist physicians at nearly every stage of the diagnostic and medication process in 10 years.

Now, nurses can use AI to remotely monitor patients with wearable devices and smartphones. You don't have to be in the same room almost anywhere in the world. Such solutions reduce costs by reducing the patient monitoring time required by caregivers. This means less hospital overhead.

In addition, by lowering human error, the method enhances patient care. Using machine learning algorithms fed by a significant quantity of data, artificial intelligence in healthcare may produce suggestions that are extremely accurate. Due of the importance AI plays in healthcare, this helps explain the field's rising importance.

Using deep learning technology, doctors are now able to detect cancer with 97% correctness. The skill is also used for other reasons, such as automatically detecting heart sounds to avoid sudden cardiac arrest or intelligently detecting skin cancer [29].

The study of pattern recognition and the computational learning theory in artificial intelligence have come up to the field of computer science known as machine learning. This algorithm is efficient at learning from a dataset and making predictions. Instead of following fixed, static programme instructions, these processes function by constructing models from sample inputs to produce data-driven predictions or decisions.

There are mainly two types of machine learning, supervised and unsupervised learning. The term "supervised learning" belongs to a process in which a supervisor doubles as an educator. Using tagged data to instruct or train a computer system is the basic definition of supervised learning. This means that a suitable response has already been given to the appropriate data. The computer is then given a new set of examples so that the supervised learning algorithm may analyse the training data (set of training examples) and offer a precise output from described or labelled data (data). Unsupervised learning is the process of teaching a computer to use unlabelled, unspecified data and giving the algorithm the capability to work on the data without guidance. In this scenario, the device's goal is to classify uncategorised data based on similarities, patterns, and variations without any prior data training.

The machine won't be trained because there is no tutor there, unlike supervised learning. As a result, the computer has a restricted capacity to independently identify the unknown structure in unlabelled data [30].

Pneumonia Detection Using Chest X-Ray Images

The Streptococcus pneumonia bacterium is usually present in a person with pneumonia, a potentially lethal bacterial infection impacting one or both lungs. One in three fatalities in India, according to the World Health Organization (WHO), are affected by pneumonia. Chest X-rays are used to detect pneumonia, and only radiotherapists with extensive training are permitted to review them. Therefore, creating an automated methodology to diagnose pneumonia may aid in quickening the illness's treatment, particularly in remote areas [31]. Due to the effectiveness of deep learning algorithms in analysing medical imaging, convolutional neural networks (CNNs) have earned a lot of interest for the purpose of categorising illnesses. In picture classification applications, pre-trained CNN models' features from large datasets are quite beneficial [32].

Enhanced Genetic Algorithm-Based Naive Bayes Classifier for Heart Disease Identification

In recent years, medical professionals have come to rely on health diagnostic systems for the recognition, diagnosis, and cure of numerous ailments. For machine learning issues requiring categorization, genetic algorithms are a key optimization strategy. Additionally, genetic algorithms can make

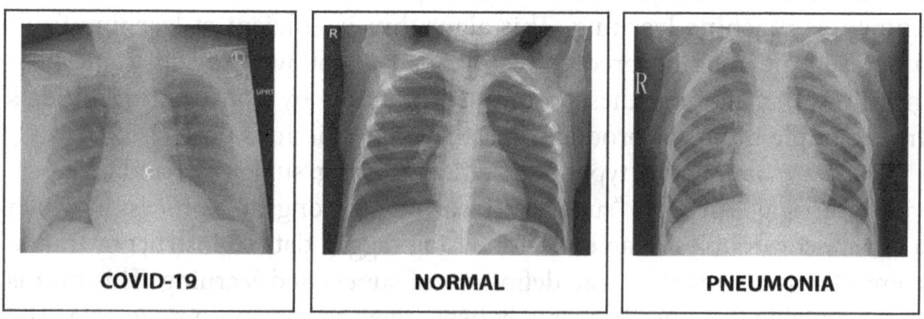

Figure 3.7 Variation in lung X-rays in different situations [35].

accurate and reliable predictions. A serious heart condition called coronary heart disease causes the blood channels that provide oxygen to the heart to constrict. In this study, we employ genetic algorithms to investigate and forecast patient cardiac conditions. The UCI machine learning store data set's heart infection data set is utilised [33].

COVID-19 Recognition Using Deep Convolutional Neural Networks
Numerous individuals have died as a result of COVID-19's fast spread around the world. Clinical trials and radiographic imaging can be used to identify the virus, which causes symptoms including fever, coughing, and aching muscles. Syndrome X-rays and computed tomography (CT) tests can be employed in the deep network to assist in the identification of the disease. Medical imaging is essential for disease analysis.

Four processes make up the process of employing a neural network to identify and diagnose illness from an image: feature mining, optimum feature selection, network training, and model presentation evaluation. There are two categories for the feature extraction stage. In the first kind, the features are obtained using image processing techniques, algorithms, and filters.

The tissue forms and textures are utilised to categorise patients among the attributes that were derived from the photos. In the second kind, the convolution network is supplied with the original pictures and their real output class as input data, and the elements are spontaneously retrieved in the final compressed layer after network training and weight modification [34].

3.11 Emerging Trends in Multimedia Systems

The use of multimedia in e-learning, personal media, assisted living, and virtual worlds is growing. New UI paradigms are used in applications, end-systems, and tools for multimedia. It's interesting to note some recent changes that can point to the general direction of the sector, even while this establishment reflects the natural process of shifting research objectives and technological innovation. I now think that some very intriguing and stand-out patterns are emerging, based on my analysis of current research in the field and conversations with other academics at various venues for multimedia research. The four main trends are as follows:

1. Increasing Media Diversity
2. Using Historical Context
3. Human-in-loop Methodology
4. Use of Feedback Control [7].

Increasing Media Diversity

In the beginning of the 1990s, the emphasis in multimedia was on visuals, and by the middle of the decade, multimedia was synonymous with video. Up until recently, audio essentially developed independently. Even the pros and cons of examining one media over several media have occasionally been discussed. However, it is now generally acknowledged that various applications and demands need the usage of various media. For example, text streams would not have been considered multimedia ten years ago. But it is now acknowledged as a crucial component of many popular multimedia applications, such as the analysis of news video [37, 38].

The body of knowledge regarding non-spoken audio, particularly musical audio, is growing. Radically varied media are now used more frequently, together with a variety of sensors that are now more affordable and diverse in their design. Infrared, motion sensor data, text in various forms, optical sensor data, telemetric data of various kinds (biological and satellite), transducer data, financial data, location data gathered by GPS devices, spatial data, haptic sensor data, graphics, and animation data are a few examples. In schedules of the most recent conferences, each of these media types is present. The current approach is to acknowledge the existence of a complex ecosystem that makes up the media space, where certain clusters spontaneously coalesce into the best subsets for a certain application. The question, What is multimedia? finally seems to be giving way to "what is the most appropriate multimedia?" in the area. Effective information assimilation and the proper use of the significant content are two major issues that result from this use of various media. The research on graphic and auditory interested models [39] represents efforts to isolate the most important information from a vast amount of duplicate material. In the study of experience sampling, the engineering method is used to generalise the interest phenomena to the whole kind of data in the context of dynamical systems. Incorporating more unique media forms seems to be a trend that will continue [40].

Using Historical Context

Research on multimedia systems differs from related fields like computer vision, image processing, and pattern recognition in that it explicitly makes use of independently represented context and history rather than merely incorporating it inadvertently. In related fields, context and history are deduced from observations of traits, learning, or training. The background and history information are used in conjunction with the media data in multimedia and is regarded as a further input data stream. It is stated that the diverse media streams aren't hired in isolation from inside the context of the precise use of multimedia data—in evaluation for inference and in adaptability for synthesis. Additionally, it clarifies how vital the surrounding surroundings are to interpretation and adaptation. The context is the present-day surroundings, while the records are the complete of the context and media alerts with inside the past. The argument for experiential computing, the paintings on metadata reuse, the usage of context for media enjoy personalization, the tries to formalise context with inside the paintings of experiential sampling, and experiential files are sometimes that satisfactory illustrate this tendency.

Human-in-Loop Methodology

This is another distinguishing trait of multimedia systems. The fundamental concept is to acknowledge that multimedia systems are mainly created with the user—the human being—in mind. Three reasons exist for the human to be involved in the system loop. The initial part of the job description is media consumer. This characteristic turned into understood with the aid of using the early compression algorithms, which took use of it with the aid of using removing perceptual redundancy in phrases of the human visible machine and psychoacoustic models. The acknowledgement of the human in the loop additionally enables the paintings at the so referred to as semantic (or sensory) gap, which attempts to attach indicators to symbols. For instance, the relevant feedback for retrieval task makes use of the human's function as a multimodal information consumer. A communicator of knowledge plays the second role. Better human computer interfaces could be created in this capacity to promote communication in the highly natural way possible. There is developing information that green structures may be created wherein responsibilities are dispensed primarily based totally on the relative strengths of people and machines, instead of completely computerized structures being always necessary. This approach is supported through the concept of experiential computing. Humans can also play the third role of affective communicators. Here, using multimedia, the main goal is to transmit ideas and feelings. This trend's primary focus is on computational media aesthetics. Understanding the computational foundations of affective communication is the goal here because doing so will aid in the evaluation and production of such affective purposes. Though early focus was on using film theory and grammar for video applications, signal processing and music theory are increasingly being coupled to handle non-speech auditory. Therefore, the fundamental trend is to acknowledge the existence of humans in the loop so as to develop systems that may take advantage of this reality. This may involve both manual intervention and suitably modifying system behaviour.

Use of Feedback Control

In traditional engineering systems, feedback control has been used rather frequently. Recently, there has been a movement toward using feedback control concepts in multimedia systems. This tendency is primarily driven by two factors. The first, as formerly mentioned, is the human with inside the cybernetics loop that dates back to Norbert Weiner's unique theories. Humans may be used to offer enter to the device due to the fact multimedia structures are created with human beings with the customers in mind. An example of this technique is the characteristic of relevance remarks in content-primarily based totally multimedia retrieval. The active capture work, in which the technology provides input to the human in the loop, is an intriguing recent spin on this concept [41].

The second explanation for this is that most system settings for media are ongoing and developing. For instance, video data from surveillance systems is continuously broadcast. In these situations, this naturally leads to the formulation of dynamical systems. The latest finding that formally establishes the value of feedback in motor control systems ought to give this trend even more steam.

Researchers may be able to attract nuanced and correct conclusions approximately clients and the efficacy of advertising campaigns with the aid of using integrating records from numerous media assets and throughout modalities. When outcomes are steady throughout numerous modalities and media reasserts, there may be more self-belief with the conclusions drawn from the records. Data from numerous modalities can offer complementary insights. For instance, [42] predicts the overall performance of musical albums and playlists the use of user-generated textual content records, metadata, and acoustic traits of songs. [43] Analyses fame branding the use of facts from Twitter, Instagram, and lab tests to better apprehend how clients interact with brands. [44] Combines records from numerous channels (Twitter and Instagram) and numerous modalities (visual picks and textual content).

The impetus for methodological innovation is just one of the many advantages that multimedia data provides for the marketing industry. Large amounts of data are being produced by customers, devices, and businesses across modalities and media sources, which emphasises the need for methodological breakthroughs that improve insights into real-world marketing difficulties.

3.12 Discussion

In theory, multimedia refers to data that spans multiple mediums. It typically refers to data that represents various sorts of media used to record details and experiences pertaining to things and occasions. Statistics, alphanumerical characters, content, pictures, audial files, and video tape are all ordinary types of data. In ordinary speech, a records set is handiest called multimedia while time-based records, such audio and video, are included. Both from a display and a semantics perspective, multimedia data differ significantly from traditional alphanumeric data. Multimedia material is quite large in terms of display and contains time-dependent qualities that need to be followed for a cohesive viewing. The presentation of a multimedia object and any following user interaction, whether it is pre-existing or created on the spot, stretch the limits of conventional database systems. A multimedia database system's capabilities and efficiency are impacted by the complexity of the metadata and information that may be derived from the contents of a multimedia item from a semantics perspective. There is still ongoing research into how to accomplish this.

Alphanumeric, graphic, image, animation, video and audio items make up multimedia data. Animatronics, video, and auditory gadgets are time-dependent relative, whereas alphanumeric, graphic, and picture objects are time-independent. Being an organised combination of audio and visual gadgets, video entities also have an underlying temporal role configuration that imposes different synchronisation requirements. A particular frame of NTSC grade video tape needs (512 x 480) pixels and 8 bits per pixel, whereas a particular frame of HDTV characteristic video tape needs (1024 x 2000) pixels and 24 bits per pixel, or 6.1 megabytes. So, even without accounting for the audio component, an hour of HDTV-quality video would require 6.6 gigabytes of storage space at a 100:1 compression ratio. If the audio and image sections have to be synced and presented in a fluid manner, using a database system for video tape gadgets display extremely hard [36].

To extract meaning from its entire content, multimedia data must undergo extensive processing due to their complicated structure. When big events are portrayed in photographs, videos, simulations, or graphics and spoken about in voiceovers, practical objects are involved in those events, which are frequently the focus of inquiry. It is frequently possible to extract information from multimedia objects that is less complicated and voluminous than the multimedia objects themselves and that can provide some hints as to the semantics of the events these objects are intended to represent. This is done by utilising cutting-edge techniques from the fields of image interpretation and speech recognition. This data is made up of features, which are used to distinguish comparable real-world events and objects across diverse multimedia files.

Multimedia data modelling examines how the logical and physical representation of multimedia items is defined and connected to one another, as well as what features have been collected from these objects and how this was accomplished [36].

References

[1] Grimes, J., & Potel, M. (1991). What is multimedia? *IEEE Computer Graphics and Applications*, 11(01), 49-52.

[2] Alty, J. L. (1991). Multimedia: What is it and how do we exploit it? Loughborough University of Technology, Computer-Human Interface Research Centre.

[3] DeRose, S. J., Durand, D. G., Mylonas, E., & Renear, A. H. (1997). What is text, really? *ACM SIGDOC Asterisk Journal of Computer Documentation*, 21(3), 1-24.

[4] Chun, D. M., & Plass, J. L. (1997). Research on text comprehension in multimedia environments. *Language Learning & Technology*, 1(1), 60-81.

[5] Subramanya, S. R., & Youssef, A. (1998, August). Wavelet-based indexing of audio data in audio/multimedia databases. In *Proceedings International Workshop on Multi-Media Database Management Systems* (Cat. No. 98TB100249) (pp. 46-53). IEEE.

[6] Kerr, B. (1999). Effective Use of Audio Media in Multimedia Presentations.

[7] Schneider, S. (2009). Audio in multimedia - its fast changing methods and growing industry.

[8] Pavithra, A., Aathilingam, M., & Prakash, S. M. (2018). Multimedia and its applications. *International Journal for Research & Development in Technology*, 10(5), 271-276.

[9] Lowe, R. K., & Schnotz, W. (2014). Animation principles in multimedia learning.

[10] Wu, Z., Xu, G., Zhang, Y., Cao, Z., Li, G., & Hu, Z. (2012). GMQL: A graphical multimedia query language. *Knowledge-Based Systems*, 26, 135-143.

[11] Godse, A. P., & Godse, D. A. (2021). *Computer Graphics and Multimedia*. Technical Publications.

[12] Guan, L. (Ed.). (2017). *Multimedia Image and Video Processing*. CRC Press.

[13] Furht, B., Smoliar, S. W., & Zhang, H. (2012). *Video and Image Processing in Multimedia Systems* (Vol. 326). Springer Science & Business Media.

[14] Wang, Z., & Zhan, X. (2016, July). Research of the Development of Multimedia Key Technology. In *2016 International Conference on Sensor Network and Computer Engineering* (pp. 438-442). Atlantis Press.
[15] O'connor, S., Waite, M., Duce, D., O'Donnell, A., & Ronquillo, C. (2020). Data visualization in health care: The Florence effect. *Journal of Advanced Nursing*, 76(7), 1488-1490.
[16] Gotz, D., & Borland, D. (2016). Data-driven healthcare: challenges and opportunities for interactive visualization. *IEEE Computer Graphics and Applications*, 36(3), 90-96.
[17] El Naqa, I., & Murphy, M. J. (2015). What is machine learning? In *Machine Learning in Radiation Oncology* (pp. 3-11). Springer, Cham.
[18] Alpaydin, E. (2020). *Introduction to Machine Learning*. MIT Press.
[19] Singh, A., Thakur, N., & Sharma, A. (2016, March). A review of supervised machine learning algorithms. In *2016 3rd International Conference on Computing for Sustainable Global Development (INDIACom)* (pp. 1310-1315). IEEE.
[20] Lodhia, Z., Rasool, A., & Hajela, G. (2017). A survey on machine learning and outlier detection techniques. *IJCSNS*, 17(5), 271.
[21] Usama, M., Qadir, J., Raza, A., Arif, H., Yau, K. L. A., Elkhatib, Y., ... & Al-Fuqaha, A. (2019). Unsupervised machine learning for networking: Techniques, applications and research challenges. *IEEE Access*, 7, 65579-65615.
[22] Usama, M., Qadir, J., Raza, A., Arif, H., Yau, K. L. A., Elkhatib, Y., ... & Al-Fuqaha, A. (2019). Unsupervised machine learning for networking: Techniques, applications and research challenges. *IEEE Access*, 7, 65579-65615.
[23] Sutton, R. S. (1992). Introduction: The challenge of reinforcement learning. In *Reinforcement Learning* (pp. 1-3). Springer, Boston, MA.
[24] Patil, B., & Vydeki, D. (2022). Health Monitoring and Management System Using Machine Learning Techniques. In *Intelligent Interactive Multimedia Systems for E-Healthcare Applications* (pp. 33-52). Apple Academic Press.
[25] Walker, W., Aroul, A. P., & Bhatia, D. (2009, September). Mobile health monitoring systems. In *2009 Annual International Conference of the IEEE Engineering in Medicine and Biology Society* (pp. 5199-5202). IEEE.
[26] Borowski, M., Siebig, S., Wrede, C., Imhoff, M. (2011): Reducing false alarms of intensive care online monitoring systems: An evaluation of two signal extraction algorithms. In: *Computational and Mathematical Methods in Medicine*, vol. 2011.
[27] Bordes, A., Ertekin, S., Weston, J., Bottou, J (2005).: Fast Kernel Classifiers With Online And Active Learning. *Journal of Machine Learning Research* 6, 1579–1619.
[28] Okamura, A. M., Mataric, M. J., & Christensen, H. I. (2010). Medical and health-care robotics. *IEEE Robotics & Automation Magazine*, 17(3), 26-37.
[29] https://spd.group/machine-learning/machine-learning-in-healthcare/

[30] Çelik, Ö. (2018). A research on machine learning methods and its applications. *Journal of Educational Technology and Online Learning*, 1(3), 25-40.
[31] Çelik, Ö. (2018). A research on machine learning methods and its applications. *Journal of Educational Technology and Online Learning*, 1(3), 25-40.
[32] Varshni, D., Thakral, K., Agarwal, L., Nijhawan, R., & Mittal, A. (2019, February). Pneumonia detection using CNN based feature extraction. In *2019 IEEE International Conference on Electrical, Computer and Communication Technologies (ICECCT)* (pp. 1-7). IEEE.
[33] Lutimath, N. M., Ramachandra, H. V., Raghav, S., & Sharma, N. (2022). Prediction of Heart Disease Using Genetic Algorithm. In *Proceedings of Second Doctoral Symposium on Computational Intelligence* (pp. 49-58). Springer, Singapore.
[34] Iraji, M. S., Feizi-Derakhshi, M. R., & Tanha, J. (2021). COVID-19 detection using deep convolutional neural networks and binary differential algorithm-based feature selection from X-ray images. *Complexity*, 2021.
[35] Candemir, S., & Antani, S. (2019). A review on lung boundary detection in chest X-rays. *International Journal of Computer Assisted Radiology and Surgery*, 14(4), 563-576.
[36] William I. Grosky, in *Encyclopedia of Information Systems*, 2003.
[37] Chua T S, Chang S F, Chaisorn L, and Hsu W, Story Boundary Detection in Large Broadcast News Video Archives – Techniques, Experience and Trends, *Proceedings of the ACM International Conference on Multimedia (ACMMM 2004)*, October 2004.
[38] TREC Video retrieval Evaluation, http://www-nlpir.nist.gov/projects/trecvid/
[39] Ma Y F, Lu L, Zhang H J, and Li M J, A User Attention Model for Video Summarization. *Proceedings of the ACM International Conference on Multimedia (ACMMM 2002)*, pp. 533-542, Juan-les-Pins, December 2002.
[40] Lienhart R, and Kozintsev I, Self-aware Distributed AV Sensor and Actuator Networks for Improved Media Adaptation, *Proceedings of IEEE International Conference on Multimedia and Expo (ICME 2004), Taiwan, June 2004.*
[41] Davis M, Editing out Video Editing, *IEEE Multimedia*, Vol. 10, No. 2, pp. 54-64, April-June 2003.
[42] Boughanmi, K., & Ansari, A. (2021). Dynamics of Musical Success: A Machine Learning Approach for Multimedia Data Fusion. *Journal of Marketing Research*, 58(6), 1034-1057.
[43] Lee, J. K. (2021). Emotional Expressions and Brand Status. *Journal of Marketing Research*, 58(6), 1178-1196.
[44] Hartmann, J., Heitmann, M., Schamp, C., & Netzer, O. (2021). The power of brand selfies. *Journal of Marketing Research*, 58(6), 1159-1177.

4

Automotive Vehicle Data Security Service in IoT Using ACO Algorithm

Sivanantham, K.* **and Blessington Praveen, P.**

HCL Technologies, Coimbatore and Crapersoft, Coimbatore, India

Abstract

This study delves into the security concerns surrounding data generated by connected cars, encompassing information such as position, engine status, speed, and more. The term "Automotive IoT" refers to an advanced network of devices, including sensors, cameras, and GPS trackers, connected to the cloud to provide real-time data for enhancing manufacturing and transportation processes. Data is transmitted through electronic control units (ECUs), controller area networks (CANs), and in-car infotainment systems. Vehicle Data Collection systems efficiently gather, convert, and transfer vehicle data to the cloud, enabling companies to develop cutting-edge applications using data-driven analytics and machine learning to enhance vehicle quality, safety, and autonomy. However, the study highlights that nearly all data in and around connected vehicles is subject to data protection laws, particularly when associated with the vehicle's registration or identification number. The integration of radar and video sensors in autonomous emergency braking is explained, emphasizing the importance of data security within self-driving cars. The study introduces the Ant colony optimization (ACO) algorithm as a means to protect car data from unauthorized access. The increasing deployment of autonomous vehicles on public highways prompts a discussion on the safety of driverless cars. The study explores various ways to attack and defend autonomous vehicles, proposing a comprehensive attack and defense taxonomy. Acknowledging the rise in vehicle theft incidents globally, the study recommends the development of an IoT-based car alarm and guard system using biometric authentication. The proposed technology, VSS-IoT, aims to provide exclusive access to authorized vehicle drivers, addressing concerns about vehicle security. Recognizing the limitations of existing security

**Corresponding author*: sivanantham.kalimuthu@crapersoft.com

Suman Kumar Swarnkar, J P Patra, Sapna Singh Kshatri, Yogesh Kumar Rathore and Tien Anh Tran (eds.) Supervised and Unsupervised Data Engineering for Multimedia Data, (93–110) © 2024 Scrivener Publishing LLC

systems for two-wheelers, the study suggests a robust Two Wheeler Vehicle Security System (TWVSS) design to enhance vehicle security and rider safety. Features like an engine immobilizer and alarm are incorporated to make the technology compatible with a wide range of automobile brands. In conclusion, the study addresses the security challenges associated with connected cars and autonomous vehicles, proposing solutions such as data protection measures, advanced security systems, and a comprehensive defense taxonomy for autonomous vehicles. The focus extends to both four-wheelers and two-wheelers, emphasizing the need for reliable security measures in the rapidly advancing automotive sector.

***Keywords*:** Data security, ant colony optimization, vehicle data, control area network CAN, electronic control unit ECU, Internet of Things IOT

Introduction

Currently, IoT is the cutting-edge technology for a number of multimedia applications, smart transportation systems, and issues with the design and operation of smart cities. The future of the smart city can include the smart transportation system (Xie, Yong, *et al.* 2017). This could be as a result of the type of content used in applying for and creating IoT apps. The dominance of internet users, the advancement of smartphone technology, and mobile communication standards have all contributed to the adoption of IoT applications in the twenty-first century (Y. Usha, and M. S. S. Rukmini 2016).

He, Wu *et al.* (2014) state that IoV promises to generate significant economic interest and research value given information and communication technology's explosive rise, drawing many OEMs, IT service providers, and researchers to the field. According to a *Business Insider* study, by 2024, according to reports, 75% of cars will have the necessary equipment to connect to the Internet. In order to improve vehicle safety and transit efficiency, future automobiles will not only sense their surroundings using internal equipment, but also connecting to other vehicles and other infrastructures, sensors (Chowdhury, Dipayan N., *et al.* 2018).

The main technologies enabling (IoT) were created concurrently with the IoT concept. According to Husni, Emir *et al.* (2016), sensor-equipped wireless network made up of widely spaced-out autonomous devices keeps an eye on the environment or the physical world. Sensor, Sensor Node, and Sensor Network are the three basic parts of the WSN.

Alvarez-Coello, Daniel, *et al.* (2021) discovered that a number of studies exist, each concentrating on distinct challenges and issues related to data from IoT sensors. There aren't many articles, nevertheless, that provide an exhaustive overview of the many methodologies. The following is a list of this paper's overall contributions:

- To describe the fundamental architecture for the fusion, processing, and Moreover, the manner in which these modules connect to the IoT sensor network.
- To provide a broad overview of various IoT sensor data analysis techniques.
- To investigate the IoT sensor output properties, including the vast volume of data from the sensors, their heterogeneity, real-time processing, and scalability concerns.
- To explain how various IoT sensor data processing techniques, including data denoising, missing value imputation, data outlier identification, and data aggregation, operate in order to address a range of issues.

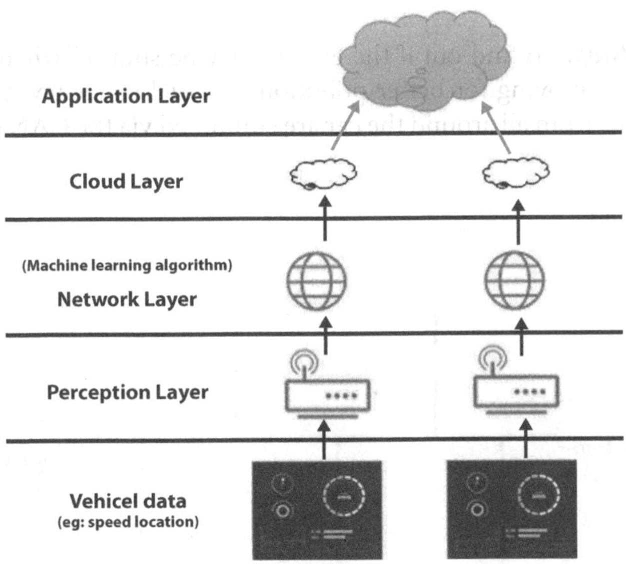

Figure 4.1 Vehicle data in IoT layers.

Electronic control unit ECU: Elshaer, A. M. *et al.* (2018): Several communication buses, including Ethernet, FlexRay, Local Interconnect Network (LIN), Controller Area Network, and Media Oriented System Transport (MOST), are used within automobiles to convey data (CAN). The CAN bus, the most well-known of these communication buses, was introduced in 1986 by BOSCH. Xiao, J *et al.* (2019) show that cars were primarily utilised for transportation at the time; data secrecy, integrity, and authenticity were not given much consideration by vehicle engineers. As a result, anyone with access to the communication bus or any connected ECU might read or send data to other ECUs.

Control Area Network CAN: Elshaer, A. M. *et al.* (2018): The reliable vehicle bus standard known as the Controller Area Network (CAN bus) can be used to connect applications on microcontrollers and other devices without the aid of a host computer. It is a message-based system that was originally developed to save copper by multiplexing electrical cabling in automobiles, though it may also be used in a variety of other scenarios. According to Jeong, Y., *et al.* (2018), since data is transmitted in a prioritised manner, the device with the highest priority can continue while the others pause. Each device sends data in frames serially. Every device receives frames, including the transmitting device.

Auto start/stop: To find out if the engine may be shut off when the automobile is not moving for better pollution and fuel efficiency, a variety of sensor inputs from all around the car are combined via the CAN bus. These

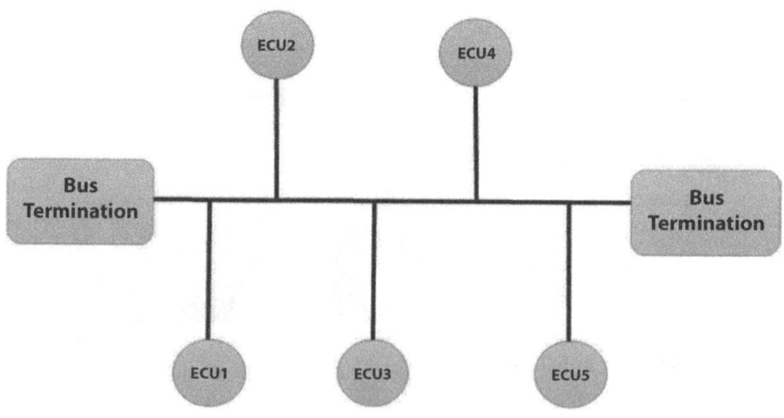

Figure 4.2 CAN bus connection.

inputs include steering angle, engine temperature, air conditioning on/off, speed sensors, and more.

Electric park brakes: Varrier, S. *et al.* (2014): The "hill hold" feature uses the tilt sensor in the car, which is also utilised by the burglar alarm, and the road speed sensors, which are used by the traction control, ABS, and engine control, to determine whether the car is stopped on an uphill. These sensors are fed through the CAN bus. Similar to this, the CAN bus transmits if the seat belts are secured so that the parking brake will automatically release when the car moves off. Inputs from seat belt sensors, which are a part of the airbag controls.

Parking assist systems: Ait Abbas, H. (2021): the transmission control unit might indicate the door when the driver engages reverse door control module and parking sensor system over the CAN bus, causing an illustration of where the curb is; the passenger-side door mirror should turn to the left. When the car is in reverse, the rain sensor transmits inputs to the CAN bus, activating the back windscreen wiper.

Global Positioning System GPS: Wang, J *et al.* (2015): to operate a fleet more efficiently and to manage a schedule that is more constrained, it is necessary to collect updates on real-time vehicle tracking, such as location, direction, speed, idle time, start/stop, and more:

- As the device changes status or direction, our car monitoring devices often give fresh GPS location updates more frequently than every two minutes.
- The equipment tracker from Track Your Truck uses satellite coverage to transmit its GPS messages, enabling you to keep track of your assets even in the most distant locations.
- Use GPS vehicle tracking for real-time mapping with automatic update, mobile tracking, and in-depth truck activity reports.

Cong, Li, *et al.* (2015) note that any asset or vehicle can have a GPS tracker installed to collect data beyond simply the object's current location. GPS vehicle tracking offers useful data for a variety of circumstances, which can be used to increase fleet compliance, efficiency, and safety.

The research summary is structured as follows. Section 4.2 discusses the current system for IoT platform used to maintain vehicle privacy data that is detailed in Section 4.3. Section 4.4 compares experimental findings for the proposed system and those from systems currently in use. Section 4.5 presents the final thoughts and the work's conclusion.

Literature Survey

Thermoelectricity with a focus on potential applications in Internet of Things (IoT) gadgets IoT develops and expands a market that is larger than ever before explained Haras, M., & Skotnicki, T. (2018). IoT nodes typically require very little energy to run, but because of their portability, localization, size, and frequently harsh working environment, powering them is a challenge. IoT has tremendous benefits, but both its governance and implementation have significant flaws explained Madakam, S *et al.* (2015). There is no universally accepted definition, universal standardisations at the architectural level are required, vendors' technologies vary, and standard protocols must be developed for better global governance, according to the literature's primary findings. Technologies that make things possible also result in some related security risks. Finally, we discussed a number of IoT-related apps that are meant to simplify our lives, explained Farooq, M. U. *et al.* (2015). There are already studies being done for its widespread adoption, but it's highly improbable that it will become an all-pervasive technology without addressing the difficulties in its development and maintaining confidentiality of the user's privacy and security.

Gokhale *et al.* (2018) explain that when everyday household appliances in our lives are connected to the internet, the setup is referred to as a "smart home" in an IoT context. IoT is more than simply a bold vision for the future. It is currently being put into practise and affects more than just technological advancement. Chattopadhyay, A *et al.* (2020) note that for the development and deployment of a secure AV, the absence of such a framework for linked autonomous systems presents a challenge. This is unlike traditional IT systems, where risk mitigation strategies and adversarial models are not as well developed as security design ideas like the security perimeter and defences-in-depth. We make an effort to identify the main AV security issues. This is done methodically by building an AV framework with security-by-design from the ground up. Therefore, identifiers are the technical challenges for AV security. According to Takefuji, Yoshiyasu (2018), because of the lack of network security expertise on the part of vehicle designers, all of these security issues exist. They have not given the security issue any thought. To safeguard against a variety of assaults, we must integrate security protection.

Elngar, Ahmed A. *et al.* (2020): Security system automation has long been a key component. The project's goal is to create and put in place a security system. This would be a system that allows control via a handheld mobile phone thanks to IOT. A vehicle system powered by IOT provides the highest levels of efficiency, convenience, safety, and dependability. Nanda, A. *et al.* (2019): IoAV must enable reliable, secure, smooth, and scalable communication between the vehicles and the roadside equipment. The IoAV platform has a lot of promise to improve transportation, including fuel efficiency, safety requirements, accident rates, and overall travel comfort. Lin, Chung-Wei *et al.* (2012) suggested a security mechanism that could be retrofitted into the CAN protocol to shield it from online attacks like replay and masquerade attacks. Because the method has a low communication overhead and does not require the maintenance of a global time, it is appropriate for this protocol. In addition, as the approach relies simply on software, its implementation won't be prohibitively expensive. According to experimental findings, our security method can deliver a high level of security without adding a significant amount of communication overhead in terms of bus load and message latency. Atoev, Sukhrob, *et al.* (2017) studied aircraft equipped with flight-state sensors, research computers, and navigational systems. Numerous aerospace applications, such as the fuel systems, pumps, and linear actuators used in aeroplanes, also make use of CAN buses.

According to Khourdifi, Y. (2019), the Ant Colony Optimization (ACO) metaheuristic, which offers a unifying framework for the majority of ant algorithm applications to combinatorial optimization problems, has been proposed. We shall refer to all ant algorithms that were applied to the TSP as ACO algorithms since they all completely fit the ACO meta-heuristic. In comparison to other methodologies already in use, the analysis section amply illustrated the usefulness of hybrid PSO and ACO approaches to disease diagnosis, described Ganji, M. F. & Abadeh, M. S. (2011). With KNN and RF, the FCBF, PSO, and ACO improved model achieves a 99.65% accuracy rating (Shang, Junliang, *et al.* 2019). The analytical part did a good job of demonstrating the value of hybrid PSO and ACO approaches to disease diagnostics in comparison to other approaches presently in use. With KNN and RF, the FCBF, PSO, and ACO recommended improved model achieves an accuracy score of 99.65%. ACO and an enhanced GA (IGA) are used to calculate AD gene order, and their effectiveness is tested using various vector distance formulas described Jing, Peng-Jie (2015). MACOED's complementary multi-objective and Pareto optimization, which boosts sensitivity and reduces false positives, is largely responsible for its success. On the other side, our updated memory-based ACO algorithm technique also contributes to raising the overall power. Singh, D. A. A. G. (2015): heuristic function produces better result compared to the classification without heuristic function. A good heuristic function is very cooperative in solving troubles by ACO. Information gain of each feature was used as a heuristic function. We compute the information gain for each attribute in the dataset.

System Design

Vehicle sensors are electrical devices that analyse several characteristics of the car and communicate information to the driver or ECU (Electronic Control Unit), based on information gathered by the sensor. Creating sound pulses, the sensors help identify nearby items. The waves show how far away the car is from the target. In most cases, the sensors contain an alarm that notifies the driver when an obstruction is present close to the vehicle. Small things, however, might not always be picked up by the sensors. This prevents your sensors from transmitting information to the computer in your engine. Your oxygen sensors may deteriorate more quickly if you use gasoline that isn't advised for your car or gasoline of inferior quality.

Vehicular Sensor Systems: The most crucial engine management sensor is the crankshaft position sensor; without it, the engine cannot function. Also, with the help of linked sensor devices offered by vehicular sensor networks (VSNs), data may be gathered to make road traffic safer and more efficient. The most popular VSN programmes also go through some security issues related to these applications. The following functionalities have been used to divide vehicular technology into three primary categories: applications for efficiency, comfort, and safety.

Wheel Speed Sensor: Typically, a Hall Effect sensor is installed on each wheel, producing a frequency that is translated into the wheel speed. Modern cruise control systems and ABS frequently employ this kind of tachometer.

Global Position System: This information can be used in autonomous vehicles to determine the best routes, driving instructions, topographic characteristics, lane mapping, and even obstacle recognition when combined with a precise map. Most modern navigation systems for vehicles use GPS; however, they lack the accuracy required for fully autonomous vehicles.

LIDAR: The LIDAR, or laser range finder system, uses a beam of light that is reflected off a revolving mirror and often has an infrared laser diode. Light is reflected back to a sensor when it strikes non-absorbing surfaces, creating a radar-like map.

Camera: Almost all autonomous vehicles include camera systems. They are used by the lane departure and lane maintaining algorithms in current production automobiles. Additionally, camera systems for purposes like reading road signs are being developed.

A multitude of data kinds are generated by the in-vehicle sensors. The speed and transmission capacity of the current CAN protocol are constrained. FlexRay and MOST, which promise fast communication speeds, are used instead of CAN because they may also have other issues like cost and compatibility.

In order to address compatibility issues and scattered data transmission, by transforming a range of message types into a message type of a target protocol, the dedicated In-VGM integrates the CAN, FlexRay, and MOST protocol and ensures reliable and real-time communication.

Ant Colony Optimization: Ant colony optimization uses an iterative process. Each iteration takes into account a range of produced ants. They each build a solution by traversing the graph from vertex to vertex while abiding by the rule that they are not allowed to pass any vertex that they have already crossed. At each stage of the solution construction, an ant chooses the next vertex to visit using a stochastic mechanism driven by the pheromone. The following vertex is chosen at random from the unexplored ones when in vertex I. In particular, j can be chosen with a probability proportional to the pheromone associated with edge if it has not yet been visited (i, j).

Algorithmic Design: Now that we know how the ants behaved above, we can create an algorithmic design. Just one food supply, one ant colony, and two alternative journey routes have been considered for the sake of simplicity. The ant colony and food source act as the vertices (or nodes) of weighted graphs that reflect the complete situation. The paths act as the edges, the pheromone levels act as the weights applied to the edges.

Assume that the graph has the form G = (V, E), where V and E are the vertices and edges of the graph, respectively. The vertices are Vs (Source vertex, an ant colony) and Vd, assuming our consideration (Destination vertex, a food source). The lengths of the two edges, E1 and E2, are respectively L1 and L2. Now, it can be assumed that the corresponding pheromone values for vertices E1 and E2 are R1 and R2, respectively, depending on their strength. Consequently, the initial probability of path selection for each ant (between E1 and E2).

Stage 1: Their ECU contains all of the data. There are no pheromones in the environment. (Algorithm design can take into account residual pheromone quantity without changing the probability shown in Figure 4.3.)

Stage 2: **Data start their search along each path equally likely.** Figure 4.4 clearly illustrates but as the curved path is longer, it takes longer for data to get to the IoT source.

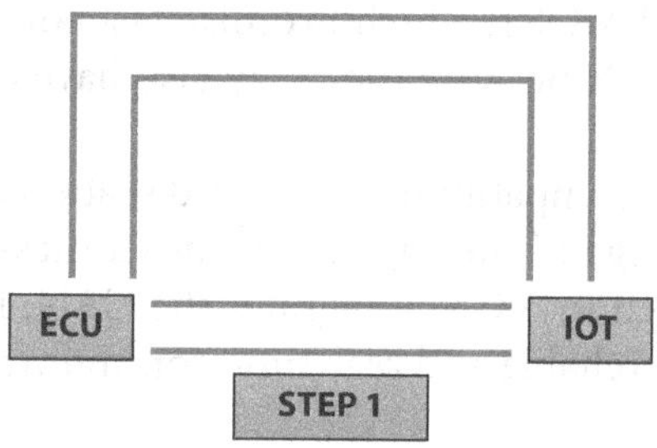

Figure 4.3 Stage 1 of ACO.

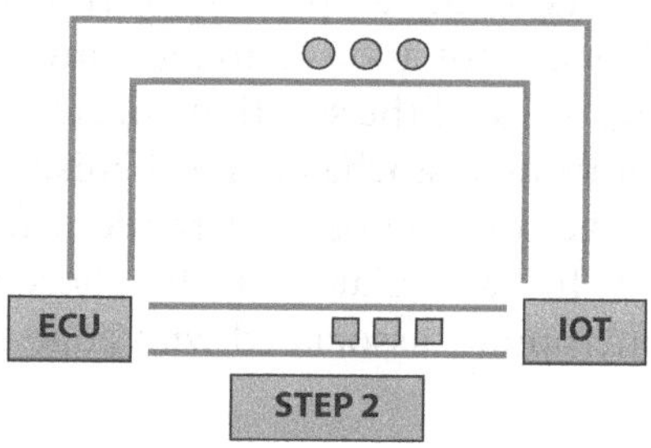

Figure 4.4 Stage 2 of ACO.

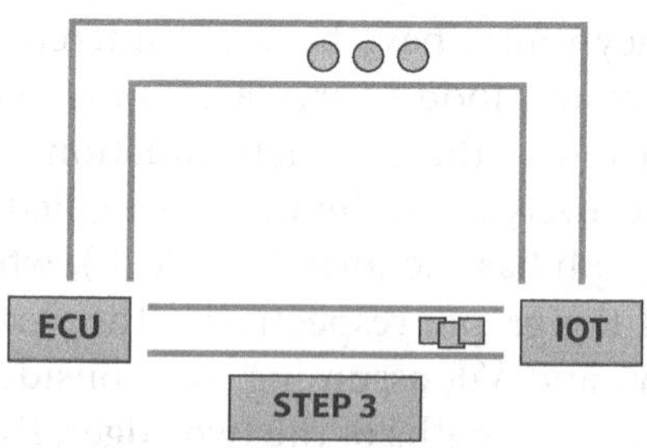

Figure 4.5 Stage 3 of ACO.

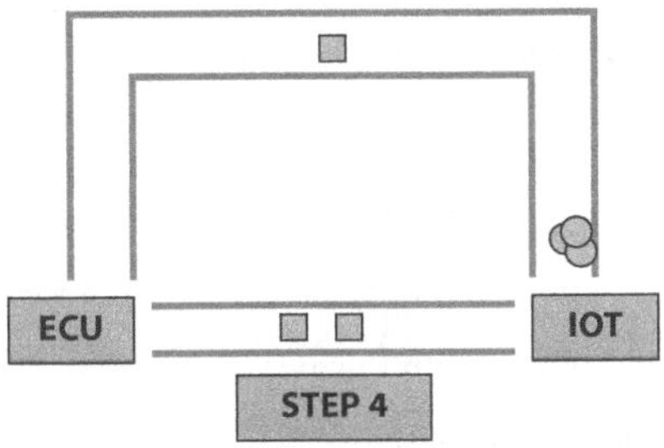

Figure 4.6 Stage 4 of ACO.

Stage 3: The shorter link allows for earlier data delivery to the ECU source. Evidently, they are now faced with similar selection problems exist here, but selection is more likely because the shorter path's pheromone trail is already there, as seen in Figure 4.5.

Stage 4: The shorter path results in a higher data return rate, and hence, higher pheromone concentrations. In addition, evaporation reduces the lengthier path's pheromone concentration, reducing the likelihood that it will be taken again. The result is, the shorter path is gradually used by the entire vehicle's ECU Data with a larger probability. As seen in Figure 4.6, path optimization has been achieved.

$$Pi = \frac{Ri}{R1 + R2}; i = 1,2$$

Accordance to path length: I = 1, 2 and "K" act as model parameters in the aforementioned update. Additionally, the update depends on how long the path is. The additional pheromone is greater the shorter the journey.

$$Ri \leftarrow Ri\frac{K}{Li}$$

Accordance to evaporation rate of pheromone: The pheromone evaporation is controlled by the parameter "v," which belongs to the range [0, 1]. Moreover, I = 1 and 2.

$$Ri \leftarrow (1 - v) * Ri$$

The [0, 1] range contains the parameter "v," which regulates pheromone evaporation. Also, I = 1, 2. During each iteration, all data are positioned at

```
Initialise the pheromone experiments and relevant settings;
While not termination do:
    Generate data_present in ECU;
Determine the fitness values related to each piece of data;
Select the best option using the available ways;
    Update pheromone trial;
End while
End procedure
```

Figure 4.7 ACO process.

the source vertex Vs. The data is then transferred from Vs to Vd after Step 1. (IoT source). Then, depending on step 2, all data make a return trip and confirm the direction they chose.

Pseudocode Ant Colony Optimization:
The above Figure 4.7 shows the pseudocode for ant colony optimization algorithm for data path from ECU to IoT. The main aim of our system is to develop automotive system in IoT platform. This proposed system will store the data of vehicle in IoT area where the data in IoT area are getting more safe and secure. Also, the data moves toward the easiest path from ECU to IoT source.

Result and Discussion

Confusion matrix: The success of the post-categorization processes was assessed using the confusion matrix. It provides examples of correctly categorised TN values that belong in a different class as well as flawlessly classified TP values, FP values that belong in one class but not another, FN values that belong in one class but not another, and FP values that belong in one class but not the other. Accuracy (ACC), precision (P), sensitivity (Sn), and specificity (Sp) scores are the most often used performance measures for categorization.

The confusion matrix, which serves as a source of measurement parameters for the classifier, has four fundamental features (numbers). The four digits are:

TP (True Positive): TP is the proportion of patients with the condition whose malignant nodes have been identified with accuracy.

TN (True Negative): The percentage of correctly recognised healthy patients is known as TN.

FP (False Positive): FP is the proportion of people who have received a false diagnosis of illness despite being in good health. Another word for a Type I error is FP.

FN (False Negative): The number of patients with falsely diagnosed health conditions is represented by the letter FN.

Accuracy: an algorithm is shown as the proportions of patients are (TP+TN) to all patients (TP+TN+FP+FN).

Specificity: Out of the total actual negative cases, it provides the percentage of negative values. In other words, what counts is the proportion of accurately discovered true negative cases Quantity of FP.

Sensitivity: The percentage of positive values out of all actually positive events is known as the TP rate (TPR).

Table 4.1 and Figure 4.8 show accuracy proposed approach comparison with existing approach, which provides a better maximum outcome than the present system. Table 4.1 states that the accuracy results of the BO, SVM, BPNN, and RF are 73.04, 74.12, 81.16, and 81.62, respectively. In comparison to other current systems, proposed system's results reveal that it achieves 88.74%, which is 6.85% higher.

Table 4.1 Accuracy.

Algorithm	Accuracy
BO	73.04
SVM	74.12
BPNN	81.16
RF	81.62
ACO	88.74

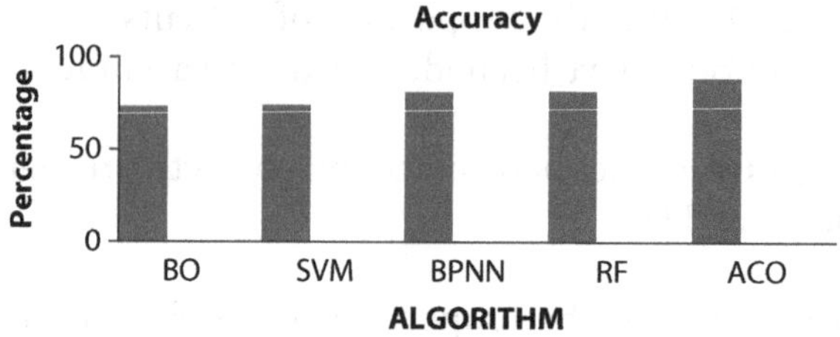

Figure 4.8 Accuracy.

Table 4.2 and Figure 4.8 show detailed explanations of the sensitivity of the proposed approach comparison with existing approaches, which offers a superior maximum result than the existing system. The BO, SVM, BPNN, and RF Sensitivity outcomes are given as 70.95, 72.35, 80.91, and 82.22, respectively. The results show that our suggested approach reaches 89.18%, which is 6.96% more than other existing systems.

Table 4.3 and Figure 4.9 show explanations of the specificity of the proposed approach in comparison with existing approaches. The indicated

Table 4.2 Sensitivity.

Algorithm	Sensitivity
BO	70.95
SVM	72.35
BPNN	80.91
RF	82.22
ACO	89.18

Table 4.3 Specificity.

Algorithm	Specificity
BO	74.06
SVM	75.88
BPNN	81.46
RF	81.01
ACO	88.32

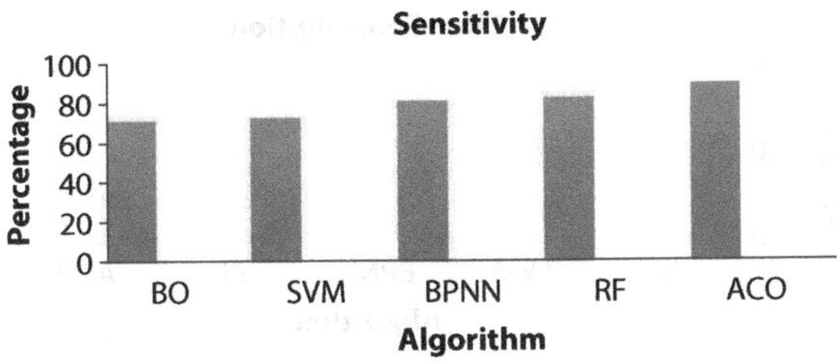

Figure 4.9 Sensitivity.

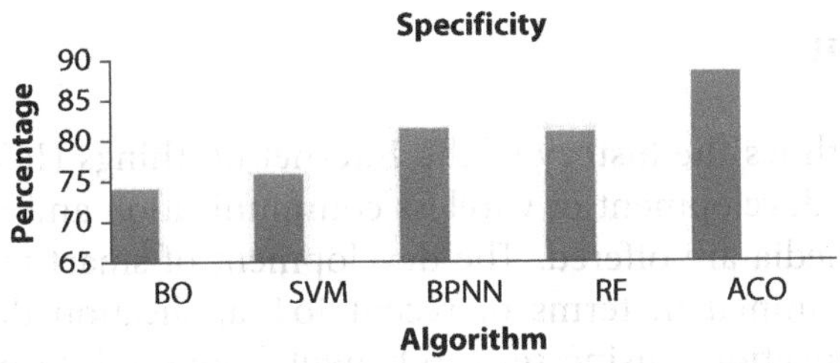

Figure 4.10 Specificity.

results are 74.06, 75.88, 81.46, and 81.01 for the BO, SVM, BPNN, and RF, respectively. The specificity results show that suggested hybrid approach reaches 88.32%, which is 7.31% more than other available strategies.
Time Consumption: When compared to all the existing systems our proposed system consumes less time to complete system with this prediction. Table 4.4 below shows time consumption of the proposed and existing system.

The outcomes of the suggested system are shown in the Figure 4.10 below. BO, SVM, BPNN, and RF are additional systems that can be used; however, ACO performs the best at time consumption.

Table 4.4 Table of time consumption.

Algorithm	Time (M.sec)
BO	61.56
SVM	63.33
BPNN	42.28
RF	38.96
ACO	29.36

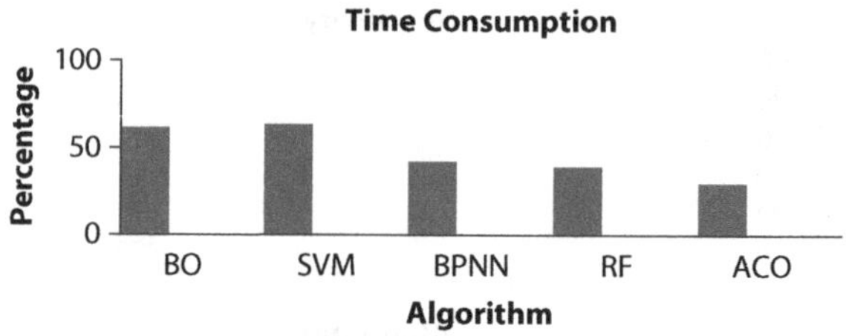

Figure 4.11 Graphical representations for time consumption.

Conclusion

The paper outlines the history of the Internet of Things (IoT). Technical details on the development of wireless communication and various communication media are offered. The development of smart transportation systems is examined in terms of recent IoT application developments. With this connection, businesses can benefit from the Internet of Things' creativity and productivity while keeping security in mind. Additionally, it facilitates the management of data and securely connected devices. Customers may get IoT security, compliance, and governance solutions from AWS in an all-inclusive, continuous, and scalable manner, as well as a defence-in-depth strategy with a range of security services. The ability of an organization IoT puts to the test the ability to manage, watch over, and secure massive amounts of data and connections from dispersed devices. These technologies improve data capture and modification. Once the data is in the cloud, it can be utilised in the future for things like assessing the health of the entire fleet of vehicles or developing machine learning (ML) models that enhance advanced driver assistance and autonomous driving technologies (ADAS).

References

[1] Xie, Y., Su, X., He, Y., Chen, X., Cai, G., Xu, B., & Ye, W. (2017, May). STM32-based vehicle data acquisition system for Internet-of-Vehicles. In *2017 IEEE/ACIS 16th International Conference on Computer and Information Science (ICIS)* (pp. 895-898). IEEE.

[2] Devi, Y. U., & Rukmini, M. S. S. (2016, October). IoT in connected vehicles: Challenges and issues—A review. In *2016 International Conference on Signal Processing, Communication, Power and Embedded System (SCOPES)* (pp. 1864-1867). IEEE.

[3] He, W., Yan, G., & Da Xu, L. (2014). Developing vehicular data cloud services in the IoT environment. *IEEE Transactions on Industrial Informatics*, 10(2), 1587-1595.
[4] Chowdhury, D. N., Agarwal, N., Laha, A. B., & Mukherjee, A. (2018, March). A vehicle-to-vehicle communication system using Iot approach. In *2018 Second International Conference on Electronics, Communication and Aerospace Technology (ICECA)* (pp. 915-919). IEEE.
[5] Husni, E., Hertantyo, G. B., Wicaksono, D. W., Hasibuan, F. C., Rahayu, A. U., & Triawan, M. A. (2016, July). Applied Internet of Things (IoT): car monitoring system using IBM BlueMix. In *2016 International Seminar on Intelligent Technology and Its Applications (ISITIA)* (pp. 417-422). IEEE.
[6] Alvarez-Coello, D., Wilms, D., Bekan, A., & Gómez, J. M. (2021, January). Generic semantization of vehicle data streams. In *2021 IEEE 15th International Conference on Semantic Computing (ICSC)* (pp. 112-117). IEEE.
[7] Elshaer, A. M., Elrakaiby, M. M., & Harb, M. E. (2018, December). Autonomous car implementation based on CAN bus protocol for IoT applications. In *2018 13th International Conference on Computer Engineering and Systems (ICCES)* (pp. 275-278). IEEE.
[8] Xiao, J., Wu, H., & Li, X. (2019). Internet of things meets vehicles: sheltering in-vehicle network through lightweight machine learning. *Symmetry*, 11(11), 1388.
[9] Elshaer, A. M., Elrakaiby, M. M., & Harb, M. E. (2018, December). Autonomous car implementation based on CAN bus protocol for IoT applications. In *2018 13th International Conference on Computer Engineering and Systems (ICCES)* (pp. 275-278). IEEE.
[10] Jeong, Y., Son, S., Jeong, E., & Lee, B. (2018). An integrated self-diagnosis system for an autonomous vehicle based on an IoT gateway and deep learning. *Applied Sciences*, 8(7), 1164.
[11] Ait Abbas, H. (2021). A new adaptive deep neural network controller based on sparse auto-encoder for the antilock bracking system systems subject to high constraints. *Asian Journal of Control*, 23(5), 2145-2156.
[12] Varrier, S., Koenig, D., Martinez, J. J., & D'Andréa-Novel, B. (2014, June). Detection of critical situations for vehicle longitudinal dynamics. In *2014 European Control Conference (ECC)* (pp. 2352-2357). IEEE.
[13] Wang, J., Rui, X., Song, X., Tan, X., Wang, C., & Raghavan, V. (2015). A novel approach for generating routable road maps from vehicle GPS traces. *International Journal of Geographical Information Science*, 29(1), 69-91.
[14] Cong, L., Li, E., Qin, H., Ling, K. V., & Xue, R. (2015). A performance improvement method for low-cost land vehicle GPS/MEMS-INS attitude determination. *Sensors*, 15(3), 5722-5746.
[15] Haras, M., &Skotnicki, T. (2018). Thermoelectricity for IoT–A review. *Nano Energy*, 54, 461-476.
[16] Madakam, S., Lake, V., Lake, V., & Lake, V. (2015). Internet of Things (IoT): A literature review. *Journal of Computer and Communications*, 3(05), 164.

[17] Farooq, M. U., Waseem, M., Mazhar, S., Khairi, A., & Kamal, T. (2015). A review on internet of things (IoT). *International Journal of Computer Applications*, 113(1), 1-7.

[18] Gokhale, Pradyumna, OmkarBhat, and SagarBhat. Introduction to IOT. *International Advanced Research Journal in Science, Engineering and Technology* 5, no. 1 (2018): 41-44.

[19] Chattopadhyay, A., Lam, K. Y., & Tavva, Y. (2020). Autonomous vehicle: Security by design. *IEEE Transactions on Intelligent Transportation Systems*, 22(11), 7015-7029.

[20] Takefuji, Y. (2018). Connected vehicle security vulnerabilities [commentary]. *IEEE Technology and Society Magazine*, 37(1), 15-18.

[21] Elngar, A. A., & Kayed, M. (2020). Vehicle security systems using face recognition based on internet of things. *Open Computer Science*, 10(1), 17-29.

[22] Nanda, A., Puthal, D., Rodrigues, J. J., & Kozlov, S. A. (2019). Internet of autonomous vehicles communications security: overview, issues, and directions. *IEEE Wireless Communications*, 26(4), 60-65.

[23] Lin, C. W., & Sangiovanni-Vincentelli, A. (2012, December). Cyber-security for the controller area network (CAN) communication protocol. In *2012 International Conference on Cyber* Security (pp. 1-7). IEEE.

[24] Atoev, S., Kwon, K. R., Lee, S. H., & Moon, K. S. (2017, November). Data analysis of the MAVLink communication protocol. In *2017 International Conference on Information Science and Communications Technologies (ICISCT)* (pp. 1-3). IEEE.

[25] Khourdifi, Y., Bahaj, M., & Bahaj, M. (2019). Heart disease prediction and classification using machine learning algorithms optimized by particle swarm optimization and ant colony optimization. *International Journal of Intelligent Engineering and Systems*, 12(1), 242-252.

[26] Ganji, M. F., & Abadeh, M. S. (2011). A fuzzy classification system based on Ant Colony Optimization for diabetes disease diagnosis. *Expert systems with applications*, 38(12), 14650-14659.

[27] Shang, J., Wang, X., Wu, X., Sun, Y., Ding, Q., Liu, J. X., & Zhang, H. (2019). A review of ant colony optimization based methods for detecting epistatic interactions. *IEEE Access*, 7, 13497-13509.

[28] Jing, P. J., & Shen, H. B. (2015). MACOED: a multi-objective ant colony optimization algorithm for SNP epistasis detection in genome-wide association studies. *Bioinformatics*, 31(5), 634-641

[29] Singh, D. A. A. G., Surenther, P., & Leavline, E. J. (2015). Ant colony optimization based attribute reduction for disease diagnostic system. *International Journal of Applied Engineering Research*, 10(55), 156-565.

5

Unsupervised/Supervised Algorithms for Multimedia Data in Smart Agriculture

Reena Thakur[1]*, Parul Bhanarkar[2] and Uma Patel Thakur[1]

[1]*Jhulelal Institute of Technology, Nagpur, Maharashtra, India*
[2]*Symbiosis Skills and Professional University Pune Maharashtra, India*

Abstract

Smart agriculture, a result of agriculture's digital transformation, has seen the development of unsupervised and supervised algorithms for managing different parts of farm operations in order to get value from a flood of data from a variety of sources. In the agriculture industry, farmers and agribusinesses face many decisions every day, each of which is complicated by a wide range of interrelated issues. Accurately estimating yields for all the crops in a plan is crucial. The only way to effectively and practically solve this issue is to employ techniques of data mining. Artificial intelligence new branch, Machine learning, offers massive possibilities to overcome numerous difficulties in the expansion of knowledge-based agricultural schemes. Through a comprehensive review of the most up-to-date scholarly literature based on keyword combinations of "crop management" and "machine learning", "soil management", "water management", and "livestock management", this chapter aims to shed light on unsupervised and supervised algorithms in agriculture. It was also noted that crop management was the primary focus. In addition, studies on both maize and wheat, as well as cattle and sheep, were the most common. In conclusion, a wide range of satellite- and unmanned ground- and air-based sensors have been used to collect high-quality data for the analysis. It is expected that this chapter will provide a functional resource for an extensive range of interested persons, raising their level of understanding of the potential benefits of employing unsupervised or supervised learning algorithms in smart agriculture and encouraging additional systematic investigation into this area. In the context of a wide range of practical settings and applications, this

**Corresponding author*: en19cs601002@medicaps.ac.in

Suman Kumar Swarnkar, J P Patra, Sapna Singh Kshatri, Yogesh Kumar Rathore and Tien Anh Tran (eds.) Supervised and Unsupervised Data Engineering for Multimedia Data, (111–132) © 2024 Scrivener Publishing LLC

chapter is intended as a technical resource for academic circles and specialists as well as decision-makers.

Keywords: Smart agriculture, unsupervised, supervised, machine learning, Internet of Things, data mining

5.1 Introduction

The backbone of the nation is agriculture because it ensures the nation's food security. It is essential to the majority of the nation's external trade. About 75% of people around the world depend on agriculture for their livelihood. We must strengthen the state of agriculture because of the necessity to boost yield in the sector of agriculture caused by the population explosion. Agriculturalists are searching for active approaches to enhance crop produce while spending less and creating healthier use of their possessions. This supports the agriculturalists brand improved conclusions and enhancement produced by bringing new cardinal knowledge into the farming sector. We may now deal with a variety of issues and overcome hurdles in the agricultural sectors utilizing deep learning techniques [1].

The foundation of every economy is the agricultural sector. In a remarkable nation like India, where the population is growing and there is typically increasing interest in food, advancements in farming division regional units are anticipated to meet the needs. Agribusiness is viewed from the traditional era taking into account the way that the ruling, and in this way, the central culture practiced in Bharat. Traditional people cultivate their harvests in their distinctive territory after which they will be able to meet their needs. This results in the creation of the common basic area unit, which is used by people, animals, and birds. The greenish environment created inside these boundaries results in strong and reinforced life. Meanwhile, through the development of advanced innovative discoveries and approaches, the agricultural arena is progressively changing.

A person's district unit has been concentrating on making phony things as a result of these major developments. The agricultural industry has been gradually declining since the development of new creative innovations and tactics. Due to these, a lot of people who work in the development industry concentrate on creating phony goods that are mixes of real goods and wretched lives. People today are not cognizant of the need of growing crops in the ideal location and at the ideal time. Due to these evolving practices, the unique climatic circumstances are also changing in opposition to essential resources like soil, water, and air, making food more perishable.

There are no suitable solutions or innovations to deal with the situation when breaking down each of these problems together with others like environment, temperature, and a few other factors. There are a few various approaches to boost agricultural economic development in India. Data will be provided by the models, affiliations, or associations among this data. Data will once again be imagined into data pertaining to historical models and potential examples. For instance, design information about crop development will encourage farmers to decide to reap occurrences and prevent it in the future.

5.2 Background

The concept "smart agriculture" describes the extensive use of Artificial Intelligence (AI), which includes large data, the Internet of Things (IoT), deep learning, and numerous additional numerical knowledge [1]. A large growth in nutrition manufacture must be attained [3] as the global population rises [2]. It is difficult for current technologies to guarantee the continual and reliable supply and superiority of food worldwide deprived of detrimental ordinary bionetworks. A brand-new cutting-edge tool for data analysis and image processing is deep learning. It has been effectively used in a number of industries, including agriculture, and has produced encouraging results. It also has a tremendous amount of potential. The management of numerous agricultural events using data gathered from many foundations has been the key to the expansion of bottomless learning-based agronomic tenders (smart agriculture) in recent times. The capacity of various intelligent systems built on AI to record, interpret, and help farmers make the best decisions at the right moment varies. Installed IoT nodes (sensors) can record data, which can then be analyzed using any deep learning technique and decisions that can be imposed on operational regions using actuators. The real-time monitoring and management of agriculture is aided by additional leading-edge technologies, such as isolated perception physical statistics, worldwide satellite broadcasting location, and computerized supercomputer regulator.

Additionally, AI-based smart agriculture can be used to schedule the best amounts of resources like water, herbicides, and fertilizer, decreasing pollution and production costs while increasing output. Less medication would need to be applied to stop the spread of plant diseases as AI can help with early identification and prevention; this considerably lowers environmental contamination [5]. For plants to be healthy, grow, and produce, agronomic inputs like water, nutrients, and fertilizers must be continuously provided [6]. Both biotic and abiotic stress may result from the lack of any of these sources. First AI can choose when to routine the proper quantity of an assumed reserve while getting hooked on justification both the current condition and forthcoming plans. The use of Deep Learning and Artificial Intelligence was examined along with the possibilities for the future. We also looked into the IoT-monitored agricultural metrics and used them as input for the deep learning algorithms to process further.

Supervised Learning

The data has already been pre-labeled and is used to train an algorithm. The model is tested with unlabelled. The algorithm is created using training data that is already known and utilized to determine the outcomes for testing data that is not labeled. Errors may occur during the manual labeling procedure. The supervised learning process discussed is shown in Figure 5.1.

Semi-Supervised Learning

The majority of the labeled data and some unlabeled data are used in semi-supervised learning for training. By keeping both labeled and unlabeled data, it lowers costs while also maintaining the accuracy of predictions. The flow of semi-supervised learning with machine learning model flow is shown in Figure 5.2.

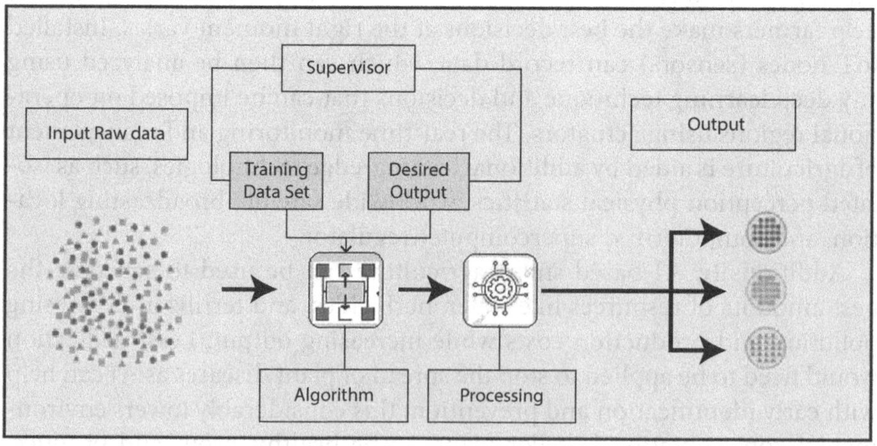

Figure 5.1 Supervised learning.

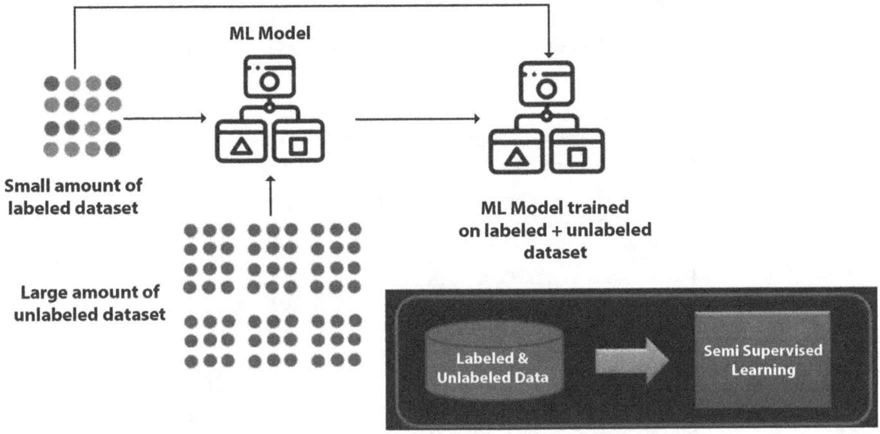

Figure 5.2 Semi-supervised learning.

- **Unsupervised Learning**

The data are unlabeled and were previously unknown. Data is grouped and organized into clusters by algorithms based on common traits and characteristics. Unsupervised learning employs clustering algorithms. The process flow from input data to output data using unsupervised learning model is shown in Figure 5.3.

Reinforcement Learning

Reinforcement learning has not used data to create models for predictions; instead, it uses observations from the outside world. Reinforcement learning with supervised, unsupervised, and hybrid model is shown in Figure 5.4.

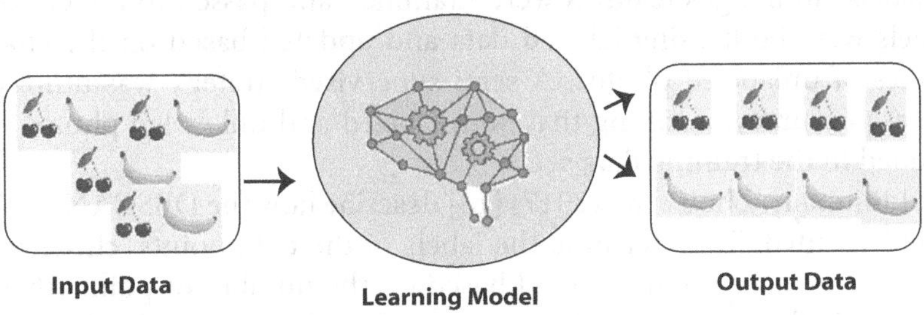

Figure 5.3 Unsupervised learning.

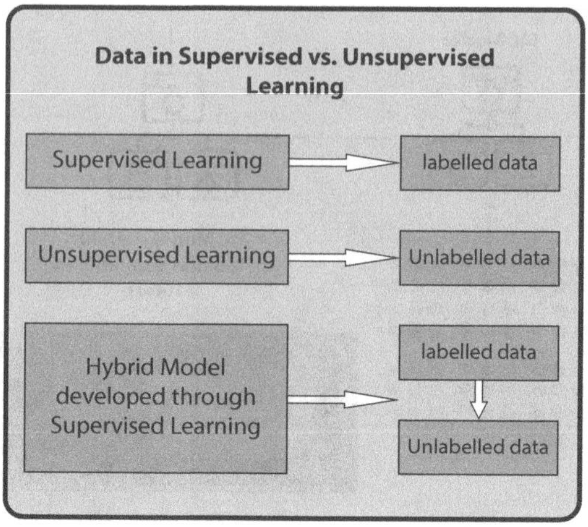

Figure 5.4 Reinforcement learning.

5.3 Applications of Machine Learning Algorithms in Agriculture

Many industries are using technology's progress to boost their bottom lines. Agriculture is one such example. Sensors and equipment are used in "smart agriculture" to collect data on the crops and produce improved results. Several agricultural enterprises use IoT, Big Data, and Cloud to analyze, assess, and manage the crops (3M 2018). Effective resource use and higher crop productivity are both aided by it. The health of the crops is tracked by sensors in the fields, which also calculate the optimal time to harvest and generate reports.

Machine learning algorithms are used in a variety of ways in smart agriculture. To discriminate between weeds and crops, Jiang *et al.* (2020) [10] give one such example. Graph convolutional network (GAN) is used to create a framework that classifies labels on photos. In order to determine the labels, an image's features were examined and passed to the classifier. Models were built using labeled data and updated based on the characteristics of unlabeled photos. A semi-supervised strategy was utilized to increase accuracy, meaning that both labeled and unlabeled photos were included in the training data set.

Additionally, Zhou *et al.* (2017) [13] describe how the DBSCAN method is implemented. To determine the labels of the data points, clustering is used. First, a core point is found based on the number of points that are closest to it. Second, a boundary is determined to separate the data points based on their proximity to and link to the core point. Outlier data points are then found, which aid in the analysis of the causes. The clusters' atypical shapes aided in the prediction of the causes of low output. For instance, some weather circumstances might have had an impact on the crop yield and produced outlier data. It might help the business owners plan ahead and come up with methods to boost output during those periods. We can perform a lot of analysis thanks to IoT because it allows us to collect a lot of real-time data using sensors in the field. It can determine how much insecticide should be used, how much water should be applied to the crops, and which crops should be cultivated in a way that benefits them depending on the weather. A variety of approaches can be applied to improve agriculture.

In agriculture, a different application of a clustering technique is described in Machica, Gerardo, and Medina (2019) [11]. The Internet of Things (IoT) facilitates the detection of irregularities in crop data. The abnormalities can alert farmers to potential issues and assist them in determining the best course of action. The use of a superimposed classification algorithm to find any anomalies in the crops is described in the study. By compiling information on crops in various regions, it seeks to identify any irregularities. It prepares models by cleaning, comprehending, and using data mining techniques.

Other applications that employ clustering methods to identify the crop exist. Zhang and Chau (2009) [12] highlight one approach that makes use of a KNN classifier to identify a plant's class using photos of its leaves. It begins by choosing a few features that can be utilized to categorize the photographs. The data points are then divided into categories using a Euclidean distance measure. A smaller distance between them denotes related data points, while a larger gap denotes less similarity. The proposed method tracked the outcomes for k binary classification issues. If there is more than one class, the problem will be broken down into binary classification problems before the suggested solution is used. In order to obtain better findings, it also employed a 10-fold cross validation technique. The data is divided by working out and challenging datasets k ages by means of an irritable authentication method known as k-fold. The train-test split with the most accurate results is used by the algorithm.

Other Applications

1. Species management

Species Breeding

In agriculture, the machine learning algorithms support precision and high-quality production. Species breeding is one of the logical and most useful in predictive breeding. This can improve the classical breeding by increasing genetic gain in the process. The method is data centric, which allows the development of the molecular markers through which the gnome can be properly captured.

The arduous procedure applied for species selection consists of observing particular patterns in the genes that are affecting how efficiently plants are using their nutrients and water. It is possible to find how well they are adapting to the happening climate change, the possibility of their resistance to any kind of illness. It is also possible to check whether the plants contain more nutrition or taste better. Deep learning and machine learning algorithms make use of huge quantities of statistics in order to examine how crops are growing in varied types of climatic changes and results in many new traits, both useful and more effective. Using the Deep Learning models a probability model could be developed for identifying the genes that provide the plant many characteristics that are beneficial in many ways for the improvement in its productivity.

The AI and Big Data methods have the capability to develop approaches for predictive breeding and therefore create many new opportunities for better smart plant breeding systems.

Species Recognition

Whereas associating leaf shade and figure is the ordinary social technique for categorizing shrubberies, machine learning can harvest additional precise and quick responses by investigating the manner construction of the greenery, which covers more information on the greenery's appearances. As an application of Machine Learning algorithms, species recognition results in helping the organizations to save species and also to detect any kind of distinct or endangered species. As per the study, there exist an astonishing 8.7 million species if identified on land and sea, out of which 7.5 million are still not identified. The challenges include intensive time and effort, lack of analytical skills, etc., where species recognition using deep learning can be a possible solution.

2. Field conditions management

Soil management

There are many complex processes and vague mechanisms in soil as it is a heterogeneous natural resource. The various components involved in this natural resource can help gain useful insights that help to predict the production and yield of the agricultural crop. Machine Learning algorithms like extreme learning machines have been evolved to be trained for detailed soil analysis, soil fertility prediction, soil quality prediction. This will no doubt contribute to precision agriculture and make the farming process more alert and fruitful in many ways.

Water Management
Agriculture's use of water affects the hydrological, meteorological, and agronomical stability. The greatest innovative machine learning (ML) requests so far are those that estimate day-to-day, weekly, or once-a-month water loss to enable additional efficient irrigation systems in addition to those that predict day-to-day condensation fact disease to support recognizing predictable climate phenomena and approximation water loss and disappearance.

3. Harvest management

Harvest Prediction
Of the greatest significance, besides well-known areas of meticulous farming, is harvest forecast, which incorporates planning and assessment of harvests, identical gather stream and petition, and yield management. Modern methods drive fine outside humble estimating based on ancient facts, integrating mainframe idea technologies to deliver data instantly and exhaustive multidimensional analyses of harvests, climate, and financial circumstances to exploit construction for agriculturalists and the overall populace.

Crop Quality
Accurately identifying and categorizing agricultural quality traits can raise product prices and decrease waste. In contrast to human specialists, machines can employ seemingly useless data and connections to expose and discover new attributes that contribute to the overall quality of crops.

Disease Detection
The most popular method of nuisance and sickness controller, both in outdoor and hot house settings, are to evenly sprig insecticides over the gathering extent. This strategy calls for large quantities of pesticides to be effective, which entails a substantial cost to the environment and the economy. When using general precision agriculture management, ML is used to target the application of agrochemicals based on the time, location, and plants that will be affected.

Weed Detection
Weeds provide the biggest hazards to crop output, excluding diseases. The biggest issue with weed control is how hard it is to distinguish them from

crops. With minimal expense and no negative effects on the environment, mainframe image and machine learning procedures can enhance the documentation and discernment of weeds. Future versions of these technologies will power weed-eating robots, reducing the need for herbicides.

Precision spraying
It is observed that crop health is affected by the watering system applied in the field. Spraying could help in preventing the infestation of pests and other diseases. Precision (also called targeted) spraying involves computer vision tasks by utilizing the target information. Some of the benefits of the technology include getting the spectral signatures of plants, soil and other materials. It minimizes the risk of plants and crops damage and maximizes the crop yield.

4. Livestock management
Livestock Production
Machine learning offers precise parameter estimation and prediction, much like crop management, to maximize the financial effectiveness of cattle manufacture systems, such as the production of bullocks and seeds. For instance, 150 days before the day of slaughter, weight prediction systems can anticipate future weights, enabling farmers to adjust the diets and environmental factors.

Animal Welfare
Today's livestock is increasingly handled as creatures who can be sad and worn out by their life cycle on a farm rather than just as food carriers. Animals' movement patterns, such as standing, moving, eating, and drinking, can determine how much stress an animal is exposed to and predict its vulnerability to diseases, weight increase, and productivity. Animals' chewing signals can be linked to the need for food adjustments.

Advantages of Machine Learning

1. Suitable time for crops
It's crucial to plant and cultivate crops at the ideal times in order to maximize their yield. It's crucial to select the correct crop for the season and soil. Otherwise, you won't receive the required outcomes owing to a mismatch.

Farmers can predict and forecast the ideal cropping season and the ideal soil and crop match with the use of machine learning. The crops that will yield the most profits can be found.

2. Crop Yield Patterns

It is crucial to the health of the crops you have planted. It is vital to find current information regarding the state of the fields, the crops, the height of the crops, and the diseased crops.

You may assess whether or not everything is being done correctly by comparing this data to your historical cropping performance. Drones and many other technological devices can be used to collect this data with the use of machine learning.

3. Water and Irrigation

It's crucial to assess the crop's water needs. Adding too little water can cause the crops to dry up, and adding too much water can completely destroy them. You must thus estimate how much water will be required this season based on prior demands.

You can reduce the crops' need for moisture with the use of machine learning. Irrigation and water management are two crucial aspects of agriculture.

4. Agribots

Costs are influenced by the use of laborers in the fields, during harvest, and throughout the entire agricultural process. When there is no work, the cost of the labor increases and accumulates.

Agribots can be used to estimate when you will require laborers on the field with the aid of machine learning, so you are aware of when you need to hire staff. When you know when you'll require skilled labor, you can avoid spending money on hiring them in advance. Skilled labor is needed throughout the last phase.

5. Farm animals

In order to breed and produce high-quality meat and other farm products, farm animals must be kept in good health. Machine learning can be used to estimate things like female animal pregnancy checks, food needs, and milking times, among other things.

Therefore, maintaining the health and productivity of the farm animals throughout the cycle is the main benefit of machine learning.

Uses of Machine Learning in Agriculture

1. Analyze Market Demand

The analysis of crop market demand in agriculture can be done using machine learning. Because they were unaware of the crop's great demand, producers occasionally cannot produce it. By predicting the demand, they can produce what will sell better and increase the value of their produce. Farmers are compelled to sell their product at a minimum support price if it remains unsold.

They are forced to accept less money and incur losses in this situation. All of these problems involving market demand can be avoided with the aid of machine learning.

2. Risk Management

Another area where machine learning might benefit agriculture is risk management. Many causes, including those external to the environment, governmental regulations, and climatic changes, might result in risks.

As a result, we can evaluate the likelihood of dangers and promptly take steps to reduce them using machine learning. Controlling the risk factors is preferable to letting the entire crop's produce spoil.

3. Breeding Seeds

Prior to planting, farmers must inspect the quality of the seeds. Breeding seeds is combining various seed varieties to create a special crop or a different species of plant.

Proper selection is required to determine which seed can be bred with which. Which seed will combine with and produce the best results can be determined with the aid of machine learning.

Breeding incorrect seeds can have severe effects and can generate crops that are unsafe for human consumption. The best results will always come from properly bred seeds. Machine learning takes the aptitude to assemble the necessary data and forecast outcomes.

4. Crop Protection

Crops must be safeguarded from a variety of threats. Crops can be harmed by poor environmental conditions, diseases, fertilizers, and even climate. Farmers have two options for protecting their crops: they may purchase crop insurance, or they can use machine learning techniques to receive daily information on the condition of their crops and potential threats to them.

A 360-degree image of the crops is available to farmers. They can learn how much fertilizer the crop needs as well as the highest amount that will not harm the crop. The crop can be well protected from all types of attacks with the use of machine learning.

5. Soil Health Monitoring

Crops cannot be planted unless the soil has been prepared. Not every type of soil is appropriate for every sort of crop. Because of soil contamination, the soil turns acidic, which affects fertility.

Finding the ideal soil is crucial in order for it to be suitable for producing crops. We can test the soil type and composition with the aid of machine learning.

6. Harvesting

Farmers have a lot of work to do during the harvesting season. Starting with the hiring of skilled labor, cutting the crops, and sending them on to the following step.

The workload of the farmers can be lightened in a number of ways with the help of machine learning. It can compile information from various sources and analyze data from previous crop seasons to create a plan of action for the farmers.

Deep Learning for Smart Agriculture

Deep learning, computer vision, image processing, robots, and IoT technology are currently considerably assisting agriculture. AI-based drone technology is very helpful for farming since it makes it easier to monitor, scan, and evaluate the crops because it produces high-quality photographs. The advancement of the crops may be followed thanks to this technique. Additionally, farmers have the option to decide when the crops are prepared for harvest. There are countless ways to describe deep learning's applications in agriculture; some of these applications are given here.

Deep learning, computer vision, image processing, robots, and IoT technology are currently considerably assisting agriculture. AI-based drone technology is very helpful for farming since it makes it easier to monitor, scan, and evaluate the crops because it produces high-quality photographs. The advancement of the crops may be followed thanks to this technique. Additionally, farmers have the option to decide when the crops are prepared for harvest. There are countless ways to describe deep learning's applications in agriculture; some of these applications are given here. Deep learning is currently being used in various smart agriculture applications, including crop cultivation, disease detection in crops, weed control, crop distribution, robust fruit counting, and yield prediction.

There are three types of learning: supervised, unsupervised, and reinforcement learning. Agricultural data is processed using supervised approaches for face detection, optical character recognition, spam email filtering, virus filtering, online fraud detection, and natural language processing. Unsupervised algorithms for anomaly detection and market segmentation are employed in sentiment analysis. Recently, technologies like artificial intelligence (AI), machine learning (ML), deep learning (DL), the Internet of Things (IoT), and robotics have been very useful in the agriculture sector to reduce labor costs, enhance crop quality, manage water and soil resources, and identify crop diseases early on.

Deep Learning Algorithms used in Agriculture shown in Figure 5.5:

1) Convolutional Neural Networks (CNN)
2) Recurrent Neural Networks (RNN)
3) Generative Adversarial Networks (GAN)

The three most often used DL algorithms are CNN, RNN, and GAN. There are numerous more DL algorithms in the subcategory, including VGGNet [4], ConvNets [5], LSTM [6,7], and DCGAN [8,9]. One synopsis could not possibly cover them all. They can be directly or indirectly generated from the three widely used DL algorithms [10]. Learning the DL algorithms in the sub-category begins with understanding the three basic DL algorithms. As a result, a detailed assessment of the DL methods in the subcategory is omitted. Many ANNs are built on the idea of backpropagation (BP), which is not the same as a deep network. As a result, it will be discussed in this section first.

Convolutional neural networks (CNN) is a deep learning method made up of a number of convolutional, pooling, and fully connected layers that

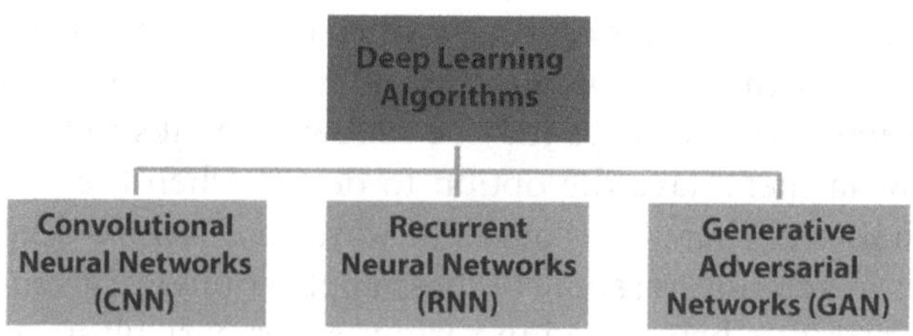

Figure 5.5 Deep learning algorithms.

has made significant advancements in speech recognition, face recognition, natural language processing, and other fields. Convolutional layers and pooling layers make up the structure for feature extraction, while fully linked layers serve as a classifier. Contrary to convolutional networks, which first transform signals into features before mapping the features to a specific target value, BP neural networks primarily map features via the network to specific values.

Convolutional Layer: Assume there are six convolution kernels and an RGB image is used as the input (X). An HW3 three-dimensional matrix represents the image size. Each convolutional layer's corresponding convolution kernel size is hw3. Convolutional layer's threshold is b. Following the convolution calculation, the size of the new image feature X is H newW new, whose convolutional layer computation procedure. The number of convolution kernels for each convolutional layer controls how many feature maps are generated or how many inputs are used in the pooling layer. The zero-padding approach, which adds a value of zero to the input vector's border to identify the edge information of a picture, has a zero-padding size of P.

Pooling Layer: In order to compress the input tensor and reduce the size of the input data, the pooling layer's task is to convert each of the input image's n by n submatrix into a distinct element value. The two most widely used pooling methods are maximum pooling and mean pooling. Maximum pooling uses the maximum of the corresponding n-n area, whereas mean pooling uses the average value of the corresponding n-n area as the pooled element value. W, H, and D make up the pooling layer's input volume, whereas W pooling, H pooling, and D pooling make up its output volume. In order to simulate how the human brain analyzes signals, CNN combines feature extraction from image processing with BP neural networks.

CNN has less parameters than deep networks because of its local perception mechanism and parameter sharing mechanism, which can reduce parameters. CNN is capable of handling high-dimensional arrays, especially when used for image classification. The most typical format for data modalities is several arrays. CNN excels in image processing, face recognition, and natural language processing because of the distinctive patterns that local weights share. Its architecture is more like a biological neural network. CNN still needs a lot of training samples, though.

Recurrent neural networks (RNN): Time series analysis, speech recognition, and linguistic homology have all advanced thanks to RNN, which can mine both temporal and semantic data. RNN is an adaption of ANN, which denotes that the input and output of the network are currently connected. The RNN can be thought of as a BP neural network whose output will be utilized as the input of the following network. The unique embodiment is that the network will retain the information from earlier calculations and homolog it to calculate the output of the current network.

Even if in theory RNN can handle time series problems, doing so in homolog is difficult because the amount of information varies and might cause gradients to vanish or explode. The Lengthy Short-Term Memory (LSTM) network enhances the recurrent neural network, which is primarily designed to handle time series issues with long intervals and high delays. The LSTM makes use of the structure of a few "doors" to selectively change the current state of the recurrent neural network. LSTM networks have been used in speech recognition, machine translation, and other fields.

Generative adversarial networks (GAN): The revolutionary aspect of GAN is in its design. Technically, it incorporates a number of the current algorithms used by BP. To generate new data and understand how the real data are distributed, a set of noise can be homologated with GAN. The structure of this network is composed of two models: a discrimination model that resembles a binary classifier [2] and a generation model to represent the distribution of the actual data. The strength of generative adversarial networks (GAN) lies in their autonomous learning of the distribution of real sample data.

Deep convolutional generative adversarial networks (DCGAN), which are widely used in image processing for tasks like image restoration from split images, dynamic scene generation, image generation, and resolution enhancement, were created as a result of the development of convolutional neural networks. DCGAN is also essential for recognising and detecting faces. Although there is always potential for improvement in GAN applications, phonological optimization of the generation model and the discrimination model are required for training a GAN, which is difficult.

Current Applications of DL in Shrewd Cultivation

Recent applications of CNN, RNN, and GAN in smart agriculture are summarized in this section.

CNN Applications in Smart Agriculture

CNN is commonly used in agricultural research because of its powerful image processing capabilities. The classification of plants or crops category, which is crucial for pest control, robotic harvesting, yield forecast, disaster monitoring, etc., comprises the majority of DL applications in agriculture. It takes time to manually detect plant illnesses. Fortunately, with the development of artificial intelligence, image processing can now be used to identify plant illnesses.

The classification and pattern recognition of leaves serve as the foundation for the majority of models for identifying plant diseases. The novel DL framework developed by the Berkley Vision and Learning Center was used to generate a model for the identification of plant diseases. For categorizing plants, a pre-trained CNN architecture called AlexNet is typically employed. According to experimental findings utilizing AlexNet from the Istanbul Technical University in 2017, the CNN architecture outperforms machine learning methods based on hand-crafted characteristics for the discrimination of chronological stages. CNN was used to supervise the classification. With the use of this method, a post-processing stage with a wide range of usable filtering algorithms was added.

RNN Submissions in Canny Cultivation

In several agricultural fields, including land cover classification, phenotypic recognition, crop yield estimation, leaf area index estimation, weather prediction, soil moisture estimation, animal research, and event date estimation, RNN has proven to be particularly beneficial for processing time series data. The goal of land cover classification (LCC), a crucial yet difficult activity in agriculture, is to identify the class that a typical plot of land belongs to. Many applications in the past relied on mono-temporal data and disregarded time-series effects in some issues. For instance, vegetation periodically modifies its spatial appearance, which can be perplexing to mono-temporal techniques. Meanwhile, biases like the weather may have an impact on mono-temporal techniques.

GAN Applications in Smart Agriculture

Although GAN is a novel type of neural network, it has already proven to be an effective technique in a number of industries, including image processing.

Datasets have frequently been enhanced using GAN. Agriculture has not seen a lot of its use. The reason they chose the content loss function over the more popular pixel-wise MSE loss was because of perceived similarity. Their algorithm was able to retrieve highly compressed images and outperformed several cutting-edge models at the time after being trained with 350 K images. This research is so fundamental that it may be used in nearly any project involving image processing, especially in the sector of agriculture where many applications are based on remote sensing photos. To enhance the realism of synthetic data, they employed a GAN-based model termed the unsupervised cycle generative adversarial network.

Agriculture Green Development

The majority of the food that is consumed worldwide is produced via crop agriculture. Examples of plant-based foods include grains, sugar, fruits, vegetables, and oilseeds. Ammonia evaporation and oxidizing nitrogen fixing caused a significant amount of waste to be lost to the environment and to leak into the soil, which resulted in an unbalanced vicious cycle. The establishment of green crop production, which would deal with the concerns of preserving food security and environmental protection, has become more challenging. For environmentally friendly input and sustainable preservation of agricultural land, a green crop production approach is crucial.

To achieve a sustainable increase in high efficiency, high value crops, this involves introducing novel crop plants, food crops, and green pesticides to an integrated soil culture control unit.

A major shift in the development of agriculture from purely intensive food production to sustainable production can be seen in the fundamental transformation of agricultural production from a traditional resource-based model with high ecological cost into increased productivity, high efficiency resource use, and poor environmental impact.

The management and creation of green products are included in the production of green crops. Soil quality and agricultural production are two factors that are crucial for the meaningful delivery of high-quality food, and both can be successfully raised by the design of the agricultural system. Animal products like milk, eggs, and meat must be produced because they include nutrients that are simpler to digest than those found in many crops. It can provide essential industrial materials for the textile and clothing industries, as shown in Figure 5.6.

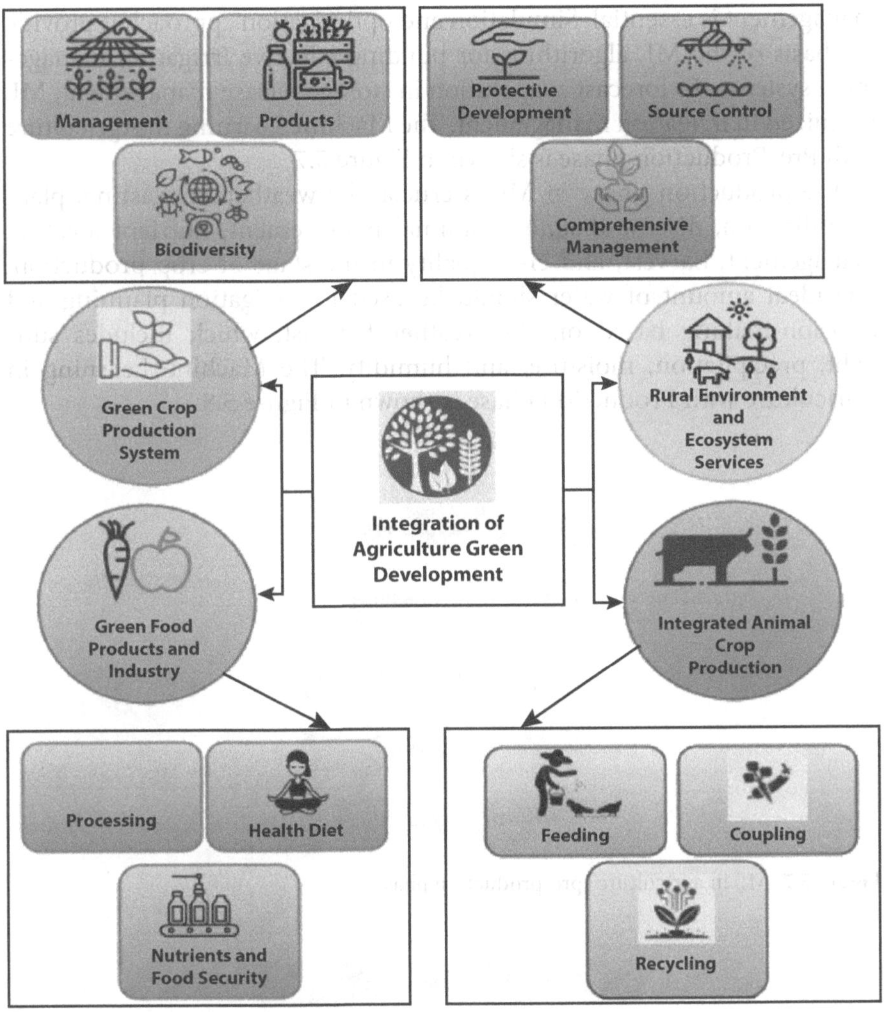

Figure 5.6 Agriculture green development.

Different Phases of ML in Agriculture

The quality and quantity of crops are significantly impacted by irrigation management. It is possible to visually analyze when, where, and how much irrigation is possible with irrigation development and management. To more accurately predict soil moisture, precipitation, evaporation, and weather, an effective irrigation system is used. In order to maintain the balance of the climatic, hydrological, and agricultural processes required for agricultural sustainability over the long term, effective irrigation management is essential. Simulation and optimization approaches provide the basis of the ML algorithms for building effective irrigation management systems. To forecast evaporation in storage release management, ML is utilized in irrigation management. The Machine Learning in Agriculture with Pre-Production phase is shown in Figure 5.7.

The production phase of ML is crucial for weather forecasting, plant identification, disease diagnosis, animal management, nutrient location management, harvest, and crop quality in the stage of crop production. The ideal amount of water should be used for irrigation planning and decision-making based on the weather forecast, which includes sunlight, precipitation, moisture, and humidity. The Machine Learning in Agriculture with Production phase is shown in Figure 5.8.

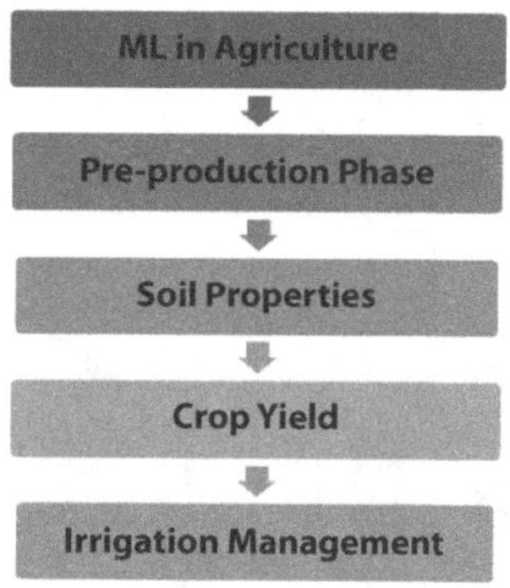

Figure 5.7 ML in agriculture (pre-production phase).

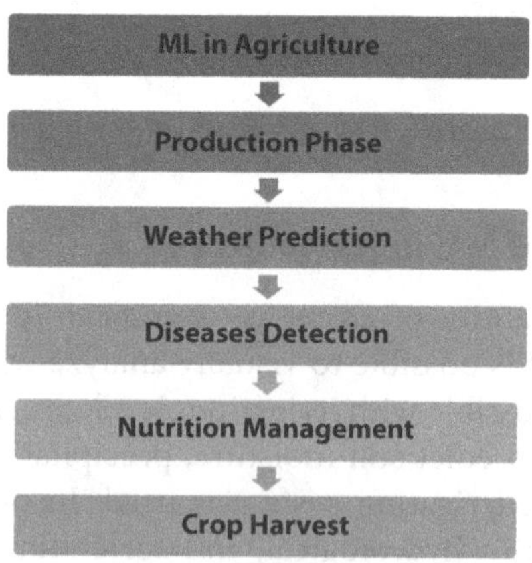

Figure 5.8 ML in agriculture (production phase).

Use of Multimedia Data in Smart Agriculture

The Internet of Multimedia Things, or IoMT, is the focus of many current studies in the field of smart agriculture [14]. With the use of IOT sensors, machine learning algorithms, and image processing, the irrigation process is improved and optimized. Better irrigation decisions are made as a result of this collaboration. As it represents the current technology changes, the multimedia data currently forms the extension services in the smart agriculture operations. The difficulty here is dealing with developments in multimedia big data processing systems and multimedia data collection techniques that are appropriate for use in smart agriculture.

References

[1] Liu, Q.; Yan, Q.; Tian, J.; Yuan, K. Key technologies and applications in intelligent agriculture. *J. Phys. Conf. Ser.* 2021, 1757, 012059. [CrossRef]

[2] Kitzes, J.; Wackernagel, M.; Loh, J.; Peller, A.; Goldfinger, S.; Cheng, D.; Tea, K. Shrink and share humanity's present and future ecological footprint. *Philos. Trans. Roy. Soc. Lond. B Biol. Sci.* 2008, 363, 467–475. [CrossRef] [PubMed]

[3] FAO. How to Feed the World in 2050; Food and Agriculture Organization of the United Nations: Rome, Italy, 2009.

[4] Kamilaris, A.; Prenafeta-Boldú, F.X. Deep learning in agriculture: A survey. *Comput. Electron. Agric. 2018, 147, 70–90. [CrossRef]*

[5] Ren, C.; Dae-Kyoo, K.; Jeong, D. A survey of deep learning in agriculture: Techniques and their applications. *J. Inf. Processing Syst.* 2020, 16, 1015–1033.

[6] Kumar, A.; Shreeshan, S.; Tejasri, N.; Rajalakshmi, P.; Guo, W.; Naik, B.; Marathi, B.; Desai, U. Identification of water-stressed area in maize crop using UAV based remote sensing. In *Proceedings of the 2020 IEEE India Geoscience and Remote Sensing Symposium (InGARSS), Ahmedabad, India, 1–4 December 2020.*

[7] Dargan, S.; Kumar, M.; Ayyagari, M.R.; Kumar, G. A survey of deep learning and its applications: A new paradigm to machine learning. *Arch. Comput. Methods Eng.* 2020, 27, 1071–1092. [CrossRef]

[8] Samira Pouyanfar, Saad Sadiq and Yilin Yan, Haiman Tian, Yudong Tao, Maria Presa Reyes, Mei-Ling Shyu, Shu-Ching Chen and S. S. Iyengar, "A Survey on Deep Learning: Algorithms, Techniques and Applications", *ACM Computing Surveys*, Vol. 51, No. 5, September 2018.

[9] Smart Farming: Data Enabling the Future of Agriculture, 2018. https://www.youtube.com/watch?v=LaMvMgdJC58.

[10] Jiang, Honghua, Chuanyin Zhang, YongliangQiao, Zhao Zhang, Wenjing Zhang, and Changqing Song. "CNN Feature Based Graph Convolutional Network for Weed and Crop Recognition in Smart Farming." *Computers and Electronics in Agriculture* 174 (2020): 105450.
[11] Machica, Ivy Kim D., Bobby D. Gerardo, and Ruji P. Medina. "Superimposed rule-based classification algorithm in IoT." *Int J Comput Sci Mobile Comput* 8, no. 6 (2019): 153-160.
[12] Zhang, Shanwen, and Kwok-Wing Chau. "Dimension reduction using semi-supervised locally linear embedding for plant leaf classification." In Emerging Intelligent Computing Technology and Applications: 5th International Conference on Intelligent Computing, ICIC 2009, Ulsan, South Korea, September 16-19, 2009. Proceedings 5, pp. 948-955. Springer Berlin Heidelberg, 2009.
[13] Zhou, Yifan, Wei Hu, Yong Min, Le Zheng, Baisi Liu, Rui Yu, and Yu Dong. A Semi-Supervised Anomaly Detection Method for Wind Farm Power Data Preprocessing. In *2017 IEEE Power & Energy Society General Meeting*, 1–5. IEEE, 2017.
[14] AlZu'bi, S., Hawashin, B., Mujahed, M. *et al.* An efficient employment of internet of multimedia things in smart and future agriculture. *Multimed Tools Appl* 78, 29581–29605 (2019). https://doi.org/10.1007/s11042-019-7367-0

6

Secure Medical Image Transmission Using 2-D Tent Cascade Logistic Map

L. R. Jonisha Miriam[1]*, A. Lenin Fred[2], S. N. Kumar[3], Ajay Kumar H.[4], I. Christina Jane[5], Parasuraman Padmanabhan[6] and Balázs Gulyás[6]

[1]Department of Electronics and Communication Engineering, Mar Ephraem College of Engineering and Technology, Elavuvilai, Tamil Nadu, India
[2]Dept of Elec. and Comm. Engg, C. S. I Institute of Technology, Thovalai, India
[3]Amal Jyothi College of Engineering, Kanjirappally, Kerala, India
[4]Mar Ephraem College of Engineering and Technology, Elavuvilai, Tamil Nadu, India
[5]Department of ECE, Mar Ephraem College of Engineering and Technology, Marthandam, Tamil Nadu, India
[6]Lee Kong Chian School of Medicine, Nanyang Technological University, Singapore, Singapore

Abstract
Secure image communication is becoming more and more important owing to stealing and content manipulation. To protect the confidential image from unauthorized access, encryption algorithms are considered. Due to the unique properties of chaotic systems, the admired encryption algorithm used is the chaos-based encryption algorithm. It deals with a 2D chaos-based encryption algorithm known as Two-Dimensional Tent Cascade Logistic Map (2DTCLM). Cascading, logistic map and tent map generate 2D-TCLM, which is applied on permutation and substitution stages to obtain an encrypted image from the original image. Simulation results show the effect of the proposed algorithm on DICOM images to obtain their corresponding encrypted and decrypted images to know the accuracy of transmission between end users. Performance metrics such as correlation, covariance, and histogram variance are analyzed to show that the transmission is possible in proficient mode.

**Corresponding author*: jonishamiriam@gmail.com

Suman Kumar Swarnkar, J P Patra, Sapna Singh Kshatri, Yogesh Kumar Rathore and Tien Anh Tran (eds.) Supervised and Unsupervised Data Engineering for Multimedia Data, (133–148) © 2024 Scrivener Publishing LLC

Keywords: Encryption medical image, transmission, 2-D tent cascade logistic map, tent map

6.1 Introduction

With the rapid advancement of information and network technology, it's becoming increasingly difficult to keep up. Every second, more and more digital photos containing various types of information are created and distributed across the networks. As a result, picture encryption, a simple picture security method, has been explored and given increasing attention. An image encryption approach transforms a digital image into an unrecognizable image that can only be reproduced with the correct key. The act of altering information using an algorithm to render it unreadable to everyone save those with particular information, commonly referred to as a key, and the process of changing information using an "encryption algorithm" into a form that cannot be decrypted without a decryption key, are both referred to as image encryption. The decryption of a picture, on the other hand, recovers the true information from an encrypted image. Image encryption techniques are divided into two categories: non-chaos selective methods and chaos-based selective or non-selective methods. The majority of these methods are customized to a certain image format, whether compressed or uncompressed, and some are even format compactible.

The color image encryption was proposed in [1], where the logistic map function was employed and the permutation algorithm performs the combined row and column scrambling. The chaotic encryption algorithm based on a logistic map was proposed in [2] for grayscale and color images; the system generates pseudo-random numbers for the scrambling of columns and rows. The dual logistic chaotic function was deployed in [3] for the encryption of color and grayscale images, while in [4], a hybrid combination of linear and nonlinear coupled lattice was utilized and found to generate proficient results when compared with the 1D chaotic system. The piece-wise linear chaotic map [5] was used to generate the pseudo-random sequence for the encryption process, while in [6], DNA complementary rule and a chaotic map were used for image encryption. The Lorentz chaotic system was coupled with the perceptron neural network architecture for the encryption of images [7], the computational complexity was found to be low when compared with the other classical encryption approaches.

The coupled two-dimensional piecewise non-linear chaotic map was utilized in [8] for image encryption and it involves three phases: diffusion, substitution, and masking. The wavelet transform coefficients were shuffled by the Fisher-Yates technique and chaotic function was used to perform encryption [9]. The integer wavelet transform (IWT) coefficients are subjected to a spatio-temporal chaotic system for encryption of images [10]. The multiple chaotic maps are used in [11] for the encryption process and provide an ideal solution to entropy-based attacks. The intertwining chaotic map was incorporated in [12] for encryption; the computational complexity was low and minimizes the impact of information leakage. An improved novel chaotic algorithm based on pseudo-random number generation was proposed in [13] for medical image encryption/decryption. In [14], a novel encryption/decryption technique based on chaotic sequences and dynamic S boxes was proposed with low computational speed. DNA rules and dual hyperchaotic map techniques are employed in [15] for the encryption of medical images, thereby ensuring a high level of security. Section 6.2 describes the medical image encryption/decryption based on hybrid mapping technique, section 6.3 depicts the simulation results with performance validation and finally, the conclusion is drawn in section 6.4.

6.2 Medical Image Encryption Using 2D Tent and Logistic Chaotic Function

Chaos-based encryption is the widely used picture encryption method across all types. This is due to the chaotic system's features of unpredictability, ergodicity, and sensitivity to start circumstances. It can produce chaotic sequences that are non-overlapping and unexpected. The classical picture encryption techniques can be cracked if the chaotic systems employed have poor performance. As a result, creating novel chaotic maps with sophisticated chaotic characteristics and employing them in the creation of new image encryption is critical. There are two general needs for the construction of chaos-based encryption systems: 1) The encryption must be invertible to get plain text during decryption. 2) The digital hardware is employed in most implementations of (discrete-time) chaos-based encryption systems, chaotic maps must be chosen that retain crucial features when digitized.

Two-Dimensional Hybrid Mapping Technique for Encryption/Decryption of Medical Images

The 2D hybrid mapping technique was formulated by the cascading of Tent and Logistic, extending the results from one-dimensional (1D) to two-dimensional (2D) function [16][17]. The suggested 2D-TCLM features complicated chaotic behaviors, according to its trajectory and information entropy analyses. With a high level of security, a novel image encryption technology known as 2D-TCLM encrypt the input medical image into a random image.

2D-TCLM is mathematically expressed as in equation (6.1),

$$\begin{cases} U_{n+1} = \begin{cases} (3+V_n)2\mu U_n(1-2\mu U_n) & \text{if } U_n < 0.5 \\ (3+V_n)2\mu U_n(1-2\mu U_n)\big(1-(1-2\mu U_n)\big) & \text{if } U_n > 0.5 \end{cases} \\ V_{n+1} = \begin{cases} (3+U_{n+1})2\mu V_n(1-2\mu V_n) & \text{if } V_n < 0.5 \\ (3+U_{n+1})2\mu U_n(1-2\mu V_n)\big(1-(1-2\mu V_n)\big) & \text{if } V_n > 0.5 \end{cases} \end{cases} \tag{6.1}$$

Where the iterative values are (U_n, V_n). μ is the control parameter, and [0, 1] is the range. The distribution of its output pairs (U_i. V_i) on 2D phase plane is described by the trajectory of a 2D chaotic map. To determine the information entropy of 2D-output TCLM's sequences, divide the output values into 256 intensities first, then apply equation (6.2) to compute the information entropy. $H_{max} = \log_2 256 = 8$ is the maximum information entropy value when all intensity levels are equal. The information entropy value is quite high when parameter u is [0.4,1], indicating good randomness. In information theory, the uncertainty of information content is measured using information entropy. It may be used to determine how random a set of data is. It has a mathematical definition (6.2),

$$H(U) = -\Sigma_i P_r(u_i) log_2 P_r(u_i) \tag{6.2}$$

U denotes a data sequence. $P_r(u_i)$ is the probability of u_i, and u_i is the i-th possible value in U. Better randomness is associated with higher information entropy value.

Logistic Map

A chaotic one-dimensional system with complicated chaotic behaviour is known as a logistic map. It is commonly used in picture encryption to generate secret keys. The following equation expresses the mathematical form of the logistic map (6.3),

$$u_{n+1} = c * u_n * (1 - u_n) \tag{6.3}$$

With ranges of (0, 4) and (0, 1), C is the control parameter and un is the starting condition. In general, the chaotic range of logistic map is restricted,

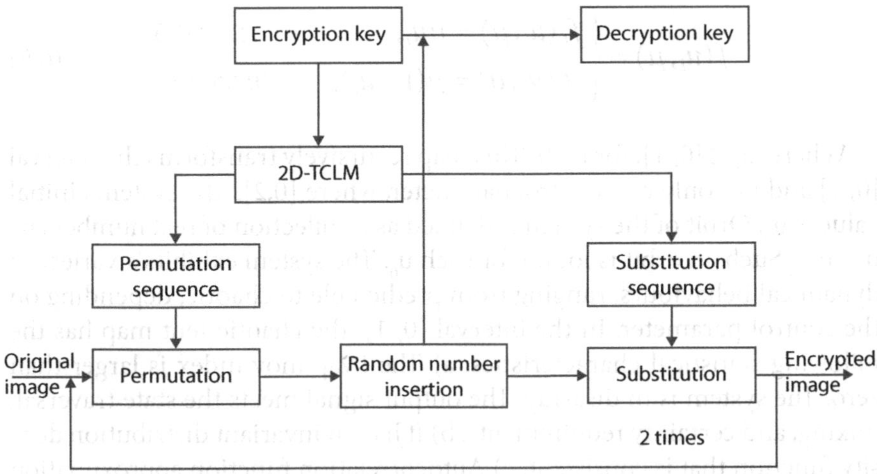

Figure 6.1 Proposed encryption/decryption methodology for medical images.

with chaotic behaviour occurring only in the range of 3.6 to 4 without periodicity. This nonlinear difference equation is designed to reflect two impacts when the population number is small: reproduction and starvation, where the growth rate will fall at a rate proportionate to the value obtained by taking the theoretical "carrying capacity" of the environment less one. The Lyapunov Exponent and the bifurcation diagram can be used to obtain this. The absence of chaotic activity is shown by the blank zone of the bifurcation diagram, which is not ideal for security purposes. Figure 6.1 shows the sequential steps for encrypting and decrypting medical photos to protect confidential information. The method uses 2D-TCLM, permutation, substitution sequences, and random number insertion. A double permutation-substitution sequence is conducted twice during encryption to increase transformation complexity. This process uses a different encryption key. Complex encryption is used to the original medical imaging to create the encrypted image. The decryption key is needed to reverse this process and rebuild the original image from the encrypted version. This technology provides a durable and secure structure to protect medical images and critical healthcare data.

Tent Map

Because the tent map is topologically conjugate, its behaviours under iteration are in this sense equivalent. Equation (6.4) gives us the chaotic tent map (6.5),

$$u_{i+1} = f(u_i, \mu) \tag{6.4}$$

$$f(u_i,\mu)=\begin{cases} f_L(u_i,\mu)=\mu u_i, & u_i<0.5 \\ f_l(u_i,\mu)=\mu(1-u_i), & otherwise \end{cases} \tag{6.5}$$

Where, $u_i \in [0, 1]$, for $i \geq 0$. This map recursively transforms the interval [0, 1] and has only one control parameter, where [0,2]. The system's initial value is u_0. Orbit of the system is defined as a collection of real numbers $u_{0,}$ $u_{1\ldots}$ $u_{n\ldots}$ Such an orbit is found for each u_0. The system exhibits a variety of dynamical behaviours, ranging from predictable to chaotic, depending on the control parameter. In the interval [0, 1], the chaotic tent map has the following statistical characteristics: a) The Lyapunov index is larger than zero. The system is in disarray. The output signal meets the state traversal, mixing, and certainty requirements. b) It has an invariant distribution density function that is consistent. c) Autocorrelation function approximation on the output rail. The chaotic sequences formed by mapping have high statistical features, although they display periodicity under finite precision. It demonstrates ergodicity as the value grows bigger. Chaotic sequences display great unpredictability as the value decreases; nonetheless, after limited repetitions, the chaotic sequence's output value is zero. This is because when using piecewise linear functions to produce chaotic mapping, the accuracy of 24 starting values is always restricted; due to computer precision limitations, the closer the number of approximates is to 1, the more likely it is to be treated as 1. As a result, the value is close to 2.

Image Cipher Generation Using 2D-TCLM

This explains how to use 2DTCLM to create a new picture encryption technique. Input is the medical image and the hybrid chaotic technique (2D-TCLM) generates chaotic sequences. The permutation and substitution process relies on chaotic sequences. The random numbers are generated during encryption stage to alter the pixel values and the same random numbers are provided during the decoding stage for decryption. The encryption technique is denoted by the letters C = Encp(P, K_e), whereas the decryption technique is denoted by the letters D = Decp(C, K_d).

Security Key

The encryption key $K_e = (u_0{}^1, v_0{}^1, \mu, u_0{}^2, v_0{}^2, a_1, a_2)$ is used in the proposed picture encryption technique. Ke's components are all in the [0, 1] range. For 2D-TCLM, there are two groups of starting values: $(u_0{}^1, v_0{}^1)$ and $(u_0{}^2, v_0{}^2)$. Equation may be used to produce two 2DTCLM parameters (6.6),

$$x_i = 0.4 + (x * a_i * 100 \bmod 0.6) \tag{6.6}$$

Where i is either 1 or 2. As a result, 1 and 2 are both in the [0.4, 1] range, ensuring that the hybrid mapping technique has an excellent chaotic outcome. It is worth noting that the decryption key is not the same as the encryption key. In the two rounds, assuming r1 and r2 are two randomly produced values in the Random Number Insertion stage, the decryption key $K_d = (u_0^1, v_0^1, \mu, u_0^2, v_0^2, a_1, a_2, r_1, r_2)$.

Permutation

Permutation involves rearranging all of the pixels in the picture. Assume that the chaotic sequence CS created by 2D-TCLM is M x N in length. It is the same size as the image. In order to acquire row and column index matrices I_r and I_c, sorting is carried out in the chaotic sequence row-wise and column-wise. The permutation of picture P is defined as follows:

$$T(m,n) = P\big(m, I_r(m,n)\big) \tag{6.7}$$

$$O(m, n) = T(I_c(m, n), n) \tag{6.8}$$

Substitution

The goal of substitution is to alter all the pixel values at random. The resultant values of permutation are reordered with size [1, MN] and then the substitution is described as follows

$$C(i) = \begin{cases} PO(i) \oplus CS(i) \oplus rv & \text{if } i = 1 \\ PO(i) \oplus CS(i) \oplus C(i-1) & \text{if } i \in [2, MN] \end{cases} \tag{6.9}$$

Where rv is a random number created during the Random Number Insertion step, and C denotes the operation outcome. Finally, reorganize C with [M, N] as the size. An original picture can be encrypted into a random-like cypher text image after two procedures.

6.3 Simulation Results and Discussion

MATLAB 2015a is utilized for the simulation of algorithms and verified on real-time abdomen CT DICOM images. In this research work, two algorithms are taken into account; medical image encryption based on wavelet transform algorithm and medical image encryption based on

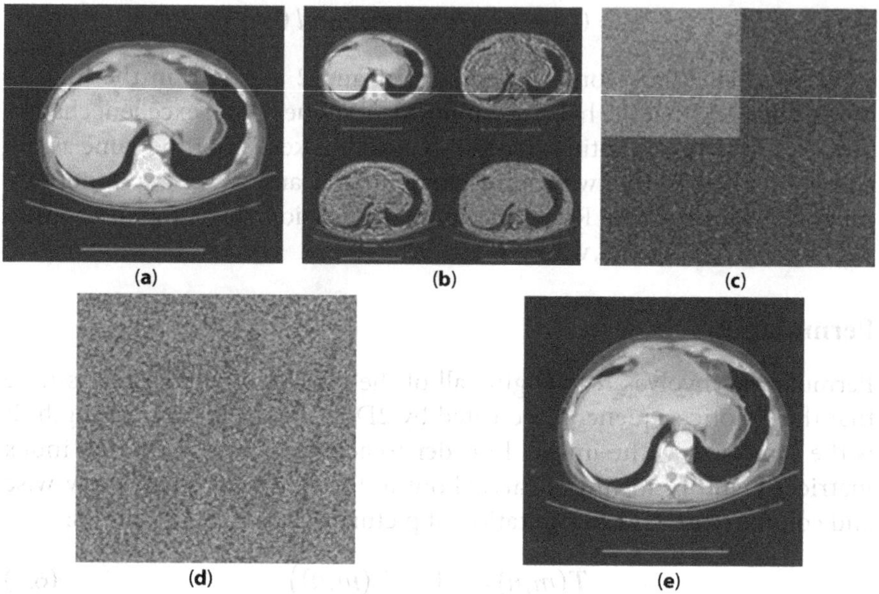

Figure 6.2 (a) input DICOM CT image (D1), (b) Haar wavelet transform output, (c) image after permutation and diffusion, (d) encrypted image, (e) decrypted image based on wavelet transform technique.

2D-Tent Cascade Logistic Map algorithm. The Haar wavelet transform is utilized here for the decomposition of input medical images into LL, LH, HL, and HH components. The permutation is carried out in the LH, HL, and HH components, and the substitution is carried out in the LL component. Figure 6.2 depicts the results of the medical image encryption using the wavelet transform algorithm. In Figure 6.2, (a) depicts the DICOM input CT abdomen image, (b) depicts the Haar wavelet transform output, (c) depicts the image after permutation and diffusion, (d) depicts the encrypted image, and (e) depicts the decrypted image.

The wavelet transform coefficients are subjected to combined column and row permutation. Initially, high-frequency components are subjected to permutation and then low-frequency components are subjected to permutation. Diffusion is carried out in the LL band. The encrypted image can then be transferred to the destination node and in the destination node, the reverse process is carried out for the reconstruction of the image.

Figure 6.3 depicts the medical image encryption results of 2D-Tent Cascade Logistic Map algorithm. In Figure 6.3, (a) depicts the input DICOM CT abdomen image, (b, c) depicts the permutation and substitution result, (d) depicts the decrypted image.

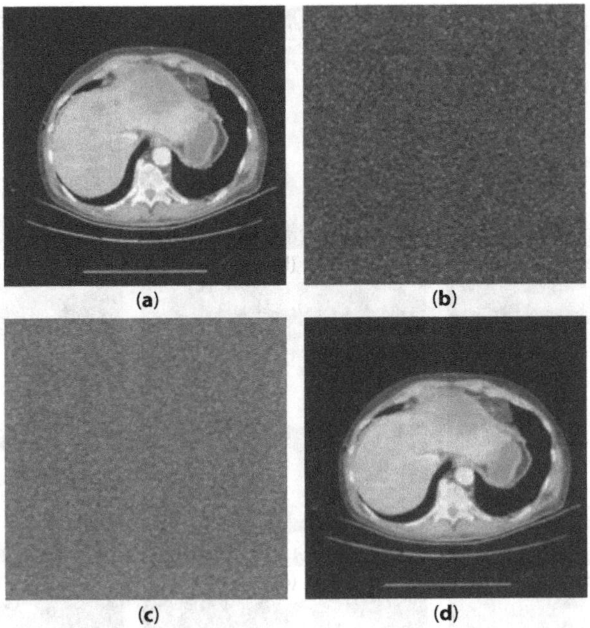

Figure 6.3 (a) input DICOM CT image (D1), (b) permutation and substitution output by 2D-Tent Cascade Logistic Map algorithm, (c) encrypted output, (d) decrypted image based on 2D-Tent Cascade Logistic Map algorithm.

Figure 6.4 depicts the results of encryption algorithm. The first column in Figure 6.4 depicts input images (D2-D5), column 2 depicts the decryption results of wavelet transform algorithm and the third column depicts the decryption results of 2D-Tent Cascade Logistic Map algorithm. The performance evaluation [17] of encryption algorithms is depicted below. The NPCR values of the encryption algorithms are depicted in Figure 6.5. Number of Pixels Change Rate (NPCR) is expressed as follows.

$$NPCR = \frac{\Sigma_{i,j} D(i, j)}{MN} \times 100 \tag{6.10}$$

Where

$$\boldsymbol{D(i,j)} = \begin{cases} \boldsymbol{0\ P(i,j) = C(i,j)} \\ \boldsymbol{1\ P(i,j) \neq C(i,j)} \end{cases}$$

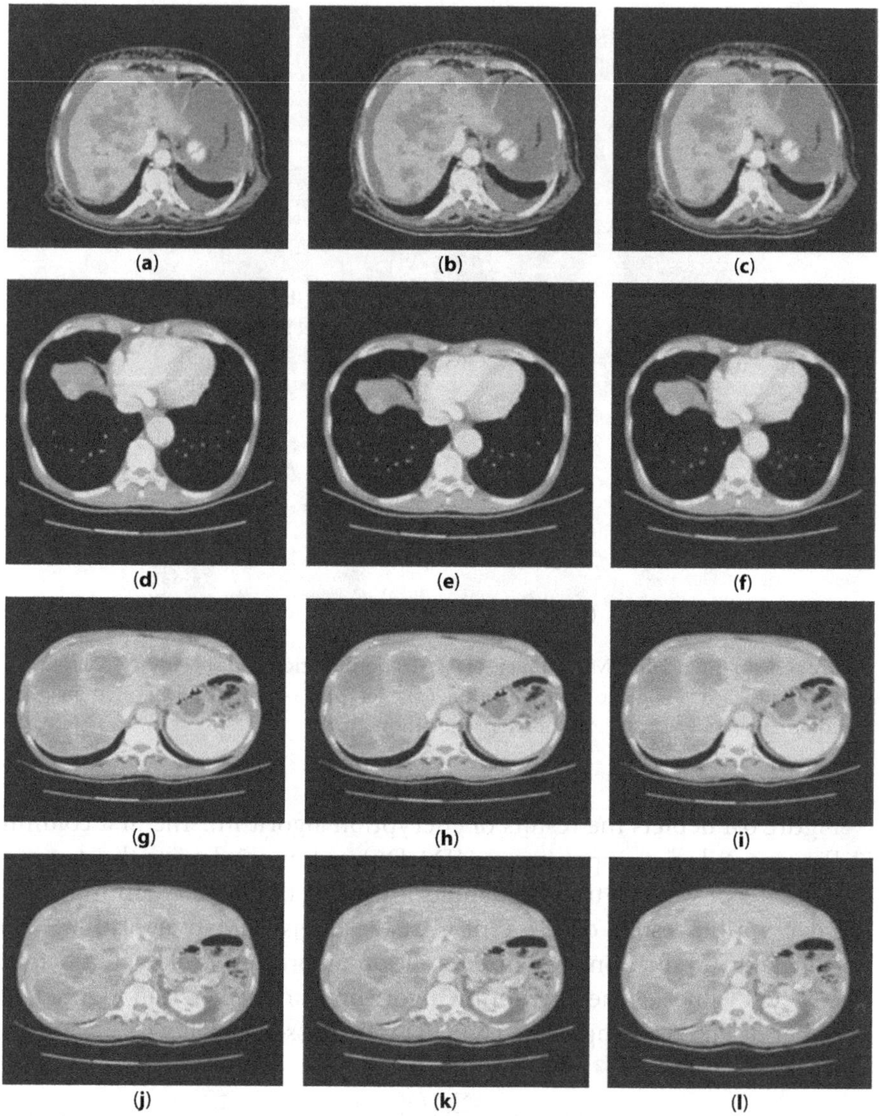

Figure 6.4 First column depicts the DICOM CT input images, second column depicts the decrypted images using wavelet transform algorithm, third column depicts the decrypted images using 2D-Tent Cascade Logistic Map algorithm.

NPCR values reveal that the medical image encryption using hybrid mapping technique is proficient when compared with wavelet transform-based one. The UACI values of encryption algorithms are depicted in Figure 6.6. The Unified Average Changing Index (UACI) is expressed as follows.

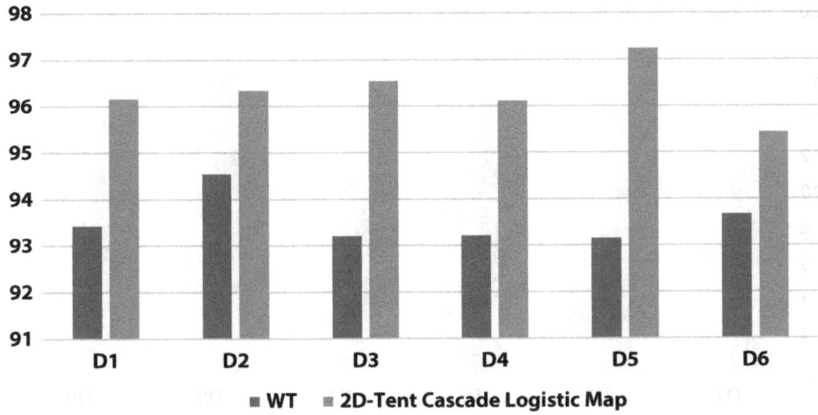

Figure 6.5 NPCR values of the encryption algorithms.

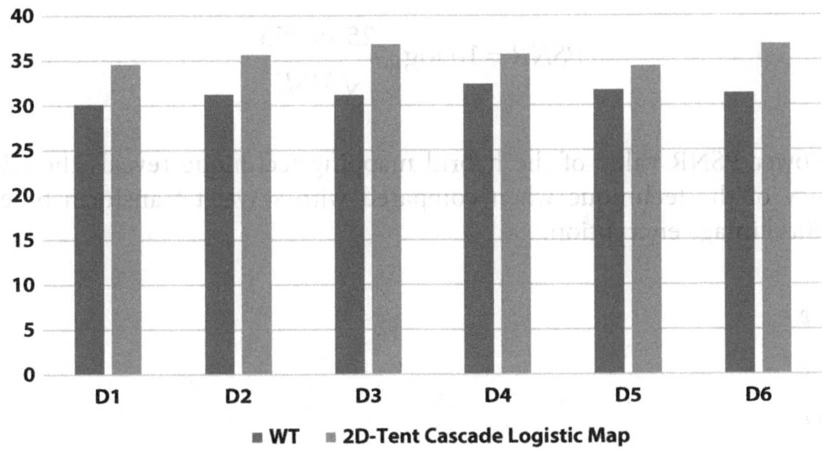

Figure 6.6 UACI values of encryption algorithms.

$$UACI = \frac{1}{MN}\left[\sum_{i,j}\frac{|P(i,j)-C(i,j)|}{255}\right]\times 100 \tag{6.11}$$

Figure 6.7 depicts that UACI values of hybrid mapping technique are superior when compared with wavelet transform–based algorithm.

The PSNR plot of encryption algorithms is depicted in Figure 6.7. A good image encryption method is expected to produce encrypted images with a low value of PSNR.

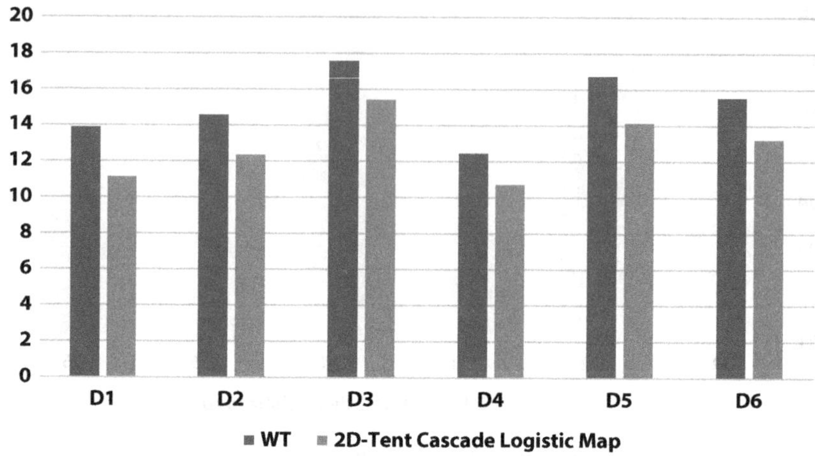

Figure 6.7 PSNR values of encryption algorithms.

$$PSNR = 10\log_{10}\frac{255 \times 255}{\sqrt{MSE}} \tag{6.12}$$

Lower PSNR value of the hybrid mapping technique reveals the efficiency of the technique when compared with wavelet transform based medical image encryption.

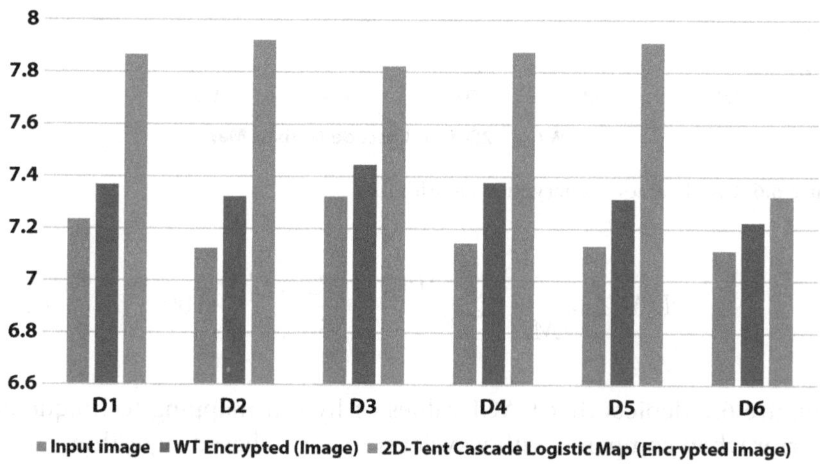

Figure 6.8 Entropy values of plan and cipher image of encryption algorithms.

The entropy values of input medical image, wavelet transform–based encryption, and hybrid mapping based encryption is depicted in Figure 6.8. The uncertainty of a random variable is measured using Entropy. Higher entropy value represents a greater level of security for image encryption.

$$E = \sum_{i=1}^{256} P(i) log\left(\frac{1}{P(i)}\right) \tag{6.13}$$

Entropy values of hybrid mapping technique are closer to 8 that indicates the proficiency of the hybrid mapping-based medical image encryption.

6.4 Conclusion

Medical image encryption role is inevitable from the security aspect in data transfer. This research work proposes a 2D hybrid mapping technique based on the tent and logistic function for medical image encryption. The algorithm was tested on real-time abdomen CT DICOM images and the results were compared with wavelet transform based medical image encryption. The validation by the performance metrics reveals the proficiency of hybrid mapping technique and the outcome of this research work paves a way towards the application for the telemedicine domain. The future work will focus on the medical image encryption/decryption for 3D medical data sets.

Acknowledgement

The authors would like to acknowledge the support provided by Nanyang Technological University under NTU Ref: RCA-17/334 for providing the medical images and supporting us in the preparation of the manuscript. Parasuraman Padmanabhan and Balazs Gulyas also acknowledge the support from Lee Kong Chian School of Medicine and Data Science and AI Research (DSAIR) centre of NTU (Project Number ADH-11/2017-DSAIR and the support from the Cognitive Neuro Imaging Centre (CONIC) at NTU. The author S.N. Kumar would also like to acknowledge the support provided by Schmitt Centre for Biomedical Instrumentation (SCBMI) of Amal Jyothi College of Engineering.

References

[1] Wang X, Teng L, Qin X. A novel colour image encryption algorithm based on chaos. *Signal Processing*. 2012 Apr 1;92(4):1101-8.

[2] Wang X, Zhao J, Liu H. A new image encryption algorithm based on chaos. *Optics Communications*. 2012 Mar 1;285(5):562-6.

[3] Pareek NK, Patidar V, Sud KK. Image encryption using chaotic logistic map. *Image and Vision Computing. 2006 Sep 1;24(9):926-34.*

[4] *Zhang YQ*, Wang XY. A symmetric image encryption algorithm based on mixed linear–nonlinear coupled map lattice. *Information Sciences*. 2014 Jul 20; 273:329-51.

[5] Liu H, Wang X. Color image encryption based on one-time keys and robust chaotic maps. *Computers & Mathematics with Applications*. 2010 May 1; 59(10):3320-7.

[6] Liu H, Wang X. Image encryption using DNA complementary rule and chaotic maps. *Applied Soft Computing*. 2012 May 1; 12(5):1457-66.

[7] Wang XY, Yang L, Liu R, Kadir A. A chaotic image encryption algorithm based on perceptron model. *Nonlinear Dynamics*. 2010 Nov; 62(3):615-21.

[8] Gao T, Chen Z. Image encryption based on a new total shuffling algorithm. *Chaos, Solitons & Fractals*. 2008 Oct 1; 38(1):213-20.

[9] Saeed S, Umar MS, Ali MA, Ahmad M. A gray-scale image encryption using Fisher-Yates chaotic shuffling in wavelet domain. In *International Conference on Recent Advances and Innovations in Engineering (ICRAIE-2014)* 2014 May 9 (pp. 1-5). IEEE.

[10] Luo Y, Du M, Liu J. A symmetrical image encryption scheme in wavelet and time domain. *Communications in Nonlinear Science and Numerical Simulation*. 2015 Feb 1; 20(2):447-60.

[11] Abd El-Latif A.A. Li L. Zhang T. Wang N. Song X. Niu X. (2012), 'Digital Image Encryption Scheme Based on Multiple Chaotic Systems', *Sens Imaging an International Journal*, Vol. 13, pp.67–88.

[12] Shatheesh Sam I. Devaraj P. Bhuvaneswaran R.S. (2012), An Intertwining Chaotic Maps Based Image Encryption Scheme, *Nonlinear Dyn*, Vol. 69, pp. 1995–2007.

[13] Gafsi M, Abbassi N, Hajjaji MA, Malek J, Mtibaa A. Improved Chaos-Based Cryptosystem for Medical Image Encryption and Decryption. *Scientific Programming*. 2020 Dec 18; 2020.

[14] Ibrahim S, Alhumyani H, Masud M, Alshamrani SS, Cheikhrouhou O, Muhammad G, Hossain MS, Abbas AM. Framework for Efficient Medical Image Encryption Using Dynamic S-Boxes and Chaotic Maps. *IEEE Access*. 2020 Aug 31; 8:160433-49.

[15] Akkasaligar PT, Biradar S. Selective medical image encryption using DNA cryptography. *Information Security Journal: A Global Perspective*. 2020 Mar 3;29(2):91-101.

[16] Pareek NK, Patidar V, Sud KK. Image encryption using chaotic logistic map. *Image and Vision Computing*. 2006 Sep 1;24(9):926-34.
[17] Ramasamy P, Ranganathan V, Kadry S, Damaševicius R, Blažauskas T. An image encryption scheme based on block scrambling, modified zigzag transformation and key generation using enhanced logistic—Tent map. *Entropy*. 2019 Jul;21(7):656.

7

Personalized Multi-User-Based Movie and Video Recommender System: A Deep Learning Perspective

Jayaramu H. K.[1], Suman Kumar Maji[2]* and Hussein Yahia[3]

[1]*Indian Institute of Technology (Indian School of Mines), Dhanbad, India*
[2]*Department of Computer Science and Engineering, Indian Institute of Technology Patna, Patna, Bihar, India*
[3]*Centre de recherche INRIA Bordeaux Sud-Ouest, 200 rue de la Vieille Tour, Talence Cedex, France*

Abstract
The internet is the prime source to watch movies and micro-videos on platforms like YouTube, Netflix and many popular websites. All these online platforms are query-based search engines which extends a burden to the user to search and find a movie or video of their choice. The problem can be solved by developing better video recommender systems that will assist users in finding more helpful content and improving their overall experience. Deep learning is the leading solution for a large volume of multimedia data for personalized recommendations based on user interests. Feature-based solutions for video recommendation systems can be broadly classified under seven different categories: 1) User Embeddings – determining a user's specific interests, 2) Representation of Item – the user's dynamic interest based on their historically accessed items, 3) neighbour-assisted representation – we find similar users history data for generating Neighbour (history) interest information, 4) Categorical representation – It is learned by classifying the user's historical items into distinct categories and recognizing their differences, 5) Collaborative representation, 6) Hybrid representation – While neighbour-assisted characterization, which defines user profile from a collaborative perspective, characterises user interest from a customised perspective at the item and category level, and 7) Using rich contents (e.g., scene, meta, motion etc.) – uses to overcome restrictions caused by the absence

**Corresponding author*: suman.maji@gmail.com

Suman Kumar Swarnkar, J P Patra, Sapna Singh Kshatri, Yogesh Kumar Rathore and Tien Anh Tran (eds.) Supervised and Unsupervised Data Engineering for Multimedia Data, (149–176) © 2024 Scrivener Publishing LLC

of specific ones. In this book chapter, we will focus in detail on the principles and deep learning solutions that exist for online video recommendations to users. We will cover in detail the overview and the literature and shall also include an experimental analysis section wherein we shall analyze the performance of the various video recommender systems on different multimedia datasets.

***Keywords*:** Video recommender system, deep learning, multimedia, artificial intelligence

7.1 Introduction

In recent years the availability of infotainment information has been tremendous. The internet is the prime part of accessing all this information. Users are facing the problem of searching for the correct information from the available data sources. Recommender systems (RS) are developed to overcome all these burdens and help the user to access the correct information. RS plays essential roles in e-commerce, and digital infotainment systems such as YouTube, Hotstar, zee5, Amazon, Flipkart, eBay, Netflix, Amazon Prime, etc., are all query-based engines. The problems are solved by improving the video recommender systems and helping users enhance their experience and find sufficient information.

Generally, there are three essential types of personalized recommender systems: 1) content-based (CB) filtering [1, 2, 3, 4], where similar items that the users liked (or searched) in the past are recommended, and similarity is obtained based on content information (metadata, tags and many). 2) collaborative filtering (CF) [5, 6, 7, 8, 9], where recommendations are made based on the information gathered from multiple user's history data and collaborative similarities of users/items, and 3) hybrid approaches [10, 11, 12, 13, 14]. CB filtering uses item feature content, but the actual performance depends on the usefulness of the feature content. CF faces a cold-start problem because instead of content analysis, it analyses the data of multiple user interactions. The hybrid approach mixes personalized and non-personalized algorithms with CB and CF models. These techniques are frequently used in a variety of industrial applications.

Nowadays, various deep-learning solutions are used to improve video and image representation. Deep learning (based on CNN feature) features replace most of the traditional (colours, words, and so on) features to improve the correctness of the representation of video/image. Representing user interest is complex because user interest is typically dynamic and challenging to analyze. At the same time, the representation of the item is relatively static. So representing the user interest in recommender systems is more critical than item representation. The diversity and fluctuations of user interest expression are not well reflected by the static and fixed-length vector size obtained from the video titles and meta-data. If you forcefully generate the recommendations by the hybrid method, you will get the worst result compared to the expected results in performance. In many cases, the unavailability of appropriate textual content in video, music, etc., further complicates the scenario.

In this chapter, we are using deep networks to study video recommendations for user interest representation. We will talk about how deep learning networks use various features collected from different user histories for generating recommendations. Input features for deep learning solutions to video recommenders can be broadly classified into seven categories, which will also be discussed in detail. Also, an analysis of different multi-user hybrid methods using early and late fusing techniques is given for more accurate results. Finally, we conduct a thorough experimental research on a real dataset of movie recommendations and evaluate how different deep learning approaches perform against it.

The remainder of the paper is arranged as follows. Section 7.2 gives a comprehensive summary of research work done in this environment. Section 7.3 introduces the different multi-user features considered for recommender systems. Section 7.4 is about the effectiveness of merging several user preference representations for video recommendation. Section 7.5 will present the data sets considered for the model evaluations, and different performances are measured and compared with prominent models. In Section 7.6, the paper is concluded.

7.2 Literature Survey on Video and Movie Recommender Systems

Deep Learning is the branch of study in Artificial Neural Networks, a novel strategy that selects moves by using policy networks and value networks to assess board positions. These deep neural networks are trained using a unique method that combines reinforcement learning from self-playing games and supervised learning from games played by human experts [16]. DL in recommender systems is a burgeoning industry [17], due to its superior performance and alluring ability to learn feature representation. Many research studies are being done on DL methods, specifically in information gathering in different ways and recommender systems. A deep learning structure is a multi-layer perceptron with numerous hidden layers. Hinton *et al.* [18] first suggested the idea of deep learning in 2006.

This section discusses convolutional neural networks, a popular deep learning model (CNN) used in recommender systems.

The CNN [19, 20] is a unique type of feed-forward neural network with pooling and convolution layers operations. It can capture both local and global features, greatly enhancing correctness and effectiveness. It works well when the structure resembles a grid-like topology for information processing. CNN is made up of one or many fully connected layers after one or many convolutional layers, just like a standard multi-layer neural network. A CNN is referred to as a multi-layer perceptron. Convolution and pool operations enable neural networks to analyze unstructured multimedia input effectively. The majority of CNN-based recommendation algorithms employ CNNs for feature extraction [15, 21, 22, 23, 24, 25].

However, several studies adopted entirely different methodologies. In his work [26], XIAOJIE CHEN uses movie stills and posters to explain films by identifying their stylistic components as an example of how to do that. Movie CNN (Convolutional Neural Network) characteristics are extracted using the programme VGG16. The VGG16 saw some changes, including removing its Softmax layer (which classified images rather than helped to describe them). A United Visual Contents Matrix Factorization model (UVMF-AES) with aesthetic awareness was developed using the VGG16 rating and output features to provide recommendations to the user(s). Techniques like negative sampling were used to optimize the procedure, and recommendations were offered at the end.

Accuracy and data sparsity are indirectly related. We can improve our model's accuracy and precision by addressing the problem of data sparsity. In [27] the authors introduced CoupledCF, a brand-new method in the neural network-based-item coupling learning model. This CoupledCF picks up explicit knowledge and further implicit knowledge. They argued that numerous conventional movie recommendation algorithms neglected complex pair linkages between and within users and items and made the assumption that item and user information are distinct and separated from each other. To obtain explicit user-movie coupling information, CoupledCF uses an NLP technique called Doc2Vec to extract the user and movie properties from review texts. To obtain this implicit information, it then generates a deep CF. It links it with the explicit user-movie information previously gathered to exhibit movie, user and movie-user couplings in an orderly manner. This model provides more accurate results than a few popular recommendation systems. Gong and Zhang [28] suggested an attentiveness-based CNN architecture for the hashtag recommendation problem that takes into consideration both public (global) and private (local) input. A hierarchical attention mechanism was developed by

Huang *et al.* [29] to expand the edge-to-edge memory network design and incorporate user histories. As a result, while creating hashtags, textual information and related user interests are integrated. A unique benchmark called HARRISON – (HAshtag Recommendation for Real-world Images in SOcial Networks), combining a CNN-based visual feature extractor with a multi-label neural network classification algorithm, was recently proposed by Park *et al.* [29]. Wu *et al.* [31] developed work on a neural image hashtagging network (A-NIH), an attention-based technique for simulating the relationship between the sequence of social pictures and hashtags. Modern recommender models for in-matrix situations include weighted matrix factorization [32] and Bayesian personalized ranking [33]. During training, both construct objective functions based on matrix factorization and discover user or item cooperation. For each individual or item, a latent vector is discovered after training. The internal interactions of latent components then predict user evaluations of the item. Finally, the top-k user recommendations will be determined based on the goods with the highest predicted ratings. The learning objective is where WMF and BPR diverge most. WMF seeks explicitly to reduce rating prediction mistakes, whereas BPR seeks to maintain pair-wise tailored ordering. The content aspects of WMF and BPR have recently been added, allowing their versions to be used to formulate suggestions for both matrix-in and out-matrix situations.

Collaborative topic regression (CTR) [34], content-based music recommender (DPM) [15], a deep learning model and collaborative deep learning [35] are examples of WMF-based models. Visual-CLiMF [44] and Visual-Bayesian Personalized Ranking (VBPR) [37] are examples of BPR-based models. Specific visual characteristics from pre-trained CNN are VBPR and Visual-CLiMF (CNN). By learning the projected reciprocal rank during optimization as opposed to the pair-wise rank, Visual-CLiMF improves VBPR. In contrast to the methods mentioned above, VideoTopic, proposed in [38], performs out-of-matrix video suggestions by simultaneously using textual and visual information, which is an early type of fusion. The accuracy of VideoTopic is significantly worse than that of CF-based models [34, 35, 36] because of the weak visual feature and limited user cooperation employed in model training. Zhou Zhao *et al.* in [39] developed a paradigm for streaming services that permit users to follow one another across various platforms. Its foundation is the concept of "homophily," which holds that people connect with and follow other people who share their interests or are similar to them and act differently in groups than they would independently. The author discusses the problem of matrices' sparsity by making the previously stated assumption. Two sub-networks of a multi-modal network are used in the research.

Table 7.1 List of papers and their summary on CNN-based recommender system.

Author and reference no.	Contribution
George Van Den Driessche, *et al.* [16]	A novel strategy that evaluates board positions using "value networks" and chooses moves using "policy networks."
Shuai Zhang, *et al.* [17]	This article thoroughly analyses the present study effort on recommender systems that use deep learning.
Geoffrey E Hinton, *et al.* [18]	The rapid, greedy method uses a stylistic wake-sleep algorithm to fine-tune the weights.
Yann LeCun, *et al.* [19]	This study evaluates various handwritten digit recognition techniques using Convolutional neural networks.
Alex Krizhevsky, *et al.* [20]	1.3 million high-resolution photos from the ImageNet training set were classified using a deep CNN into 1,000 separate classes.
Xue Geng, *et al.* [21]	A recommender can swiftly suggest images based on feature similarity by translating the many user-image networks.
Donghyun Kim *et al.* [22]	In this study, researchers proposed an original recommendation model for raising the accuracy of rating prediction. This is convolutional matrix factorization (ConvMF) that is based on CNN and probabilistic matrix factorization (PMF).
Yogesh Singh Rawat *et al.* [23]	This study suggests a deep neural network that, based on an image's context and content, may predict a variety of tags for it.
Chenyi Lei *et al.* [24]	Some user-centric tasks, like picture recommendations, necessitate accurate representations of images and user preferences and intent regarding images. This work uses a deep learning approach to address what is known as hybrid representations.

(*Continued*)

Table 7.1 List of papers and their summary on CNN-based recommender system. (*Continued*)

Author and reference no.	Contribution
Suhang Wang, *et al.* [25]	This study introduces a paradigm for suggesting POIs that use visual material, called Visual Content Enhanced POI recommendation (VPOI).
Xiaojie Chen, *et al.* [26]	The authors proposed work that recommends the different data visuals using content matrix factorization.
Quangui Zhang, *et al.* [27]	This research paper proposed a unique non-IID learning-based CoupledCF for collaborative filtering.
Yuyun Gong *et al.* [28]	This work presented a unique architecture with an attention mechanism.
Haoran Huang, *et al.* [29]	Introduced the new method of edge-to-edge memory network design and incorporated user histories.
Minseok Park, *et al.* [30]	The authors present the dataset (HARRISON) as a standard for hashtag recommendations for real-world photographs on social media.
Wu *et al.* [31]	This paper presented a brand-new technique called Voting Deep NN with Associative Rules Mining - VDNN-ARM that can be utilised to address hashtag recommendations in multi-label.
Yehuda Koren, *et al.* [32]	In this study, the item rating patterns characterise both things and users. A recommendation is made when item and user factors are highly compatible.
Steffen Rendle, *et al.* [33]	In this study, researchers introduce the maximal posterior estimator (BPR-Opt), a general optimization criterion for personalised ranking that comes from a Bayesian analysis of the issue. Additionally, they offer a general learning approach for BPR-Opt model optimization.

(*Continued*)

Table 7.1 List of papers and their summary on CNN-based recommender system. (*Continued*)

Author and reference no.	Contribution
Chong Wang *et al.* [34]	It provides users and items with an open interpretation of latent architecture and can make recommendations for both newly created works and works that have already been published.
Hao Wang, *et al.* [35]	This study may resolve the sparsity issue by using additional data, such as item-specific content.
Sujoy Roy *et al.* [36]	The authors introduce a novel approach to learning latent component representation for films in this paper that is focused on simulating the emotional bond between user and item.
Ruining He *et al.* [37]	In this article, researchers suggest a scalable factorization technique to include visual information in predictors of people's attitudes. Then they apply this model to a variety of sizable, real-world datasets.
Qiusha Zhu *et al.* [38]	This study focuses on a user-profile and cold-start modelling method called VideoTopic.

Convolutional Neural Networks (CNNs) have been implemented in recommender systems to perform collaborative filtering and content-based recommendation, among other duties. Table 7.1 presents an overview of several prevalent concepts.

7.3 Feature-Based Solutions for Movie and Video Recommender Systems

This section will discuss the various feature-based solutions and their representations. Figure 7.1 shows the various methods used in video recommendation systems.

Introduction

All the existing methods come under three categories: Content-based representation (CB), Collaborative-based representation (CF), and Hybrid Representation. The Matrix factorization method on online scalable CF

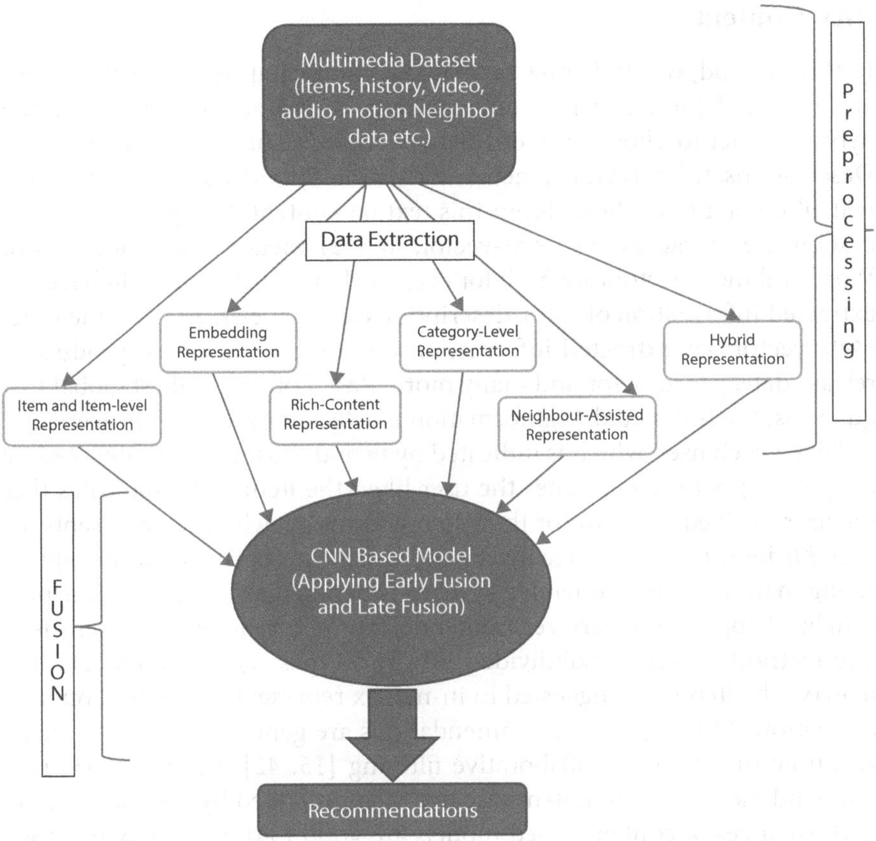

Figure 7.1 Movie and video recommender systems.

algorithms was proposed by Huang *et al.* [8]. A flexible updating technique is considered for implicit input from diverse user activities. The CF method encounters a cold-start problem while buying new products is not advised in the recommender system because they have not yet been introduced to user engagement. To come out of this problem, CF recommends new videos based on the similarity of previously accessed videos by users. It can evaluate the item similarity by video content analysis (including tags, audio, subtitles, and additional content features).

For instance, Deldjoo *et al.* [1] introduce the CB recommender system that extracts useful video features, including lighting, scenes, motion, and colour. In specific hybrid methods, CF and CB are combined into one framework. For instance, a multi-task rating aggregation strategy was suggested by Zhao *et al.* in their publication [22]. He claimed that by considering several sources of information, a rating problem produced many fused ranking lists.

Rich Content

In this method, we study how textual and contextual rich content features are extracted for video recommendations. These are important for the hybrid model to choose the out-matrix recommendation performances. Descriptions, titles, reviews, meta information for videos and many others will all come under these. From this textual content, two pieces of information are extracted: 1) word-vector, and 2) meta-vector information. Word and meta vectors are built for every video. Word vector will have the extracted information of titles, descriptions and reviews. At the same time, Meta vector has extracted information on language, country, producers, release date, genre, actor and many more. Based on the highest global frequencies, the full metadata information is selected for further processing.

Given each user, which is indicated by m and the total items denoted by n, $x_{ij} \in \{?, +\}$, where + denotes the user liked the item and ? indicates that the user disliked the item (or they do not know it), where x_{ij} represents ith user jth item of implicit feedback, and finally, it transformed to implicit rating matrix for recommended systems is denoted as $X = 0, 1^{mxn}$. The personalized top k items are recommended for the randomly chosen user. The method is further subdivided into two types: 1) In-matrix, 2) Out-matrix. The items are suggested in in-matrix representation based on user evaluations [40, 41]. The recommendations are generated based on items and user similarity of collaborative filtering [15, 42]. In out-matrix recommendations, the top k items are not recommended by anyone, and the performances of content-based models are good [34]. In-matrix methods are used in Weighted matrix factorization [32] and Bayesian personalized rankings [33].

Latent Representation

Latent representation is also known as user embedding; the user interest is represented in a static vector and provides comprehensive user interest profiling. Deep network-based methods use such recommender systems. During training, User embedding is learned and defined as $L^U = \left[l_1^U l_2^U, \ldots l_N^U\right] \in R^{dxN}$, where L^U is user embedding learned, N and d denotes the total available number of users and embedding size. Therefore, the user i th latent is represented by l_i^u. Embedding is one of the traditional ways to represent user interest. The use of it in latent factor models is common [32]. For instance, SVD++ [43] integrates neighbourhood and latent factor models into a single framework, and another item-item similarity of item factors is introduced to the model.

Item Representation

We use embedding notions to represent items. The items are embedded in the latent space in this instance. We extract visual features for each video d_j from the high-dimension content f_j^v. By learning the embedding matrix, E_j is converted to a lower dimension, as in eq. (7.1).

$$v_j = E_j f_j^v \tag{7.1}$$

where v_j denoted as d dimensional vector and $v_j \in R^d$. Each video can be categorized into one or more groups, which is represented by the vector $f_j^c \in M^{T_C}$, where $M = \{0, 1\}$ and the maximum number of categories is denoted by T_C. Learning the embedding matrix, E_c converted it to lower dimensions shown in eq. (7.2).

$$c_j = E_c v_j^c \tag{7.2}$$

where c_j is a d dimensional vector and $c_j \in R^d$. Finally, we perform element-wise-sum, i.e. $x_j = v_i + c_j$, to fulfil the item's representational result, and $x_j \in R^d$ also d dimensional vector.

Item-Level Representation

It is a learning-based approach that provides reliable predictive interest representation based on viewing history. The attention mechanism served as inspiration for this, which decides the most promising part of a given task. We introduced Item-Level Interest Representation.

The historical video for jth user is denoted by $It_j = it_{j1}, it_{j2}, \ldots, it_{jT_j}$. The jth user total number of historical videos are denoted as T_j. The visual feature vector is denoted by f_{jt}^v, which is associated with tth video it_{jt}. We use the transform matrix E_v' to reduce to a lower dimension.

$$v_{jt}' = E_v' * f_{jt}^v \tag{7.3}$$

where, $v_{jt}' \in R^d . v' = \left[v_{j1}', v_{j2}', \ldots, v_{jT_j}' \right]$ used to describe a user's interest from an item's perspective. For a given candidate video vd_i, a two-layered network computes the attention score in the manner described below:

$$\beta(j,t,i) = W_{\beta\sigma}\left(W_{1\beta}v'_{jt} + W_{2\beta}x_i + W_{3\beta}\overline{v'} + b_\beta\right) \tag{7.4}$$

The average feature vector of all past videos is denoted by $\overline{v'}$.

$W_3\beta$, $W_2\beta$, $W_1\beta$, $W_\beta \in R^{dxd}$, and the parameters that need to be learned are denoted as b_β are $\in R^d$. The sigmoid activation function is denoted as σ(·). The normalized item-level attention score is given as follows:

$$\tilde{\beta}(j,t,i) = \frac{\exp(\beta(j,t,i))}{\sum_{t=1}^{T_j}\exp(\beta(j,t,i))}. \tag{7.5}$$

Ultimately, the *j*th user item level is represented as follows:

$$u_j^J = \sum_{t=1}^{T_j}\tilde{\beta}(j,t,i)v'_{jt}. \tag{7.6}$$

Category-Level Representation

We find many disadvantages in item-level representation. In the first place, item-level representation is generated from content characteristics, so there is a semantic gap across semantics and content features. Second, because many objects have the same qualities, it will clearly distinguish each item for user interest representation. The user can access one of them having the same properties by chance.

The category-level representation is introduced to get more advantages. This is mentioned in the paper [24], which raises the concept. It says that instead of content features, the category is considered and which is more closely related to semantics, and video features are represented in a quantized manner.

For each user historical item, one category vector is created $\left\{f^c j1,\ldots,f^c_{jT_j}\right\}$ and the category distribution vector is calculated as $u_j^c \in R^{T_c}$, where the maximum number of categories is indicated by T_c. The high dimensional category distribution vector reduced to low dimension by the projection of another embedding matrix *C* is as follows.

$$u_j^C = Cu_j^c \tag{7.7}$$

The *j*th user categorical representation is denoted by $u_j^C \in R^d$.

Neighbour-Assisted Representation

Generally, user-based CF for the target user finds the neighbours' user (similar behaviour) and uses the history of neighbours to imply the target user. Let j represent the user j's historical video, and $|\mathbb{V}_j \cap \mathbb{V}_o|$ represents the maximum number of overlaps between users and the familiarity across users j and o. Then it calculated the nearest neighbour user L by selecting more overlaps and comparing them with historical videos.

Where $z_{j1}^N,\ldots,z_{jL}^N$ denotes neighbour embedding. The attention score of the given candidate's video v_i is calculated by a two-layered network as follows:

$$\alpha(j,l,i) = W_{\alpha\sigma}\left(W_{1\alpha}u_{jl}^N + W_{2\alpha}x_i + b_\alpha\right) \tag{7.8}$$

Where the model parameters W_α, $W_1\ \alpha$, $W_1\ \alpha$, $W_\beta \in R^{dxd}$, and $b_\alpha \in R^d$ respectively. $\sigma(\cdot)$ is how the ReLu activation function is written. It is better than the sigmoid function. The normalized attention score using a soft matrix is given as follows:

$$\tilde{\alpha}(j,t,i) = \frac{\exp(\alpha(j,l,i))}{\sum_{l=1}^{L}\exp(\alpha(j,l,i))}. \tag{7.9}$$

Finally, this score is used to weigh the Neighbour to calculate neighbour-assisted representation.

$$u_j^N = \sum_{l=1}^{L}\tilde{\alpha}(j,t,i)u_{jl}^N. \tag{7.10}$$

A user-assisted representation calculates other neighbour users and simultaneously learns all users assisted representations.

Collaborative Representation and Hybrid Representation

In the section mentioned earlier, we mentioned different kinds of user-interest representation, Rich-content representation is represented by u_i^{R-c}, u_i^{I-t} represents item-level, u_i^{N-a} Neighbour-assisted representation, u_i^{L-a} Latent representation, and u_i^{C-a} Category-level representation. The category and item-level user interest representation characterizes interest like in CBF. The neighbour-assisted representation uses the aspect of the Collaborative filtering approach. We combined and created the Hybrid method from these previous CBF and CF methods. The user i is represented in $Z = 5$ kinds of, where $\{u_i^z\}_{z=1}^Z$ denotes the interest representation of user i of Z categories. Which can be represented as $u_i^1, u_i^2, u_i^3, u_i^4, u_i^5$ are alias of $u_i^{R-c}, u_i^{I-t}, u_i^{N-a}, u_i^{L-a}, u_i^{C-a}$.

7.4 Fusing: EF – (Early Fusion) and LF – (Late Fusion)

This section looks at the effectiveness of merging several user preference representations for video recommendation. The fusing strategies are considered EF and LF. For EF, we also investigate various fusion functions.

Early Fusion

Prior to the user and item interaction, an EF model unifies several user profile representations. The u_i^* is the final user representation, $\{u_i^z\}_{z=1}^Z$ is fed into a fusion function.

$$u_i^* = f\left(\{u_i^z\}_{z=1}^Z\right) \tag{7.11}$$

where f is denoted as a fusion function. and $u_i^* \in \mathbb{R}$.

The fusion function f is a variable and delicate function. For experimentation, we are using four different types of fusion functions, the Attention, Total, Maximum, and Feed Forward neural networks. The following defines each of these.

- Max Fusion: we got inspired by Convolution Neural Network (CNN), a mainly used and popular Max Pooling method. In this case, it selects the highest value from each multiple-user interest representation. It is denoted as follows.

$$u_i^* = max_{z=1}^Z u_i^z \tag{7.12}$$

- Sum Fusion: It is used in SVD++ [23]. For Multiple-user interset, it performs the element-wise-addition operation.

$$u_i^* = \sum_{z=1}^{Z} u_i^z \tag{7.13}$$

- Attention Fusion: The Total (SUM) function averages several user interests, and the Maximum (MAX) function selects the highest values across all dimensions. Both of these functionalities represent opposite extremes. Between the two extremes, we can actively distribute the weights across the several user profile representations. To learn the weights by employing the attention approach. Specifically, the multiple-user interest $\{u_i^z\}_{z=1}^{Z}$ is represented in keys and values and item x_j is represented as *query*. The attention function(AF) is defined as follows.

$$AF(A,B,C) = softmax\left(\frac{AB^T}{\sqrt{d}}\right)C \tag{7.14}$$

where query $A \in \mathbb{R}^{n_A*d}$, key $B \in \mathbb{R}^{n_B*d}$, values $C \in \mathbb{R}^{n_C*d}$ and $n_B = n_C$. The mechanism for many heads of attention repeatedly uses the basic attention function, which is also used in this research:

$$\begin{aligned} u_i^* &= [hd_1;\ldots;hd_h]W^o \\ hd_i &= Attention\left(AW_i^A, BW_i^B, CW_i^C\right) \end{aligned} \tag{7.15}$$

where attention head is denoted as h, and in this paper, we used $h = 4$ and parameter metrics learned is denoted as $W_i^A \in \mathbb{R}^{d_h*d}, W_i^B \in \mathbb{R}^{d_h*d}$, values $W_i^C \in \mathbb{R}^{d_h*d}$ and $W^O \in \mathbb{R}^{d*d}$.

FFNN - Feed-Forward Neural Network: Non-parametric functions are maximum and total fusion. For applying deep learning techniques for multi-user interest representation, one layer of FFNN is learned and fused. Particularly, specifically, we initially join them by

$$u_i = \left[u_i^1, -u_i^2, -\ldots, -u_i^K\right], \tag{7.16}$$

where concatenation operation is denoted as $[-]$, and u_i^* is obtained by training one layer FNN as follows.

$$u_i^* = W_c^T u_i, \tag{7.17}$$

where FNN is expressed by $W_c \in \mathbb{R}_K d^*d$.

From the above, all we obtained u_j^* is denoted as the final interest representation. The last interaction between the user and items is defined in mathematical form.

$$a_j = u_j^* \odot x_i \tag{7.18}$$

After performing the product operation, we eventually employ a multilayer perceptron where an element-wise product is indicated by the symbol $\odot$.

$$\hat{y} = \varnothing(a_i) \tag{7.19}$$

where MLP is represented by $\varnothing(\cdot)$. The predicted matching score is defined by $\hat{y}$.

Late Fusion

Here, multiple user interests are not combined. Instead, we make use of them to connect with items. Between each user representation u_i^k and item representation x_i, we performed element-wise product operations:

$$a_j^k = u_j^k \odot x_i \tag{7.20}$$

for each $\{a_i^z\}_{z=1}^Z$, we obtained the corresponding matching score $\hat{y}^k = \varnothing_k\left(a_i^z\right)$ trained separate MLP $\varnothing_k(\cdot)$. The definitive matching score is obtained as $\hat{y}$ is:

$$\hat{y} = \frac{1}{Z}\sum_{z=1}^{Z} \hat{y}^z \tag{7.21}$$

the performance of the LF is better because more parameters learn in it.

Loss Function

The binary-classification method is one of the main methods used in this paper since we are curious about the CTP – (click-through prediction) method. The following is a definition of a sigmoid cross entropy loss function.

$$Loss_{\theta} = -(y\log\sigma((\hat{y})) + (1-y)\log(1-\sigma(\hat{y}))) + \lambda \,||\,\theta\,|| \quad (7.22)$$

The $y \in 0, 1$ expression indicates if the user clicked the video or not, model parameters are represented by θ, the sigmoid function is indicated by $\sigma(\cdot)$, and the strength of L2 regularization is controlled by hyper-parameter λ.

7.5 Experimental Setup

This section introduces the datasets considered for the experiments, evaluation models and methods, experimental settings and results of in-depth analyses.

Datasets Description and Evaluation Metrics

The MovieLens 10M [44] dataset is used for empirical studies. Table 7.2 describes the MovieLense 10M datasets and mentions different index data

Table 7.2 Statistics of MovieLense 10M dataset.

Index	Train	Test
# Users	51001	46692
#Video	10380	9830
#Rating	10000054	9988676
#Category	19	19
#Positive Data	1216527	268917
#Negative Data	5781953	1398369
Positivity Density	0.22%	0.06%
Rating Density	1.34%	1.38%

and train and test sample data taken for the experiment. Due to copyright restrictions in full-length videos, we downloaded the trailers and finally checked whether they belonged to the full-length videos. For the mismatched trailers, we used available video clips instead of full videos from YouTube. Of the 10,682 videos available in the MovieLens 10M database, 10,380 were downloaded. Using CNN on the trailer, a 4,000-dimensional vector of visual features is provided. Each movie belongs to one or more categories. The interaction is split into two parts: training takes up 80%, and the remaining 20% is used for testing. The dataset is converted to a rating of 5; if the rating is 5, then it is 'yes'; otherwise, it is converted to 'no'.

Implementation and Evaluation Metrics

Here, we used the Area under the curve most popular method as a metric:

$$Accuracy = \frac{1}{P}\sum\nolimits_{j=1}^{P} \frac{1}{\left|Q_j^+\right|\left|Q_j^-\right|}\sum\nolimits_{q_i \in Q_j^+}\sum\nolimits_{q_m \in Q_j^-} \delta(\hat{y}_j, q_i > \hat{y}_j, q_m)$$

Where user j may click the video v_i. The predicted matching score is denoted by $\hat{y}_j, v_i$. The user j clicked the video or not, and the indicator function is denoted by V_j^+ or V_j^- and $\delta(\cdot)$. We also select Precision-I, Recall-I, and NDCG-I to quantitatively assess the Top-K suggested results because CTP results can be used to generate. For MovieLens-10 M, I is specified to have a value of {5, 10}.

Performance Analysis

Performance Analysis of Different Fusions functions

- Preparations - All the methods are performed in TensorFlow on an AMD GPU. For all the processes, we used the below-mentioned hyper-parameters:

  - Training – In this experiment adopted stochastic optimization: Adam [52] for training and the batch is set to size = 128. For the best performances, L2 regularizations are tuned in the scale of $[10^{-7}, 10^{-6}, 10^{-5}, \ldots, 1]$ and the weight for MovieLense 10M is set to 1×10^{-7}.
  - Network Structure: Different numbers of historical videos are also different. The TensorFlow model, which

accepts the batch size, is the same length. So we padded with zero those for others to ensure it has the same length. For the MovieLense 10M, both historical video length and L number of neighbours are set to 20. The YouTube-Net, NCF, Deep-FM and Wild&Deep are set to 64 ← 128 ← 256.

- Latent (Embedding Size) – is tested for all [8, 15, 24], and for embedding size 64, the experimental results are provided. Each item has a connection to the visual characteristics vector and content.
- Performances – The performances are analyzed in Table 7.3 and Table 7.4. In learning-based methods, the performance is good in content-based filtering (CBF). Here Pre-I, Rec-I, and N-I are indicated as Precision, Recall and NDCG at I. We perform statistical tests, and the findings show that all measures have improved statistically ($p < 0.05$ for t-test).

According to the experimental analysis N-5 and N-10 and overall accuracy (AUC) metrics in this approach regularly and considerably beats these solid baselines, demonstrating that the suggested model is robust and reliable for many movie recommendation scenarios.

- EF and LF Strategies –

The output of this model for the MovieLense 10M dataset using several fusion algorithms are shown in Table 7.3, where $z \in \{Max, Sum, AF, FFNN\}$, where the Max, Sum, AF and FFNN are indicating Total,

Table 7.3 Different fusions functions performances with late fusion model.

Fusion	Pre-5	Pre-10	Rec-5	Rec-10	N-5	N-10	AUC
EF-Max	0.32	0.276	0.279	0.436	0.673	0.686	0.679
EF-Sum	0.328	0.275	0.283	0.437	0.677	0.675	0.685
EF-AF	0.327	0.278	0.28	0.435	0.678	0.684	0.683
EF-FFNN	0.328	0.276	0.282	0.435	0.678	0.683	0.685
Late Fusion	**0.329**	**0.2761**	**0.4218**	**0.5968**	**0.6798**	**0.6861**	**0.6867**

maximum, Attention Function and Feed Forward Neural Networks. The *EF* (*z*) is denoted as an Early fusion of *z*. For MovieLense 10M, the early fusion sum gives better results for other functions. In most metrics functions, the sum and max are better than AF and FFNN. Late fusion's overall performance is better compared to other early fusion techniques. Table 7.3 explains the different performances compared with the EF functions and LF functions for various metrics. The LF model gives the best performance results compared to other EF functions.

Multi-User Interest Performance Analysis

Table 7.4 shows the results of multi-user interest representation (MUI). Here EIN, IIN, NIN, CIN, C, IR, RC and hybrid representation are denoted as Embedding, item-level, neighour, category, collebrative, item, rich contents and hybrid representation. The best outcome obtained is denoted in bold. On the dataset, the performances on Pre-10, Rec-5, and Rec-10 of MUI-IIN and MU-EIN are comparable to or slightly superior to those of MU-Hybrid, and MUI-CIN perform worse than MUI-Hybrid. In this model, performance is better in all metrics and second best in Pre-{5,10}, and Rec-{5, 10} metrics. Based on the pre-5 and pre-10 metrics model achieving approximately 3.92% improvement in performance for the MovieLense 10M dataset. Based on AUC the DIN is the second best compared to MUI-hybrid and about ~3.21% in terms of Rec-5. For DIEN ~3.1% for Rec-10. However, our approach regularly surpasses these two

Table 7.4 Multi-user interest performance analysis.

Models	Pre-5	Pre-10	Rec-5	Rec-10	N-5	N-10	AUC
MUI-EIN	0.3199	0.3196	0.4199	0.5967	0.676	0.6755	0.6707
MUI-IIN	0.3214	**0.3229**	**0.4297**	**0.5971**	0.6766	0.6798	0.685
MUI-NIN	0.2936	0.3131	0.4182	0.5831	0.6493	0.6664	0.6637
MUI-CIN	0.2789	0.2857	0.2335	0.2385	0.6429	0.6548	0.638
MUI-C	0.3284	0.2757	0.4201	0.5971	0.6757	0.6826	0.6839
MUI-IR	0.3189	0.2687	0.4109	0.5817	0.6742	0.6816	0.6658
MUI-RC	**0.3299**	0.2771	0.4208	0.5941	0.6771	0.6838	0.6803
MUI-Hybrid	**0.3294**	**0.2861**	**0.4218**	**0.5968**	**0.6798**	**0.6861**	**0.6997**

robust baselines, demonstrating that our suggested MUI-Hybrid is reliable and effective for a variety of video recommendation scenarios.

Performance of Deep Learning-Based Recommenders on MovieLense10M Dataset

The different deep learning models considered for the performance comparison are discussed below, and Table 7.5 will show the different performance compared with different Deep Learning Models.

- Bayesian Personalized Ranking (BPR) [33] – For the same user, a pair-wise rating system determines the relative worth of two items.
- Content-based filtering (CBF) [45] – A user's previously seen video feature vectors are averaged to provide a user interest vector. Based on the closeness between a user interest and an item characteristic vector, a prediction score is computed.
- SVD++ [43] - a hybrid model and is considered a special case to build the mentioned IIN; the focus is replaced by an average grouping.
- WD – (Wide & Deep model) [46] - comprises two principal parts: the deep and wide model. The linear broad model is one, and the nonlinear deep neural model is the other.
- Deep-FM [47] - It automatically learns the cross features components from factorization machines and replaces the wild parts of the Wild & Deep Model.
- NCF – (Neural collaborative filtering) [48] is a DL-based recommendation. NCF will learn both item-level and user-level embedding with the help of the network (i.e., with performances of the element-wise product between items and users) and do item and user-level concatenation using feed-forward layers.
- Deep Interest Networks (DIN) [49] - for modelling user interest, it adaptively learns user interest with the help of historical behaviours concerning actual items.
- Deep interest evolution network (DIEN) [50] - an upgraded DIN network that captures dynamic interest evolving. They removed batch normalization in DIN and DIEN to increase the performance.

Table 7.5 Performance comparison with different deep learning model.

Models	Pre-5	Pre-10	Rec-5	Rec-10	N-5	N-10	AUC
BPR	0.3045	0.2587	0.2522	0.3972	0.6591	0.6675	0.6672
CBF	0.1982	0.1834	0.166	0.2931	0.5164	0.5481	0.5457
SVD++	0.3224	0.27	0.2708	0.4161	0.6789	0.6851	0.6771
WD	0.3229	0.2721	0.271	0.4191	0.6711	0.6781	0.6831
Deep-FM	0.3218	0.2702	0.2678	0.418	0.6732	0.6809	0.6818
NCF	0.3281	0.2687	0.2741	0.4253	0.677	0.6822	0.6851
DIN	0.3272	0.2818	0.4209	0.5654	0.6751	0.6858	0.6994
DIEN	0.3263	0.2812	0.2789	0.4327	0.6748	0.6853	0.6961
YouTube-Net	0.3186	0.269	0.2664	0.4161	0.6681	0.6764	0.682
MUI - Hybrid	**0.3294**	**0.2861**	**0.4218**	**0.5968**	**0.6798**	**0.6861**	**0.6997**

- YouTube-Net [51] two neural networks, one for ranking and the other for generating candidates. In this model, they used a ranking network for experimental studies.

7.6 Conclusions

In this book chapter, we have presented personalized multi-user movie recommendations in which the model incorporated click-through prediction techniques for user interest. This paper includes the methods of Embedding, Rich-content, Item representation, category representation, Neighbor-assisted, and hybrid methodologies. We also presented the rich content features used when no single feature is available, and many features are available. We studied how to use different fusion techniques to get maximum user interest representation for good performance. This model can be further applied for richer data, such as audio, motion and colour.

Along with this suggested user interest, from the perspective of the user's social cues, demographic profiling and representations be very valuable in providing advice for further research. Plans call for social cues to strengthen the suggested user interest representation with neighbour assistance. For additional work, it is better to use multi-dimensional fusion to describe the videos and by consideration of data sparsity and accuracy.

References

[1] Yashar Deldjoo, Mehdi Elahi, Paolo Cremonesi, Franca Garzotto, Pietro Piazzolla, and Massimo Quadrana. Content-based video recommendation system based on stylistic visual features. *Journal on Data Semantics*, 5(2):99–113, 2016.

[2] Justin Basilico and Thomas Hofmann. Unifying collaborative and content-based filtering. In *Proceedings of the Twenty-First International Conference on Machine Learning*, p. 9, 2004.

[3] Marco Vanetti, Elisabetta Binaghi, Barbara Carminati, Moreno Carullo, and Elena Ferrari. Content-based filtering in online social networks. In *International Workshop on Privacy and Security Issues in Data Mining and Machine Learning*, pp. 127–140. Springer, 2010.

[4] Jieun Son and Seoung Bum Kim. Content-based filtering for recommendation systems using multiattribute networks. *Expert Systems with Applications*, 89:404–412, 2017.

[5] Yehuda Koren, Steffen Rendle, and Robert Bell. Advances in collaborative filtering. *Recommender Systems Handbook*, pp. 91–142, 2022.

[6] John S Breese, David Heckerman, and Carl Kadie. Empirical analysis of predictive algorithms for collaborative filtering. arXiv preprint arXiv:1301.7363, 2013.

[7] Shumeet Baluja, Rohan Seth, Dharshi Sivakumar, Yushi Jing, Jay Yagnik, Shankar Kumar, Deepak Ravichandran, and Mohamed Aly. Video suggestion and discovery for YouTube: taking random walks through the view graph. In *Proceedings of the 17th International Conference on World Wide Web*, pp. 895–904, 2008.

[8] Yanxiang Huang, Bin Cui, Jie Jiang, Kunqian Hong, Wenyu Zhang, and Yiran Xie. Real-time video recommendation exploration. In *Proceedings of the 2016 International Conference on Management of Data*, pp. 35–46, 2016.

[9] Yali Du, Meng Fang, Jinfeng Yi, Chang Xu, Jun Cheng, and Dacheng Tao. Enhancing the robustness of neural collaborative filtering systems under malicious attacks. *IEEE Transactions on Multimedia*, 21(3):555–565, 2018.

[10] Xin Dong, Lei Yu, Zhonghuo Wu, Yuxia Sun, Lingfeng Yuan, and Fangxi Zhang. A hybrid collaborative filtering model with deep structure for recommender systems. In *Proceedings of the AAAI Conference on Artificial Intelligence*, vol. 31, 2017.

[11] Qinglong Li, Xinzhe Li, Byunghyun Lee, and Jaekyeong Kim. A hybrid cnn-based review helpfulness filtering model for improving e-commerce recommendation service. *Applied Sciences*, 11(18):8613, 2021.

[12] M Sandeep Kumar and J Prabhu. Hybrid model for movie recommendation system using fireflies and fuzzy c-means. *International Journal of Web Portals (IJWP)*, 11(2):1–13, 2019.

[13] Bisheng Chen, Jingdong Wang, Qinghua Huang, and Tao Mei. Personalized video recommendation through tripartite graph propagation. In *Proceedings of the 20th ACM International Conference on Multimedia*, pp. 1133–1136, 2012.

[14] Andrea Ferracani, Daniele Pezzatini, Marco Bertini, and Alberto Del Bimbo. Item-based video recommendation: An hybrid approach considering human factors. In *Proceedings of the 2016 ACM on International Conference on Multimedia Retrieval*, pp. 351–354, 2016.

[15] Aaron Van den Oord, Sander Dieleman, and Benjamin Schrauwen. Deep content-based music recommendation. *Advances in Neural Information Processing Systems*, 26, 2013.

[16] David Silver, Aja Huang, Chris J Maddison, Arthur Guez, Laurent Sifre, George Van Den Driessche, Julian Schrittwieser, Ioannis Antonoglou, Veda Panneershelvam, Marc Lanctot, *et al.* Mastering the game of go with deep neural networks and tree search. *Nature*, 529(7587):484–489, 2016.

[17] Shuai Zhang, Lina Yao, Aixin Sun, and Yi Tay. Deep learning based recommender system: A survey and new perspectives. *ACM Computing Surveys (CSUR)*, 52(1):1–38, 2019.

[18] Geoffrey E Hinton, Simon Osindero, and Yee-Whye Teh. A fast learning algorithm for deep belief nets. *Neural Computation*, 18(7):1527–1554, 2006.

[19] Yann LeCun, L´eon Bottou, Yoshua Bengio, and Patrick Haffner. Gradient-based learning applied to document recognition. *Proceedings of the IEEE*, 86(11):2278–2324, 1998.

[20] Alex Krizhevsky, Ilya Sutskever, and Geoffrey E Hinton. Imagenet classification with deep convolutional neural networks. *Communications of the ACM*, 60(6):84–90, 2017.

[21] Xue Geng, Hanwang Zhang, Jingwen Bian, and Tat-Seng Chua. Learning image and user features for recommendation in social networks. In *Proceedings of the IEEE International Conference on Computer Vision*, pp. 4274–4282, 2015.

[22] Donghyun Kim, Chanyoung Park, Jinoh Oh, Sungyoung Lee, and Hwanjo Yu. Convolutional matrix factorization for document contextaware recommendation. In *Proceedings of the 10th ACM Conference on Recommender Systems*, pp. 233–240, 2016.

[23] Yogesh Singh Rawat and Mohan S Kankanhalli. Contagnet: Exploiting user context for image tag recommendation. In *Proceedings of the 24th ACM International Conference on Multimedia*, pp. 1102–1106, 2016.

[24] Chenyi Lei, Dong Liu, Weiping Li, Zheng-Jun Zha, and Houqiang Li. Comparative deep learning of hybrid representations for image recommendations. In *Proceedings of the IEEE Conference on Computer Vision and Pattern Recognition*, pp. 2545–2553, 2016.

[25] Suhang Wang, Yilin Wang, Jiliang Tang, Kai Shu, Suhas Ranganath, and Huan Liu. What your images reveal: Exploiting visual contents for point-of-interest recommendation. In *Proceedings of the 26th International Conference on World Wide Web*, pp. 391–400, 2017.

[26] Xiaojie Chen, Pengpeng Zhao, Yanchi Liu, Lei Zhao, Junhua Fang, Victor S Sheng, and Zhiming Cui. Exploiting aesthetic features in visual contents for movie recommendation. *IEEE Access*, 7:49813–49821, 2019.

[27] Quangui Zhang, Li Wang, Xiangfu Meng, Keda Xu, and Jiayan Hu. A generic framework for learning explicit and implicit user-item couplings in recommendation. *IEEE Access*, 7:123944–123958, 2019.

[28] Yuyun Gong and Qi Zhang. Hashtag recommendation using attention based convolutional neural network. In *IJCAI*, pp. 2782–2788, 2016.

[29] Haoran Huang, Qi Zhang, Yeyun Gong, and Xuan-Jing Huang. Hashtag recommendation using end-to-end memory networks with hierarchical attention. In *Proceedings of COLING 2016, the 26th International Conference on Computational Linguistics: Technical Papers*, pp. 943–952, 2016.

[30] Minseok Park, Hanxiang Li, and Junmo Kim. Harrison: A benchmark on hashtag recommendation for real-world images in social networks. arXiv preprint arXiv:1605.05054, 2016.

[31] Wu, Y. Li, W. Yan, R. Li, X. Gu, and Q. Yang, Hashtag recommendation with attention-based neural image hashtagging network, in *Proc. 25th Int. Conf. Neural Inf. Process. (ICONIP), Siem Reap, Cambodia*, Dec. 2018, pp. 52–63, doi: 10.1007/978-3-030-04179-3_5.

[32] Yehuda Koren, Robert Bell, and Chris Volinsky. Matrix factorization techniques for recommender systems. *Computer*, 42(8):30–37, 2009.

[33] Steffen Rendle, Christoph Freudenthaler, Zeno Gantner, and Lars Schmidt-Thieme. Bpr: Bayesian personalized ranking from implicit feedback. arXiv preprint arXiv:1205.2618, 2012.

[34] Chong Wang and David M Blei. Collaborative topic modeling for recommending scientific articles. In *Proceedings of the 17th ACM SIGKDD International Conference on Knowledge Discovery and Data Mining*, pp. 448–456, 2011.

[35] Hao Wang, Naiyan Wang, and Dit-Yan Yeung. Collaborative deep learning for recommender systems. In *Proceedings of the 21th ACM SIGKDD International Conference on Knowledge Discovery and Data Mining*, pp. 1235–1244, 2015.

[36] Sujoy Roy and Sharath Chandra Guntuku. Latent factor representations for cold-start video recommendation. In *Proceedings of the 10th ACM Conference on Recommender Systems*, pp. 99–106, 2016.

[37] Ruining He and Julian McAuley. Vbpr: visual bayesian personalized ranking from implicit feedback. In *Proceedings of the AAAI Conference on Artificial Intelligence*, vol. 30, 2016.

[38] Qiusha Zhu, Mei-Ling Shyu, and Haohong Wang. Videotopic: Content based video recommendation using a topic model. In *2013 IEEE International Symposium on Multimedia*, pp. 219–222. IEEE, 2013.

[39] Zhou Zhao, Qifan Yang, Hanqing Lu, Tim Weninger, Deng Cai, Xiaofei He, and Yueting Zhuang. Social-aware movie recommendation via multi-modal network learning. *IEEE Transactions on Multimedia*, 20(2):430–440, 2017.

[40] Paolo Cremonesi, Yehuda Koren, and Roberto Turrin. Performance of recommender algorithms on top-n recommendation tasks. In *Proceedings of the Fourth ACM Conference on Recommender Systems*, pp. 39–46, 2010.

[41] James Davidson, Benjamin Liebald, Junning Liu, Palash Nandy, Taylor Van Vleet, Ullas Gargi, Sujoy Gupta, Yu He, Mike Lambert, Blake Livingston, *et al.* The YouTube video recommendation system. In *Proceedings of the Fourth ACM Conference on Recommender Systems*, pp. 293–296, 2010.

[42] Yifan Hu, Yehuda Koren, and Chris Volinsky. Collaborative filtering for implicit feedback datasets. In *2008 Eighth IEEE International Conference on Data Mining*, pp. 263–272. IEEE, 2008.

[43] Yehuda Koren. Factorization meets the neighborhood: a multifaceted collaborative filtering model. In *Proceedings of the 14th ACM SIGKDD International Conference on Knowledge Discovery and Data mining*, pp. 426–434, 2008.

[44] F Maxwell Harper and Joseph A Konstan. The movielens datasets: History and context. *ACM Transactions on Interactive Intelligent Systems* (TIIS), 5(4):1–19, 2015.

[45] Michael J Pazzani and Daniel Billsus. Content-based recommendation systems. In *The Adaptive Web*, pp. 325–341. Springer, 2007.

[46] Heng-Tze Cheng, Levent Koc, Jeremiah Harmsen, Tal Shaked, Tushar Chandra, Hrishi Aradhye, Glen Anderson, Greg Corrado, Wei Chai, Mustafa Ispir, *et al.* Wide & deep learning for recommender systems. In *Proceedings of the 1st Workshop on Deep Learning for Recommender Systems*, pp. 7–10, 2016.

[47] Huifeng Guo, Ruiming Tang, Yunming Ye, Zhenguo Li, and Xiuqiang He.Deepfm: a factorization-machine based neural network for ctr prediction. arXiv preprint arXiv:1703.04247, 2017.

[48] Ayush Singhal, Pradeep Sinha, and Rakesh Pant. Use of deep learning in modern recommendation system: A summary of recent works. arXiv preprint arXiv:1712.07525, 2017.

[49] Guorui Zhou, Xiaoqiang Zhu, Chenru Song, Ying Fan, Han Zhu, Xiao Ma, Yanghui Yan, Junqi Jin, Han Li, and Kun Gai. Deep interest network for click-through rate prediction. In *Proceedings of the 24th ACM SIGKDD International Conference on Knowledge Discovery & Data Mining*, pp. 1059–1068, 2018.

[50] Guorui Zhou, Na Mou, Ying Fan, Qi Pi, Weijie Bian, Chang Zhou, Xiaoqiang Zhu, and Kun Gai. Deep interest evolution network for click-through rate

prediction. In *Proceedings of the AAAI conference on Artificial Intelligence*, vol. 33, pp. 5941–5948, 2019.
[51] Paul Covington, Jay Adams, and Emre Sargin. Deep neural networks for YouTube recommendations. In *Proceedings of the 10th ACM Conference on Recommender Systems*, pp. 191–198, 2016.
[52] Diederik P Kingma and Jimmy Ba. Adam: A method for stochastic optimization. arXiv preprint arXiv:1412.6980, 2014.

8

Sensory Perception of Haptic Rendering in Surgical Simulation

Rachit Sachdeva[1]*, Eva Kaushik[1], Sarthak Katyal[1], Krishan Kant Choudhary[1] and Rohit Kaushik[2]

[1]*Institute of Technology and Management, New Delhi, India*
[2]*CS and Mathematics Department Data Analytics Program University of Illinois, Springfield, USA*

Abstract

The essential ideas behind haptic technology, including haptic interface and haptic rendering methods, as well as its application to surgical simulation, medical education, and other diverse topics, are presented in this paper. In empirical psychology and physiology, this refers to the sense of contact. The process of analyzing and developing capabilities in response to user interactions with virtual entities is elaborated as haptic rendering. Haptic may indicate haptic transmission, haptic perception, and haptic technology. Humans and other animals can respond to one another by using their feelings through haptic technology. Haptic perception is the process of recognizing objects through touch. Haptic implies tactile response, which means it delivers feedback in the state of sensation as we may sense the material properties and motions of virtual objects devised by a computer.

The use of haptic technology in the medical profession has proven extremely beneficial, and it has a wide range of applications in many different industries. By providing effective exchange via virtual reality, it helps to ease the surgeon's obligations. It amplifies a person's experience in the virtual environment. The haptics ability ranges from computer graphics to psychophysics, cognitive science, and neurosciences.

Keywords: Haptic technology, surgery, kinesthetic, sensor, actuator

**Corresponding author*: frenkrachiit@gmail.com

Suman Kumar Swarnkar, J P Patra, Sapna Singh Kshatri, Yogesh Kumar Rathore and Tien Anh Tran (eds.) Supervised and Unsupervised Data Engineering for Multimedia Data, (177–188) © 2024 Scrivener Publishing LLC

Introduction

Haptics rendering is an approach involving forces via a force-feedback device. Using it, we can easily facilitate a user to connect, sense and utilize virtual objects. It improves a person's experience in a virtual environment. The way people convey ideas and interact with computers has changed, thanks to haptic. The current refinements privilege to revise and enhance the fictitious computer-induced entities in a way that stimulates a cogent sense of tactile. Numerous force feedback haptic devices are used in incision simulation and medical education to accomplish haptic technology, which allows the user to enter data to the computer and obtain sensory information about a particular part or body area [1]. The haptic rendering pipeline, shown in Figure 8.1, generates tactile input for virtual environments. Figure 8.2 visualizes surface convolution, a computational procedure applied to potentially significant surfaces of the subject or system.

The haptic rendering could further be classified into three vital stages:

- Collision detection stage
  Load the attributes of the 3D entities from the database and get collision detection to resolve which virtual objects clash.
- Force computation stage
  It computes the collision forces, force smoothing and force mapping.
- Tactile computation stage
  Generate the contact feedback element of the simulation and the calculated consequences are counted to the power vector sent to the haptics result display. The haptics rendering channel includes a more diminutive standardized architecture corresponding to its replica [2].

Here, an actuator and detector that exchange data between the user and the computer and either give pulsating or external forces that make up the haptic system. Actuator receives scheduling calls via the Application Programme Interface (API) and Product functioning methods.

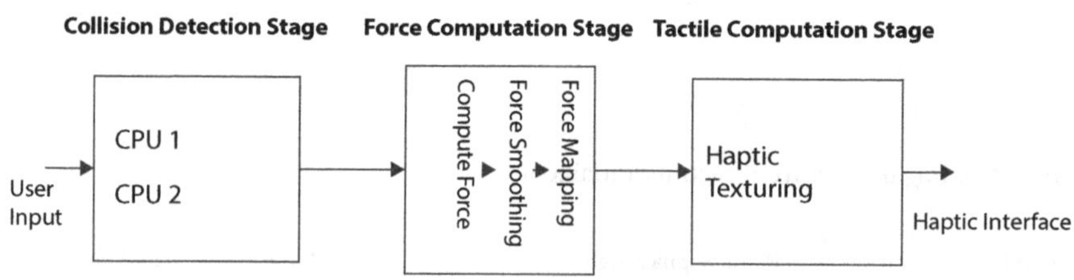

Figure 8.1 Haptic rendering pipeline.

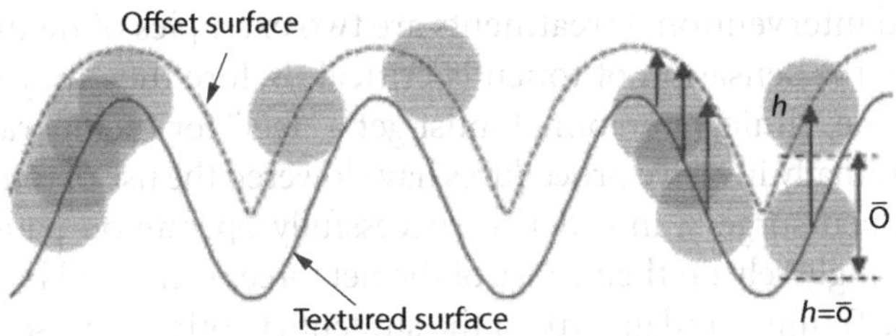

Figure 8.2 Surface convolution.

These calls limit the call of a particular haptic programme. The control circuitry then passes this management system information to the actuator after passing it to the OS whenever the user interacts with haptic devices [3]. Haptic interfaces can take many different shapes, such as computerized connection that attach a person's finger to the screen such that anytime the user moves their fingers, the motion is translated into actions on the screens by sensors, which also deliver the appropriate feedback. Furthermore, haptic technology plays a significant part in the healthcare industry, with simulation and medical apprenticeship being two of the most common applications. Using haptic rendering techniques, haptic technology can detect collisions between simulated organs and haptic equipment like surgical instruments. Feedback on the developed energy is sent to the user. Based on how they interact with the bodily parts, various instruments used in the medical industry for operations such as cystoscopy, colonoscopy and minimally invasive surgery are stated below.

Methodology

Touch aids us in determining size, structure, and weight, as well as orienting oneself in space. In medicine, touch is essential for good clinical practice.

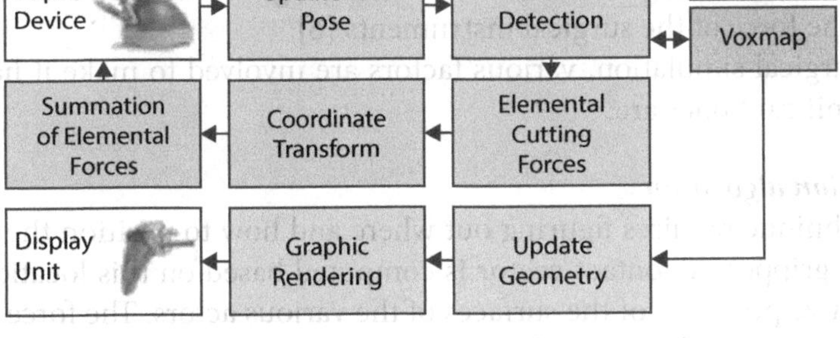

Figure 8.3 Components of haptic rendering algorithm.

Surgical and interventional treatments are two examples of medical procedures where the sensation of touch is critical. Before they may safely perform medicine, clinical personnel must get a "feel" for the operation.

Since minimally invasive procedures have lowered the use of touch in comparison to open surgery, in order to successfully operate on patients, clinicians increasingly rely on their sense of the net forces generated by tool-tissue interactions. Training and growth of the student's haptic motor sensorimotor system are required for training for a specific technique. In a suitable haptic device, users may feel torques. The union forces creates coupling moments created at the equipment end, for example, can be felt by the user [4].

Haptic modeling algorithms detect surgical instrument interactions with artificial organs and display force reactions by organs to users using haptic hardware. Viscous elasticity, anisotropy, inconsistency, time and rate dependency in substantial characteristics of organs are some of the challenges in creating a haptic device for tangible feedback. Two approaches based on their functionalities, particle-based technology and finite element technology, are employed to solve the aforesaid challenges and provide relevant tactile input [5]. As shown in Figure 8.3, the haptic rendering algorithm comprises several critical components that work together to create a realistic and engaging touch experience within a virtual environment. The method's core is the representation of geometry, which describes virtual objects and their surfaces.

Particle-based models

The connecting points of the tissue are linked together by spring-like equipment. Each point has its location, acceleration, and velocity, and moves under the impact of the operating instrument's forces.

Infinite-element modeling

By segmenting the model into surface or volumetric portions, the deformation states of the organ are calculated, formulating each element's properties and combining them to calculate the organs' states of deformation under the force of the surgical instruments [6].

In surgical simulation, various factors are involved to make it happen. The significant ones are:

- ***Collision algorithm***

The technique requires figuring out where and how to position the haptic device's gripper. A contact vector is computed based on this location and the relative positions of the surfaces of the various actors. The force vector is then shown on the haptic device.

- ***Haptic and visual loops interaction***

A graphical program refreshes the frame buffer 30–60 times per second on average. However, to provide a reliable and steady haptic feeling, a haptic application must refresh the depiction of forces to the haptic device 1,000 times per second or more. The user will see interruptions in the animation if the frequency of a graphical program is less than 30Hz. In a haptic application, the user notices force discontinuities and a reduction in quality when the system refreshes at a frequency below 500-1,000Hz.

Projection over surface

The placement of the projection tip of the 3D pointer or proxy on an object's surface will allow succeeding phases to determine if the proxy and the area are in touch. The cell Locator class of VTK is used to find the superficial point nearest to the proxy. This is a class that allows you to locate cells in 3-dimensional space [7]. In Figure 8.4, is shown the projection-tracing algorithm. This figure may show a computational procedure for tracing projections in image processing or computer graphics. Tracing projection algorithms helps analyze and manipulate visual data in many applications.

Here, FindClosestPointWithinRadius is a function that searches for the nearest point within a radius.

- ***Contact detection***

Distance between the meeting site or SCP and the proxy is evaluated to see if a contact has happened. If the distance is modest and the proxy moves in the contradictory direction of the surface's normal vector, it will be assumed that the proxy is in touch with the object, and the distance between the two places will define the proxy's penetration range in the volume [8].

- ***Computation and rendering of forces***

The response force that the haptic device must exert when contacting the proxy on a surface is estimated as the last step. Hooke's law is used, which states that the force is proportional to the displacement. Figure 8.5 depicts Hooke's Law. Hooke's Law, a fundamental physics and materials science principle, defines how force affects spring-like materials. Formula: $F = -kx$, where F is force, k is spring constant, and x represents displacement.

```
cell Locator -> SetDataset(Surface);

cell Locator -> BuildLocator();

cell Locator → FindClosestPointWithinRadius(posProxy, radius, posSCP, cellId, subId, dist);
```

Figure 8.4 Algorithm used for tracing projection.

F = −K · x

Here,

x = | penetration module |. Normal vector

K: Rigidity constant

hdSetDoublev(HD_CURRENT_FORCE, F+Fd):

F d = −b · v

Figure 8.5 Hooke's Law.

The figure may show this Law's proportional and linear nature, stressing its importance in elastic material mechanical behavior.

- A dampening effect is also used to increase the haptic sensation. The force signal is filtered by the damping. The usual damper equation is:
- Where, v is the end effector velocity, while b is the damping constant. The force is then sent to the haptic device.

Background Related Work

Hayward, V, [9]: Beginning in the early 1990s, a haptic interface allows a new sensory display modality to transmit information while applying controlled forces to the surgeon's hand. The haptic interfaces take into account the user's position in order to detect when and whether contacts happen as well as to gather data for calculating the proper interaction force. They have focused their attention on the force response algorithm for rigid objects. Because of non-negligible deformations, the possibility of self-strike, and the overall complexity of modeling, complement object response modeling introduces a new level of complexity that results in factually significant and varied areas of contact. At that time Tactile rendering aiming to give users the ability to handle, manipulate, and touch virtual things via a haptic link was enough.

Salisbury *et al.* [10]: A point-based haptic rendering method to mimic catheter and duct particle interactions. The connection between the laparoscopic forceps and the duct as well as the catheter was generated using the ray-based haptic interaction technique, where the forceps were modeled as connected line segments. They helped advance laparoscopic surgery. Cholecystectomies, appendectomies, and hernia repairs are some of the most common laparoscopic procedures. As gallstones are made of cholesterol, bile salts, and calcium, if blocked the outlet of the gallbladder can cause pain in the abdomen.

Lin *et al.* [11]: Integration of haptic interfaces into a training programme that replicates minimally fatal operations. Haptic Rendering uses mathematical simulations of surgical tools to find collisions with the aid of organ simulation models, during spoof sessions, calculates and reflects the forces of user interactions in real time. Haptic Recording, where measured properties of organs were recorded, and Haptic Playback where advanced approaches for user interactions use force feedback to direct a user during a training session. In the laparoscopic training system a pair of tactic devices provide the user with the reaction forces while they are using the real instruments and virtual organs. Laparoscopic tools occasionally include a new actuator attached to the handle to provide force feedback to the user for tissue grabbing.

A K Peters *et al.* [12]: The virtual simulation connected to the world in three broader terms: Haptic communication is the way that people and animals respond to one another by touching. The process of identifying objects through touch is known as haptic perception, and haptic technology, which is tactile feedback, or feedback delivered through touch, enables users to physically experience the movement of virtual things that a computer generates for them. They created a Haptic Interface that aids in providing haptic feedback to the user, to allow users to manipulate an object in the virtual environment They created a single sensory receptor for the entire body and provided haptic feedback in response to the body's movements. They divided the feedback received from the haptic devices into kinesthetic and tactile.

Application

Anesthesia: Needle simulation is a hot issue with many applications in clinical operations such as biopsies, injections, neurosurgery, brachytherapy cancer treatment, and regional anesthesia. We concentrate on local anesthesia (LA) since training possibilities are limited and virtual reality-based (VR) LA emulators are unavailable. To achieve sufficient physical skills for efficient completion of such tasks, RA needs extensive theoretical understanding and repetitive practice. As a result, we employ haptics to fix the problem. A force sensor and a distance measure are mounted to an LA needle in a non-intrusive manner. The Simulation Open Framework Architecture's (SOFA) FEM algorithms will be used to model soft-tissue deformations. Several needle bending techniques are now being adopted and assessed [13].

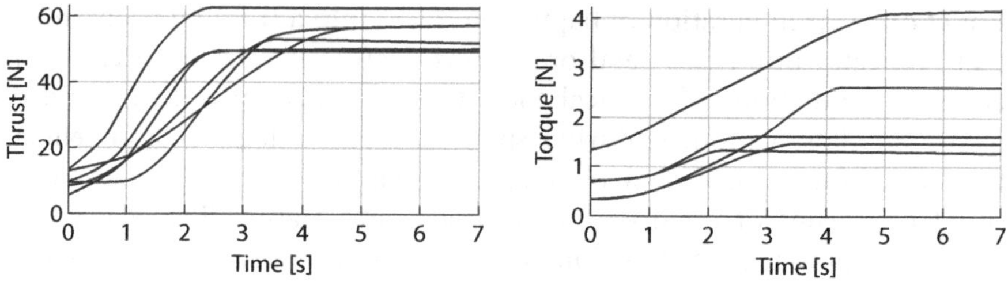

Figure 8.6 Thrust and torque prediction in glenoid reaming.

Case Study

Glenoid Reaming

In shoulder joint replacement procedures, glenoid reaming is a difficult bone-machining procedure. Due to its inherent intricacy, glenoid reaming makes an ideal target for haptic-augmented surgery simulators. Various point shell and voxmap resolutions were used for the visual-haptic glenoid reaming simulation trials. Accurate prediction of thrust and torque in glenoid reaming, as illustrated in Figure 8.6, adds to better surgical planning, lower intraoperative risks, and better overall outcomes for patients having shoulder joint replacement procedures.

Using this technique, a clinical CT scan of a human scapula was utilised to create the voxmap model, which was then segmented and upsampled to the required resolution. Running times similar to Tab are feasible because the execution time of VPS approaches depends on the sampling resolution of voxmap and point shell structures. The approach permits haptic modeling of bone cutting procedures to incorporate high-fidelity, micro-resolution bone models. Table 8.1 shows the standard variation of running times for different resolutions. The standard deviation is a statistical way to measure how spread out or different a set of numbers is. In terms of running time, it means how far the performance times are off from the mean or average running time.

Table 8.1 Standard deviation of running time in different resolutions.

	Voxmap resolution		
Point shell resolution	128^3	256^3	512^3
128^3	0.27 (0.10)	0.29 (0.10)	0.35 (0.70)
256^3	0.28 (0.10)	0.29 (0.10)	0.71 (0.35)
512^3	0.41 (0.09)	0.35 (0.11)	0.76 (0.36)
1024^3	0.41 (0.08)	0.46 (0.10)	0.95 (0.35)
2048^3	1.18 (0.16)	1.28 (0.17)	1.80 (0.46)

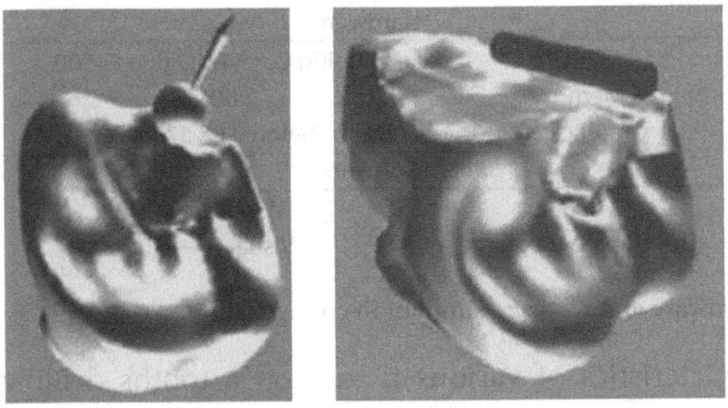

Figure 8.7 Tooth's burring cross section. Dental instruments are necessary for numerous dental procedures and tooth health. Dentists use the dental mirror to see inside the mouth and the probe to identify cavities and problems on the tooth's surface. Plaque and tartar are removed by the scaler, improving oral health. Dental drill instruments vary by task, such as cavity preparation. Teeth are held and removed with forceps. Thin dental probes detect gum pocket depth to assess mouth health. A and b represent the tooth's surface structure, which includes cuspids, incisors, and other elements that form and function it. The tooth's complicated geometry makes it worthwhile in various oral functions. These dental tools help dentists diagnose, treat, and maintain oral health. Dental instruments are necessary for numerous dental procedures and tooth health. Dentists use the dental mirror to see inside the mouth and the probe to identify cavities and problems on the tooth's surface. Plaque and tartar are removed by the scaler, improving oral health. Dental drill instruments vary by task, such as cavity preparation. Teeth are held and removed with forceps. Thin dental probes detect gum pocket depth to assess mouth health. A and b represent the tooth's surface structure, which includes cuspids, incisors, and other elements that form and function it. The tooth's complicated geometry makes it worthwhile in various oral functions. These dental tools help dentists diagnose, treat, and maintain oral health.

This is the first instance in which micro-resolutions for bone machining simulation have been made possible. This makes it possible to incorporate micro-CT bone pictures into simulations and more precisely model the structural characteristics of bones while performing haptic computations.

Haptic Rendering in Dental Surgical

The interaction force between dental tools and teeth should be accurately reflected by the haptic depiction in dental surgical simulations. Figure 8.7 depict the structure of a tooth and some dental instruments, respectively. A tooth contains a tiny amount of geometry on its surface and a variety of tissues inside, as depicted in Figure 8.7. The following is a list of the functions of a dental surgery training system:

- Practice common surgical procedures, such as exploring dental orifices, preparing teeth, and observing the physical

Hardware	
CPU	Intel(R) Core(TM)2 duo E4500
Memory	2.00 GB
Graphic card	Geforce FX 5700LE
Software	
OS	Windows XP
Developing language	Visual C++ 6.0

Figure 8.8 Hardware and software simulation configuration.

characteristics of various tissues on a tooth's drilling cross section.

- Provide accurate haptic feedback: The system should be able to feel the smallest geometries on a tooth's surface, from fossa on the occlusal surface to shape of the cusp, and it should be able to distinguish between the physical characteristics of crumbing tissue and toned tissue during exploration operations.

The co-located haptic-visual augmented reality platform's physical prototype is erected on top of a partially silvered mirror. The operator can see visual data about the virtual scene and feel force information thanks to the display and force-feedback device. The display-space of the virtual object may be viewed and combined with the original moment through the partially silvered mirror.

Future Scope

The advancement of the exciting touchless haptics technology has the potential to significantly increase the precision and effectiveness of operations. This stimulation can be used in physical therapy for patients who have had a stroke or surgery that requires rehabilitation to restore the use of their motor system. Multiple programmes trying to reach the output simultaneously may raise security issues since they may crash, whether due to a hacker, interference with other signals or ultrasonic waves, or some other factor. The translation or measures of the answer are of concern when this input is concealed or camouflaged [14].

New degrees of realism, safety, and cost effectiveness in medical training and military are made possible by this technology.

Result

It is essential to use the haptic device to concurrently record and show haptic feelings during surgical procedures. There is a lot of interest in the haptic display of compliant objects for Minimally Invasive Surgical Simulation and Training (MISST), haptic recording and playback principles. By utilizing a robotic arm's kinematic and novel characteristics, from to the end, alone, researchers in robotics have, to some extent, succeeded in obtaining the tractable characteristics of objects. Haptic playback can make use of the force field theory that robotics researchers established for guiding mobile robots and leading robot arms in the presence of impediments.

Conclusion

Medical staff can be trained more effectively using VR-based healthcare simulations than the current method, which focuses mostly on patient interaction. This is similar to how flight simulators assist pilots in their training. Integrating haptics into MISST seems essential because MIS techniques call for manipulating the organs with tools while touching, feeling, and feeling them. Although developing realistic simulations is technically difficult, recent developments in electromechanical technology may make this possible and open up new possibilities. Simulators for a variety of medical operations have been developed in recent years by an increasing number of research labs and businesses. Medical professionals and technicians work closely together to advance haptics-integrated technologies utilized in the medical field. We anticipate that using medical simulations for training will dramatically improve patient care.

Acknowledgement

We thank Mr. Rohit Kaushik** research scholar, University of Illinois, USA, for guiding us. His contribution and highly valuable feedback markedly enhanced our manuscript.

References

[1] Meng, Yan, no. "Apply Haptic Rendering for Intubation Simulation." *International Journal of Engineering and Technology*, vol. 7, no. 3.16, 2018, p. 61, https//doi.org/10.14419/ijet.v7i3.16.16184.

[2] "Imitating Soft Skin for Haptic Outfit Wearing." Basic Computer Clothes and Non-Reality for Taxpayers We See, 2015, runners 570–601, https//doi.org/10.1201/b18703-26.

[3] Wang, Dangxiao, *et al.* "Examination of Haptic Delivery styles." Haptic donation reproduction Good Deception, 2014, pp. 117–130, https//doi.org/10.1007/978-3-662-44949-3_5.

[4] Wang, Dangxiao, *et al.* "Haptic Offering Simulation Good Deception." 2014, https//doi.org/10.1007/978- 3-662-44949-3.

[5] Wei, Lei, and Alexei Sourin. "Haptic Provisioning of Haptic Mixed goods." *2010 International Conference on Cyberworlds, 2010*, https//doi.org/10.1109/cw.2010.12.

[6] Hannaford, B, and R Leuschke. "Provision of Multi Finger Haptic bias." Haptic picture, 2008, runners 67–82, https//doi.org/10.1201/b10636-6.

[7] "Giving Strategies." Haptic picture, 2008, pp. 157 - 157, https//doi.org/10.1201/b10636-10.

[8] Hou, Xiyuan. "Sustainable Haptic Offering in the Visible terrain." https//doi.org/10.32657/10356/61783.

[9] Hayward, V. "Physically-Based Haptic Synthesis." In Haptic Rendering, 2008, pp. 297–309, https//doi.org/10.1201/b10636-17.

[10] Salisbury, K., Conti, F., & Barbagli, F. (2004). Survey haptic rendering: Introductory concepts. *IEEE Computer Graphics and Applications*, 24(2), 24–32. https://doi.org/10.1109/mcg.2004.1274058

[11] Lin, Ming C., and Miguel A. Otaduy. A.K. Peters, Haptic Rendering Foundations, Algorithms, and operations, 2008.

[12] A.K. Peters, Haptic Rendering Foundations, Algorithms, and operations, 2008.

[13] Seungmoon Choi, and Hong Z. Tan. "Haptic Offering- piecemeal from Visual Computing - refers to the factual Haptic Distribution of Local Design." *IEEE Computer Graphics and Applications*, vol. 24, no. 2, 2004, runners 40–47, https//doi.org/10.1109/mcg.2004.1274060.

[14] Preusche, Carsten, *et al.* "Haptic Delivery and Control." Haptic Personal Vision Basic and Applications, runners 411–426, https//doi.org/10.1007/978-3-7643-7612-3_33.

9

Multimedia Data in Modern Education

Roopashree*, Praveen Kumar M., Pavanalaxmi, Prameela N. S. and Mehnaz Fathima

Sahyadri College of Engineering & Management, Mangaluru, India

Abstract

The multimedia learning environment includes various components to facilitate learning. Only part of the criterion applies to hardware and software. Multimedia combines graphics, video, sound, text, and animation to produce a powerful educational tool. Good education still needs to be improved in developing nations. Various methods, including multimedia technology, have been explored to increase access for most people in underdeveloped nations. Digital learning materials with multimedia components enhance information processing and encourage effective mental representations in pupils. Digital learning resources convey text, image, video, and audio content. Technology in education encompasses the use of new tools and techniques and the development and use of efficient learning management systems, information dissemination, feedback, and performance evaluation. Online education platforms have emerged due to the use of multimedia data in traditional classroom-based teaching and learning. Online learning is popular due to its time and data access flexibility. Effective sharing of high-quality educational resources promotes self-learning. Teachers primarily require access to learning materials that can assist pupils in developing concepts in multiple ways to meet their particular needs. This chapter highlights the diversity of multimedia data utilized in modern schooling. The article highlights the difficulties in integrating multimedia data in several school sectors

Keywords: Education, physical education, multimedia, ICT

**Corresponding author*: rupsknown2u@gmail.com

Suman Kumar Swarnkar, J P Patra, Sapna Singh Kshatri, Yogesh Kumar Rathore and Tien Anh Tran (eds.) Supervised and Unsupervised Data Engineering for Multimedia Data, (189–216) © 2024 Scrivener Publishing LLC

Introduction to Multimedia

A multimedia is a form of communication that uses content in the form of text, audio, animations, video, or images in a single presentation when compared to traditional mass media which uses printed material and audio recordings [1]. Animated videos, video podcasts, and audio slideshows are examples of multimedia. This also forms the building base of other technologies, hardware, and software, as well as the effective interaction of communication applications.

Multimedia forms a new mode in computer science by combining various media content into one computer usage. This makes the computer useful for entertainment and education along with business purposes.

Multimedia technologies in education act as a supplement to the existing curricula for further encouraging and enhancing curriculum development.

The Basic Elements Used in Multimedia for Education

Multimedia includes five different components, through which students get more freedom to express and exchange their creative ideas. The five different elements of multimedia are explained below.

Text

Text, in general, gives critical information. Text enacts as the anchor that connects all the other elements in multimedia. A well-written multimedia text enhances communication. The most extensively used type of written or spoken communication is text, which is a collection of predetermined words or symbols. The majority of multimedia uses it. Applications can be integrated with various media in a remarkable and significant way to present information and convey mindsets. Word processing software is built on text, which is also the core data source for many multimedia tools. In fact, the transformation of a book into a computerized form is necessary for many multimedia applications.

Sound

Sound is used to highlight and emphasize the transition. Educators can present a huge amount of information in a single go when the screen display and sound are synchronized. This method is used in different ways, all of which rely on the spoken explanation of the complex image which is on display. When used innovatively, imagination is stimulated by sound; when used inappropriately, it becomes an annoyance or hindrance. Students must be allowed to have their imagination without having any imagination bias and avoid getting influenced by any video which is inappropriate. One main advantage of sound files is that they can be stopped and restarted easily.

The best technique to draw attention is through audio since adding sound to a media application allows consumers to access information that would be hard to share through other means. Red Book audio is one of the many audio formats that are available today. It is employed with multimedia applications and is the foundation for the best sound that is being produced. Another audio sound format is Windows Wave, which can contain any kind of sound that can be recorded by a microphone and can only be played on computers running the windows operating system. The Musical Instrument Digital Interface (MIDI), which is essentially a specification created by musical instrument makers, is the last type of audio sound that may be used. MIDI can only hold audio data in the form of musical notes.

Video

Video is one of the most powerful tools of information since it allows the learner to understand things visually. This is the ability of the learners to choose and interact with the digital video content which opens up the possibility of using digital video content in education. There are a few instances in which the students who are studying specific concepts or processes may encounter a scenario where it appears to be more complex when taught solely through the use of images and diagrams or through text. In such cases, theoretical concepts can be represented with aid of the quality video [2].

If the content of the video is relevant to the complex concepts with the proper information it can pique people's interest. Video is used for the demonstration of the complex concepts which is in text. For example, when learners are studying the specific complex concepts from the notes, a short video of the teacher can be inserted which emphasizes the key points at a key time; alternatively, the readers or learners can be instructed on what to do next. However, video cannot replace the physical lecture in the classrooms; it can be only a supplement to the textual information.

Video can be used to convey information that is too expensive or difficult to convey in another format, or to recreate the incidents later. For example, chemical reactions are volatile and students cannot be exposed to them in real life or in medical surgery; students can understand them better through a video before going into actual practice. A video is a useful tool for e-learning since it makes it easier to demonstrate tools and processes in practice.

Animation

Animation is useful to demonstrate the information to learners in smaller chunks that they can digest easily. When animations are given with user input for different variables, students will get different versions of it.

Animations are mainly used for demonstration purposes or to illustrate a concept [3]. Animations are drawing-based and videos are of real life. There are two different kinds of animation:

1) Cel-based animation, 2) object-based animation. Cel animation is one that has multiple drawings; each drawing is slightly different from the others. When these drawings are shown in rapid succession they appear to be in motion, such as the engine's crankshaft operation. Object-based animation (also known as slide or path animation) means that the object is moved across the screen. The object remains unchanged. Learners can make use of object animation to demonstrate a point. For example, imagine a Gettysburg battle map with the representation of troop movement.

An animation is a collection of images that give the impression of motion. Digital animation is used in multimedia. Digital animation can be divided into two categories in general: Animations in 2D (2 dimensions) and 3D (3 dimensions). Basic items can be animated in two dimensions. On the screen, these things move and are placed in various settings or positions. The term "3D animation" describes the process of turning still images into moving three-dimensional digital objects. Examples of animations include whirling and zigzagging across the screen. Animations depend heavily on the size and kind of animated visuals because they frequently involve graphics. Animation can be made in a variety of methods.

Graphics

Graphics is one of the most creative options for learners. This can be drawings, photographs, spreadsheet graphs, and CD-ROM images, or are taken from internet sources. With the help of a scanner, hand-drawn work can also be included. According to Standing [4], "the capacity of recognition memory for pictures is almost limitless." The reason behind this is that cortical skills are required for images, including dimension, form, texture, color, line, visual rhythm, and, most importantly, imagination [5, 6].

Graphics are the digital representation of non-text data, such as a diagram, charts, or pictures, and they provide appeal to multimedia applications. They support the use of animated still images to illustrate concepts. Bitmaps (paint graphics) and vector (draw graphics) are the two types of graphics that are employed. Bitmap images are actual pictures that can be taken with tools like cameras or scanners. Computers can draw vector graphics because they just need a little amount of memory. Different types of picture formats exist, including the captured image format and the format used when storing images.

Educational Requirements

Using multimedia tools in the classroom is a difficult, complex task but it is rewarding. All the available multimedia elements, including text, animation, video, sound, and graphics, are already present in most libraries in some form or another. Students have access to an almost limitless amount of information. This kind of exploration will lead to discoveries, but the story is over unless the knowledge is learned. Knowledge gained will be like knowledge forgotten until there is an opportunity to apply the discoveries and demonstrate the same.

Giving learners the chance to create their documents in multimedia has several benefits in education. Learners go with their own information from four perspectives: (1) as researchers, they must be able to select and locate the information which is needed to understand the concepts which are chosen; (2) as authors, they must know the intended audience and how much information must be given to readers to understand the concept; (3) as designers, learners must know to choose the suitable media to share the concepts; and (4) as writers, they must know the format in which the information has to be fitted.

It is difficult to find out the technical specification of the machines used by the readers to know which is the best multimedia medium that can be used. Depending on the concepts and technical requirements proper multimedia elements can be chosen. To apply the previously mentioned principle to all visuals, digital media elements must be consistent, relevant, and congruent which is effective and presented. Whatever the most recent technological advancement, instructional design principles remain applicable. When using visuals for aesthetic purposes, for example, caution is required. Misrepresentation of information of a single visual element will become a content barrier and impede learning, even if the program as a whole follows instructional design principles.

Computer Interface – Human

Multimedia applications are easy to use with little training or self-education like any other application, tool, or appliance. There must be good interfacing for the interaction of humans and computers. Television Producers, Publishers of books, and music set the standards for computer-based publications. With the advancement in high-definition displays, the demand for computer-based multimedia is going to increase continuously.

Access, Delivery, Scheduling, and Recording

To use multimedia content in real time the access time to the computer must be at less than a second. There must be a provision to deliver the information at a later time through scheduling as in a TV broadcast channel. Learners may get the benefit from delivery based on demand with scheduled delivery. Students in open learning ways can request their multimedia unit to schedule their learning time at their free available time. Users may want to save sessions or learning experiences for later reference.

Interactivity

To be credible as a learning medium, multimedia which is computer-based must have good interactivity, like classroom exercises or laboratory experiments. Educationists have demonstrated that the participation of the student in learning material will make few learnings easier and will make retaining more permanent. This process also includes the creation of virtual reality which makes it easy for the complex process to be understood. It is the sole responsibility of the application engineer to incorporate interactivity. Interactivity can be incorporated only if the network can deliver sound very quickly or a moving picture; the network must be able to communicate two-way so that the application design will have human interaction.

Resources and Classroom Architecture

The technology required for classroom instruction is a bit complex [7]. The classroom requires a slide projector, overhead projector computer, networks, display tools like TV, and projector screen. Until recently the classroom used to have only a blackboard and table for the teachers. Now the classroom requires maintenance which is expensive and also requires security since new equipment is included in the classrooms. Figure 9.1 depicts an example of an educational environment based on multimedia. The classrooms are fitted with standard presentation equipment which will also include a complete explanation of what is included and what is not.

Advantages of Multimedia in Education

A multimedia is an effective tool for improving personal communication. This enables better storytelling and gives good narration ideas to people so that they can explain them to other people. Making multimedia content is an excellent method to keep the audience engaged and help them understand your content more efficiently. Advantages include:

- A shift in student and teacher roles.
- Enhanced self-esteem and motivation.

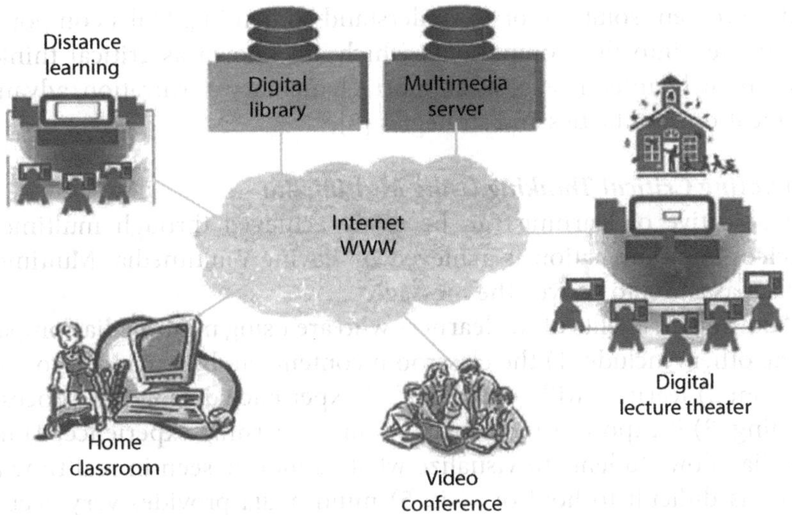

Figure 9.1 A typical educational environment based on multimedia. [1]

- Technical abilities.
- Difficult task completion more efficiently.
- Increase in collaboration with peers
- Increased reliance on outside resources.
- Audience attention/improved design skills

Disadvantages of Multimedia in Education

The disadvantage of multimedia is that users find it difficult to interact with their content. People have limited ways to interact with the text, images, and sounds on a website. It does not provide them with the same experience as visiting a physical store.

- Multimedia content production is much more expensive than any other type of production because it involves more than one medium.
- Multimedia production demands the use of an electronic device, which can be costly.
- Because multimedia requires electricity to function, the cost of using it rises.

Usage of Multimedia for Improving Critical Thinking

Thinking is the major activity required for a human being to interpret and process information. Human beings think in order to take decisions, to find a problem solution, or to understand something. Skills components are divided into five components which are known as critical thinking skills, namely: inference, basic support, elementary clarification, advanced clarification, and tactics and strategies [8].

Promoting Critical Thinking Using Multimedia

The objective of learning can be easily achieved through multimedia. Efficient communication is achieved by having multimedia. Multimedia will act as a tool to convey the message.

Additional benefits of the learners who are using multimedia compared to the others include: 1) the classroom content can be expanded to a new horizon; 2) learners will get diversified experience during this process of learning; 3) it exposes the students to direct learning experience; 4) multimedia allow students to visualize what cannot be seen in real time and which is difficult to hold or visit; 5) multimedia provides very accurate and up-to-date information; 6) it improves interest among the learners and motivates them by giving attractive display material; 7) it improves the ability of the learners to cultivate their imagination and to create creativity and innovation by thinking critically; 8) multimedia improves the efficiency of the learning; 9) multimedia will solve the problem if critical thinking among the learners is improved [9].

Traditional Learning Approaches

The traditional approach to education is teacher-centric and encourages the teacher's dominance in the classroom environment. Here, teachers use the memorization technique of drill and rote. With this approach, kids learn through memorization and repetition.

Traditional teaching methods, where the teacher is solely in charge of the learning environment and manages the classroom, are obsolete. The teacher, who also conducts class lectures, serves as the student's instructor and is the one who determines what and how to teach, and is in charge of all duties and powers.

The purpose of teaching is to help students learn; the more a student learns, the more effective a teacher is in their job. One of the traditional methods of instruction is the classroom, where the teaching process primarily takes place. Students in a full class sit together in the classroom to learn the material that teachers present, and they acquire knowledge through practice.

Features of traditional teaching methods:

- Teacher-centric classrooms
- Knowledge is provided by teachers. Teachers take the role of knowledge transferer.
- Chalk and talk methods are widely used.
- Mainly focuses on well-organized classrooms.
- Main concern is to make students ready for the examination rather than analyzing the concept.

The classroom environment has changed in recent years; students are not considered target listeners but rather they will take an active role in their education. They will speak up and ask questions about what is being taught by the teacher. The methods and styles of instruction have evolved over time. Interactive methods have taken the place of the old school of education that relied on memorization and recitation.

Advantages of Traditional Learning

- ***Active education***
  The college life experience of a student can be enhanced in traditional campus life by having contact with professors and instructors. In contrast, there aren't many options for online education. On campus, students can schedule in-person meetings with their professors to talk about a project, the class, or their performance.

- ***All subject areas or courses cannot be trained in multimedia mode***
  Online courses can only take a student so far if they are thinking about specialization in the area of film producing, biology, agriculture, nursing, and music. While it is simple to complete some of the required coursework for these specializations online, classes with labs, practical sessions on clinical instruments usage, or performances must be taken on a traditional campus. For such specialized courses, the resources required are provided using traditional teaching methods.

- ***Library Access***
  The school or college library should be constantly lively with pupils working together, studying, and conducting experiments and writing research for papers on the projects. Without accessing the research materials students are unable to realize the potential within them.

- ***Activities outside of the classroom***
  There are some educational opportunities that are unique to the school. These include activities at school, field trips, and various clubs in which students can participate. They will learn valuable life lessons from each of those experiences that they can apply.

- ***Keeping interpersonal connections***
  Throughout their time in college, students get involved with a variety of people. Making meaningful connections that will likely last for years is one advantage of attending an on-campus university. The majority of the college experience will be spent working on numerous group and individual projects that require students to interact with their classmates. One way to maintain interpersonal connections at a university is through the creation of various clubs, meetings for the preparation of exams, and the exchange of study materials. Keeping those connections on campus is quite simple.

Drawbacks of Traditional Learning

Although people want to follow a system, they are always constrained by their own inclinations to do otherwise. The egregious incidents that take place in conventional schools are a clear indication of this.

- **Expensive:** Traditional learning centers typically offer less affordable education because they require more resources, which drives up course costs.
- **Lack of flexibility:** College and university students find it harder to study because of the rigid schedules. The schedule must be used by the students to plan their regular classes, and they must keep track of attendance. Due to the students' mandatory attendance at school, they are unable to demonstrate their talents.

- **Cost of commuting:** The traditional educational system includes the costs of commuting to schools and lodging costs while attending classes. While going to and from the class, the cost of transportation will increase.

Multimedia-Based Learning Approach

A type of computer-assisted instruction called multimedia learning employs two modalities simultaneously [10]. In contrast to the conventional classroom practice of lecturing to students or having them read aloud, the use of visual learning (videos, pictures, written text, and animations) and vocal learning as separate networks for sending content is innovative. Although a teacher can deliver multimedia lessons, computers running software are frequently used to do so.

Virtual learning environments are an alternative to conventional learning settings. Virtual schools are becoming more prevalent worldwide as they provide a novel approach to education. The remote learning platform, which includes exams, course materials, assessments, themes, and other tools outside of the teaching space, includes a virtual class as one of its components.

Due to the fact that most scholars practice a variety of applications in this field, mainframe learning can be just as effective as traditional learning. E-learning, in its broadest sense, refers to all educational contexts that make significant use of ICT. The e-learning platforms' technical features cater to the needs and preferences of the students while also meeting their educational requirements. To do this, there must be a strong relationship between the pedagogical, technical and technological aspects.

Cognitive learning, which originated as a critique of behaviorism a few decades ago, defines learning as the process of looking for information that has been stored in memory after initial information processing, mental image formation, and abstract processing. The traditional model of education places a strong emphasis on the teacher's reflections, the transmission of knowledge, abstract symbols, targeted applications, finalizations, and predetermined structures.

Although the information is fundamentally objective and self-regulating of the student's awareness, the student nonetheless acquires it subjectively through processing, constructions, and personal interpretations. Unlike knowledge, learning is influenced by support materials, independent and cluster working circumstances, strategies used, and various forms of expression and communication during this internalization process.

Based on the knowledge-technology relationship, anchored learning supported by multimedia is a style of learning that makes it easier for students to practice problem-solving abilities. Multimedia has been activated and made more interactive through the use of computers in education. In the context of computer-assisted training, it is believed that interactivity is important.

Advantages of Multimedia in learning:

- **Greater comprehension**
  One benefit of multimedia learning, according to research, is the capacity to link oral and graphical representations of content, which is important for a deeper understanding and supporting the application of education in other frameworks.
- **Better problem-solving skills**
  A sizable portion of the human brain is dedicated to the processing of visual information. As a result, adding images, sound, and animations to texts helps to stimulate brain activity. Students are more attentive and retain more information. Students are more adept at identifying issues and coming up with solutions when learning occurs in a multimedia environment as opposed to one where textbooks serve as the only source of instruction.
- **Improvement in constructive feelings**
  According to psychologist Barbara Fredrickson, feeling good makes it easier for individuals to see more opportunities in their existence. The convention of multimedia in instruction has an impact on the student's attitude during the learning process.
- **Extensive knowledge of access**
  Due to smartphones, computers, the internet, and tablets, scholars are better equipped with the information they require. Most students with access to the internet acquire the required information online, according to their requirements. Sharing knowledge and taking part in class discussions become easier when evidence is as accessible as it is today.
- **Exploring world**
  With the help of multimedia, children can discover places they would never have traveled to. In a geography class, students can research different cities from around the globe, the

tallest mountains, and the most perilous jungles. Today, students in science classes can explore space and other planets. Dissecting rare animals and learning about various habitats is simple for biology students who are using a multimedia learning environment.

Drawbacks of Multimedia Learning

Since producing multimedia content requires a lot of time and has a limited amount of storage space, this technology might not be suitable for everyone. The following are some additional drawbacks of multimedia:

- **Information avalanche:** Information overload is one of the biggest issues with multimedia. A person is more likely to feel overloaded by the amount of information available the more time they spend online. Additionally, studies have demonstrated that the simultaneous use of multiple media reduces productivity.
- **Reduced interaction:** Users find it challenging to engage with its content. There are few opportunities for people to interact with the text, images, and sounds on a website. It doesn't provide them with the same experience as going to a physical store.
- **Takes up a lot of time:** A variety of content types can be produced using multimedia as a resource, but this takes a lot of time. While they could have been exercising or spending time with friends and family, people frequently spend hours on their phones or computers.
- **Intensive resources:** It takes a lot of resources to use multimedia. It uses up space on a computer and can draw a lot of power as a medium. The overall price of multimedia is amplified by this.
- **Requires significant investment:** Investment in multimedia is significant. This applies in particular to musicians, singers, videographers, and other people with special talents.
- **Market dependency:** Although multimedia can be a very useful tool, there are some drawbacks as well. Due to the materials needed for development, multimedia is typically exclusive.

Applications of Multimedia in Education

Usage of Multimedia in Learning During the Pandemic

The COVID-19 pandemic compelled educational communities around the world to declare the end of face-to-face teaching in schools/colleges and to turn to "online teaching and learning." As a result, both teachers and students encountered numerous difficulties and had to bridge the gap between their expectations and reality. Due to the changed teaching and learning environment, there is a growing need among teachers and students for new technology.

The multimedia platform has played an essential role during the global emergency COVID-19 pandemic circumstances for disseminating critical information throughout the world. Using a variety of multimedia types to accurately communicate the facts one can avoid the spreading of fake news and material can be updated periodically. It has become crucial to manage information during pandemics to guarantee that public health remains the government's top priority.

Online distance learning technique was first introduced during the outbreak situation across the globe as the standard operating procedures to the public. These were imposed by WHO as well as respective countries' governments. The growth of Information and Communication Technology (ICT) has significant effects on the educational system.

The use of multimedia by students and faculty in schools and colleges has been on the rise for the purpose of online learning by adapting online learning tools such as Microsoft and Google Meet applications. Depending on the goals, each application offers a varied level of multimedia.

In the current challenging environment, technology and communication are the cornerstones for the improvement of the economy and people's lives. The government's primary commitment is to lessen and close the digital gap in society in order to strengthen its economy. The result is that people around the world can benefit from high-quality internet and remain connected.

ICT development is fueled by a variety of causes, including improved coverage, enhanced capabilities, rising data demand, and smartphones. Due to the pandemic, multimedia makes it simpler for employees to work from home.

For instance, the adoption of 5G and broadband in every nation enables the population to benefit from better living conditions. The use of multimedia during an outbreak helps organizations save time, cut costs of expenditure and stabilize their financial and operational positions. For the purpose of preventing disease, proper knowledge of the COVID-19 pandemic is essential.

Students rely on collaborative learning (CL) in a learning environment to enhance their performance. This is a learning platform that promotes students' CL and allows them to communicate freely with their peers and subject experts. This study examines how college students use social media to address the crucial idea of CL during the COVID-19 pandemic. Utilizing the previously existing internet technology, online education platforms have facilitated the continuation of education.

In this situation, multimedia components have offered a wide-ranging learning environment to include people in conversations about educational subjects among peers and in interactions between students and teachers. The teacher's activity and commitment to teaching may be nourished, renewed, and supported by resources.

Resources can be divided into three categories: cognitive resources (such as images and/or theoretical tools used to work with teachers), social resources (such as a discussion on a forum), and material curriculum resources (such as textbooks, digital curriculum resources, manipulable objects, and calculators).

Approach the GSuite and consider its possibilities, particularly for managing virtual classrooms: ICT incorporation into the introduced educational approaches; creating a learning chunk (educational segment) using the best methodologies and technologies involving the students in a trainer-led activity in a virtual classroom.

The course was offered via the GSuite platform. All the materials and resources have been shared in a course that has been set up on the Classroom App. Google Forms has been utilized to ask for some tasks, whereas GMeet has been used for synchronous activities.

The first approach to train the faculties to enhance skills and abilities in the adaptation of ICT tools was to gauge students' knowledge of their fundamental ICT abilities and skills. For this purpose, teachers administered an admission test that was prepared using Google Forms and shared on Classroom. To be more precise, this was the learning tool they employed during the Covid emergency.

The Impact of Training

(i) Teachers gained comfort developing courses, distributing files, links, and Google Drive materials, assigning homework, and sharing a window or a screen.

(ii) Methodologies for teaching and learning should be active and student-centered. Students and instructors should have a mutually beneficial connection, and the teacher should act more as a mentor than as a source of information.

- Learning materials from textbooks are converted into electronic books (e-books).
- Newspapers, publications, and scholarly journals converted to web platforms.
- Laboratory activities such as practical experiments, research activities continued on software simulation laboratory applications, and virtual labs.
- Social interactions continued on videos on YouTube, Google Meet, Microsoft Teams, and the Zoom app.
- Cognitive resources using sharing platforms to manage working groups to facilitate cognitive learning.
- E-training increased ICT capabilities and abilities, and as a result, more conscious use of ICT helped with better lesson preparation and resource management.

Resources Useful for Teaching in the Online Platform

- Organizing and planning software for learning chunks
- All the social learning resources
- Cloud software is used to exchange educational resources between teachers and other teachers, teachers, and students, and students and students laboratory tasks, social media apps (Google Meet, Zoom, Microsoft Teams) were used.
- Virtual laboratories are required to conduct virtual experiments and better understand the subjects.

Finally, if students, faculties, and researchers are aware of and make efficient use of all the ICT and multimedia resources then the Covid-19 pandemic definitely supports teachers' professional growth without harming their physical health.

Solving Issues with a Computer Using Hypermedia Games

Multimedia adventure games can be thought of as information sets with predetermined questions and possible questions pathways. The number of potential paths, the degree of sophistication and difficulty, and the complexity of the solutions to predetermined questions or problems all vary in this type of game typically.

The use of adventure games for problem-solving strategies is supported by the following factors:

1. **Support and help**: The interactive nature of these games allows the computer to provide the students with feedback, assistance, and support. Children in this learning environment probably still require some guidance from a teacher.
2. **Adjusting to a range of reactions**: Games that are well-made offer a wide range of possible responses. One of the crucial factors in determining the degree of cognitive demand in these games is the range of responses. There are numerous approaches to solving problems. One benefit is that students are presented with a variety of response options, allowing them to respond from various points of view. From a less positive perspective, this required element of providing potential solutions may restrict students' creativity.
3. **Effectiveness of time**: The majority of games are well made and offer the option to save the data at any time and come back to it later.
4. **Learning through experience**. Computer games provide countless opportunities for problem-solving experimentation. In a very short amount of time, the students can experiment with the various options. In practice, it is challenging to offer this kind of learning through trial and error over an appropriate period of time, and it is frequently impossible to test various hypotheses in the fields of science.
5. **Commitment and enthusiasm**. Children adore these games because they put everything in a meaningful context within a captivating fictional world that appears to be alive and well.

The coordination of a variety of difficult and related skills is required when solving problems. These skills include:

- Recognizing the type of information that is pertinent for the solution and understanding and representing the problem
- Collecting and arranging
- Creating and managing a strategy or plan
- Reasoning, testing hypotheses and making decisions

- Using a variety of tools for problem-solving, keeping an eye on fixes, and assessing outcomes.

Collaborative Learning

With multimedia, information can be accessed from any corner of the world for better teaching and learning experience. The current generation of teachers/learners is surrounded by new technologies. They are highly connected with digital platforms and the internet in order to stay in touch with friends/family, for knowledge acquisition, or to find information whenever they want.

Multimedia plays an important role in the teaching/learning process. Collaborative learning has always been recommended as it motivates learners to learn from each other. Collaborative learning is a promising approach to acquiring knowledge. Multimedia can be used as a means to foster this collaborative learning process.

The use of multimedia helps in creating a platform for teachers/learners to have active discussions on curriculum, debates, and different approaches to finding a solution to any given problem. Collaborative learning using multimedia allows students to ponder the learning objective and to collectively take decisions on problem-solving. It encourages teachers/learners to not only share knowledge and information but also help and support each other. A learner, therefore, has a better cognitive approach to the subject.

With the help of multimedia, national and international teacher/learner networks can be created to exchange teaching/learning methods. This network community can create, edit or distribute content on any subject. The content can be wikis, blogs, podcasts, and a world digital library (manuscripts, maps, rare books, audio files, recordings, films, prints, images, and drawings). Journals can be published on a certain topic. It can be open to the public domain for readers to post comments. Audio and video files can be created and distributed or shared with the peer community. All this can be downloaded when the need arises. They are easy to create, share and consume. The students can choose from the digital resources available for reference learning. Teachers/learners can be the end users or source producers. It provides easy access to education for research and information at the tip of our fingers. The use of multimedia in teaching/learning makes the entire process interesting and interactive.

A student can post about their project, and get a review from global learners. Peer communication is encouraged where the members can post questions or ideas. The classroom activities can be stored. The students who remain absent can access them whenever they want. Also, the teacher can assess the student's work. They can keep a track of the assignments and projects and evaluate and contribute to the work, by giving useful information or by making corrections.

When students learn in groups collaboratively, there is an improved outcome. Students work together, interact, and become open to different perspectives. They work in groups, mutually searching for solutions or to understand a concept.

In collaborative learning, students can search, research a topic, analyze, discuss and gather the information needed. It challenges their thinking competencies towards having critical thinking, reflecting on a subject, and problem-solving methods. They can evaluate each other's work and thereby encourage peer review.

Collaborative learning works well for all types of students. When top achievers give elaborate explanations on a presented topic, it results in asking more questions which only deepens the existing knowledge base. It creates a sense of motivation to learn and to encourage their classmates to learn. All this leads to better peer tutoring, practice, assessment, correction, and overall development. Collaborative learning demands responsibility, patience, and persistence but the outcome is that it develops a community of active and critical students that are mutually involved to participate and grow intellectually.

Use of Multimedia for Assessment and Examination

Tests are usually conducted to evaluate a student's performance or skill. The global pandemic has challenged the vulnerabilities that exist in conventional assessment/examination methods. Digital assessment, computer-based digital assessment, e-assessment, and online assessment techniques can be implemented using multimedia to conduct examinations and evaluate a learner's knowledge outcome. They create better assessment ways to help understand where students who are having trouble with the material are having issues.

It becomes an alternative approach to the traditional pen-paper method. The tests can be conducted online with the help of the internet or a computer-based facility. The assessment can include multiple choice questions, online and offline task submissions, descriptive and objective writing, etc. With this method, the process of conducting tests, assessments, and evaluations becomes much easier. Proctoring solutions could be provided to avoid cheating in examinations. Integrating the Web, digital video, sound, animations, and interactivity, in the assessment tools can make assessment design and implementation more efficient, timely, and sophisticated.

Multimedia can be used for summative or formative evaluation during examinations. Depending on their preferred learning methods, formative assessment enables students to demonstrate their learning in a variety of ways. Examiners can now conduct better formative assessments thanks to technology, especially with the use of classroom response systems (CRS). A CRS is a tool in which each student has a portable device that connects to the computer of the teacher. The pupils respond to the examiner's questions by posting their own on their devices. The answers may then be shown on a graph so that students and the assessor may observe the proportion of students who provided each response and conduct analysis.

Summative tests or projects with predetermined grading scales are more prevalent in classrooms and are designed to be easier to grade. The ability to provide students with rapid feedback on their responses is a big advantage of using multimedia during the assessment process. Students are able to gauge their performance in the classroom when they receive these replies, which can either inspire them to do better or boost their self-assurance. Different learners can demonstrate what they learned more effectively using different summative assessment methods, such as digital presentations, movies, and others that the teacher or student may come up with. Teachers can upload graded tests online so students can access them.

Grading is an examiner-led activity that is interlinked with evaluation or assessment. Here the examiners grade or mark the answer scripts online or on the computer facility. Multiple choice assessments can be manually marked or auto-marked. On the completion of the exams, the results can also be uploaded and stored. With the help of multimedia, evaluation becomes easier.

There are several advantages to using the multimedia-based examination.

1. Convenience: Students do not have to travel to a particular place to give the examinations. They can give their examination from any remote place.
2. Integrity: The integrity of the assessment/examination is maintained. The proctoring solutions make it a highly secure process.
3. Scalable: A large number of students can attend the examinations from different locations.
4. Evaluation: This mode of proctored assessment and evaluation gives less scope for human error.
5. Time: The entire process consumes less time and is easy.

There are a few disadvantages with respect to using multimedia in the assessment or examination process. They are as follows:

1. Usability issues during the exam
2. Increased stress level due to unfamiliarity with e-exam systems
3. Inadequate functionality.

Physical Education Using Multimedia

The effectiveness of many physical education lessons can be greatly enhanced by the video teaching method. It presents education through images, animations, and sounds. The use of images and videos in the classroom not only enhances but also increases the convenience of instruction. Employees who live distant from their place of instruction or who have limited time can also use this method effectively. Using different technologies, analysis of the activities of teachers and students can be performed in video teaching methods. These analysis results can be utilized to improve the efficiency of teaching and learning. The use of interactive teaching methods and multimedia technologies in physical education classrooms can increase students' interest in learning and increase the effectiveness of their learning. In order for learning and evaluation plans to be based on interactive electronic resources, teachers must implement modern learning theories. Physical education has various restrictions when compared to other academic fields. These restrictions include the type of equipment, the size of the facility, the surrounding environment, and the weather; all of them have an impact on the teaching process. Due to the disparities in physical education instruction, it is essential to employ a rich media teaching system to enhance the quality of physical education instruction. The shortcomings of traditional physical education teaching can be perfectly replaced by the rich network teaching system [11].

Multimedia and interactive instruction can enhance one another and improve learning by strengthening its scientific foundation. The annealing algorithm is used to evaluate the effectiveness of interactive multimedia on physical education by building a model. This multimedia is based on the traditional method itself but receives input from all sensory channels. Teaching effects of PE classes are studied using the said algorithm. People from different background are chosen to create the model. Evaluation subjects chosen are students, peer teachers, experts, and lecturers themselves. Students can evaluate if the teaching serves their purpose of learning and how the teaching contributes to their development. A peer teacher evaluates the knowledge of the subject a teacher is handling, his teaching style and teaching methods used. An expert hired by the management can evaluate the performance of the teacher on a regular basis. Teachers can self-evaluate their teaching methods to obtain the results. Evaluation indicators are to be decided to create the evaluation model. Results of learning, interactive sessions handled by the teacher, and resources used can be the indicators to evaluate the effectiveness of multimedia teaching. The feasibility of the model developed based on the annealing algorithm is verified through a comparative study. The results of the comparison show that the evaluation model has high processing efficiency and results in the improvement of students' PE learning [12].

A multimedia tennis training system is designed to improve the learning process and to make teaching effective. 5G Internet of Things technology can be used for the production of the multimedia system. The multimedia education system prepares the students to learn effortlessly; creating curiosity among them inspires their own initiative to learn. It also supports the reform and growth of education. These systems have remote management of students learning by the teacher, structure assignments more scientifically, and provide students with greater receptivity to teachers' plans. Prior to designing the system requirement analysis needs to be done to ensure the need for developing the multimedia-based system. Users of the multimedia teaching system can peruse lesson resources, proposal summaries, instruction films, and instruction images, and engage in virtual messaging and question-and-answer sessions, while supervisors can carry out information organization tasks through the multimedia teaching system [13].

Liu G and Zhuang H have proposed an assessment prototype based on the random number forest algorithm. The teaching level of the PE network is analyzed and evaluation of the instruction outcome is done using the random forest algorithm and quality evaluation index. A multimedia instruction evaluation index prototype can be created by thoroughly analyzing the four components in accordance with the evaluation objectives. The components involved are instructors, learners, instruction courseware, and education platform. The evaluation system defines the teaching process, the effectiveness of the teaching, and the assessment methods used. Evaluating indicators are chosen from different categories such as education approach, content, instructor's excellence, capability, technique, and effectiveness [14].

Zhao M. suggested a data fusion approach to improving the teaching mode which is based on a multimedia network. It also optimizes the comparable node clustering algorithm based on K-means to make it more appropriate for the teaching monitoring of flipped classrooms in college physical education. Results of the evaluation of physical fitness, learning interest, and skill enhancements are tabulated in a paper. Comparative analysis is also done based on the obtained result. The result showed improved enthusiasm among students for the new education model suggested [15].

Lian S. has used BP neural network algorithm to estimate the appropriate information of badminton major students in an institute. A comparison of physical fitness and performance measurements are done before and after the experiment. The outcomes of the experiment demonstrate how effectively using multimedia technology to teach badminton can raise student interest and happiness in the sport while also enhancing their physical fitness and badminton performance [16].

Gu Y. discussed the benefits of the Internet of Things on college pupils' volleyball and table tennis skill learning. The teaching quality and efficiency of PE teachers can be improved by integrating IoT and PE. The author has built a teaching mode of IoT and volleyball spiking technology. He also combined two modes of technology to teach table tennis to analyze its effectiveness on the same [17].

Computer-Assisted Instruction (CAI) multimedia uses computers as its primary teaching tool. It supports teaching and learning using the computer technology which can be used to store, process and present the information to teachers and students. CAI is the blending of educational content from multiple media, giving students a vibrant, engaging, convenient, and adaptable user interface, completing various teaching activities via human-computer interaction, and optimising the learning process and goals [18].

A multimedia-based model developed for PE has three main parts: physical teaching platform, teachers' module and students' module. Many platforms are used to connect teacher and student such as CAI software, virtual reality system, PowerPoint resource, video demonstration, etc. The teachers' module includes teaching plan, designing teaching process, selection of multimedia, and collection of course content. The students' module comprises classroom learning platform, online learning platform, scheduling learning activity and giving feedbacks of teaching quality to teachers. Results of the evaluation are presented through a graph to draw a conclusion that the proposed method can enhance the effectiveness of PE and encourage student interest in physical education [19].

The use of multimedia network technology is essential to increasing the effectiveness of instruction, piquing student interest, developing their capacity for innovation, and expanding the scope of their learning. In order for multimedia information to naturally link with one another and develop into an interactive, new type of computer system technology, it refers to the integrated use of computer technology to deal with a wide range of media information, such as text, sound, graphics, photos, animation, and video. Multimedia technology is nothing but an information processing technology, a human-computer interaction technology, and a technology to integrate different media with different applications. The technology developed for teaching purposes should be multidimensional, capable of enlarging and expanding the information available. The information available could be integrated into a single piece of information; different systems available should be able to integrate to create multimedia information. It should have an interaction capability whether it may be human–to–human or human–to–machine. The information used should be in digital form so that it can be processed or stored in a computer system [20].

When employing educational technology, we should pay more attention to how the tools and apps are used, how capable they are in the information acquired, how users and tools interact, and the beneficial effects of their use. Teachers should use software tools that should have educational value, improve student involvement in learning, are easy to use, and involve interaction capability. They need assessment tools as well to monitor the development of student interest and behavior towards physical education.

Business English Learning Using Multimedia

Yanyan Xin used data mining and multimedia technologies to assess the effectiveness of business English instruction. In the beginning, the association rule recommendation method employing data mining is used to the multimedia data that are gathered throughout classes. Indicators for evaluating the quality of teaching in colleges and universities are made based on collaborative filtering algorithms in association rules. Next, genuine university teaching data is utilized. The developed method is examined using business English as an example. The algorithm's use is tested, and the College Business English teaching methodology is assessed. Finally, it is concluded that data mining technology has the potential to become more widely used and can characterize and assess effective teaching behavior [21].

The competence of Business English majors can be improved by combining multimedia networks with field practice. Online teaching hours can be extended by employing multimedia networks as a teaching tool, allowing for more personalized instruction. Teachers could design their own assessment methods and give tasks to students based on their study pace. Multimedia networks offer multi-interactive strategies that encourage student collaboration and communication. Multimedia networks could be used to design and offer teamwork and communication instruction to students. A computer-sssisted language learning system focuses on enhancing instructional methods, instructional resources, and instructional environment [22].

Multimedia courseware benefits from display integration, hyperlink selection, human-computer interaction functionality, the richness of large-capacity storage, and ease of high-speed transmission, among other things. It is capable of realising the integrated integration of science, art, and technology in the classroom. The flexible use of multimedia in corporate English instruction has produced outstanding teaching results, and higher education has always placed a strong emphasis on the student-centered, teacher-led teaching paradigm. The teaching contents in Business English teaching should be multidimensional based on teaching requirements [23].

The issue of employing multimedia teaching tools to teach Business English at higher education institutions is discussed by Olena Karpova. The use of multimedia tools in teaching business English in its modern forms, methods, and strategies has been taken into consideration. The author has described the elements, idiosyncrasies, and classroom applications of the multimedia method. Research techniques like surveys, exams, quizzes, educational experiments, and statistical math techniques have all been used. According to the author, multimedia technology is a subset of pedagogical technology that denotes the arrangement of a learning process that mixes conventional forms, instructional strategies, and methodologies with multimedia resources and products. The components of the newly introduced multimedia have been identified as interactive methods and techniques, multimedia tools, and multimedia goods [24].

Zhang B. has studied the creation and development possibilities of a system for teaching business English that is built on computer multimedia technology, collects teaching data using computer vision technology, and then teaches using virtual reality. In order to give machines the same visual abilities as people and even the capacity to "think," computer vision primarily investigates ways to employ video-sensing devices and computers to replicate the human visual system for the collection and processing of external visual input. In order to develop new teaching techniques for business English subjects, analyze the teaching purpose, content, and viability, and investigate the challenges and needs of students in business English subject learning to determine the educational methods in a smart way, computer vision technology is connected to the teaching of business English courses through virtual teaching design and research. The methods used include questionnaires, experiments, interviews, and literature reviews. This article also sets up a virtual hypothesis experiment to objectively analyze the development prospects of educational methods in an intelligent environment in business English teaching from the aspects of curriculum teaching, classroom effects, and learner efficiency; it then summarizes the areas that require improvement. The techniques mentioned are explained using Maya and other software's multidimensional design functions [25].

Despite its many drawbacks, multimedia technology has allowed language teachers to become more effective teachers of English. Even though language classes use multimedia technology, there are still interactions between students and professors because the aural, visual, and textual effects on students increase their attention. It replaces computer sound and visual picture analysis for the teachers' instructions. This gives students very little time for interaction. It fails to take into account how students think on the spot, boosting their capacity to learn and correct problems. Although students in a class utilizing multimedia technologies are able to swiftly absorb the material, their ability to think abstractly is constrained, and their ability to reason logically is lost. The use of multimedia technologies is a pricey and ineffective way to teach English [26].

Conclusion

Multimedia has many benefits that makes learning engaging. It can inspire creativity in teachers and students so that they can use it to teach or learn with the aid of its elements. With the aid of multimedia, learning has become much simpler. Multimedia can help our educational system become better.

Some of the obstacles mentioned in the various articles include teachers' lack of resistance and confidence to adapt, their beliefs and attitudes regarding the use of multimedia technology in the classroom, their lack of ICT skills and fundamental knowledge, their lack of financial support, administrative, and, technical support and their lack of a physical environment. These barriers make it difficult to use multimedia in education.

Depending on the type of multimedia tool, target groups, deployment strategies, technology components, and, application area the learning outcomes and evaluation methodologies of the multimedia tools will vary. The advancement of technology will also increase the learners' enthusiasm.

References

[1] Asthana, A. (2008). Multimedia in Education. In: Furht, B. (eds.) *Encyclopedia of Multimedia*. Springer, Boston, MA. https://doi.org/10.1007/978-0-387-78414-4_140.

[2] Reiber, L. P. *Computers, Graphics, & Learning*. Dubuque, IA: Wm. C. Brown Communications. Inc., Brown & Benchmark (1994).
[3] Mayer, Richard E., and Richard B. Anderson. "Animations need narrations: An experimental test of a dual-coding hypothesis." *Journal of Educational Psychology* 83, no. 4 (1991): 484.
[4] Standing, Lionel. "Learning 10000 pictures." *Quarterly Journal of Experimental* Psychology 25, no. 2 (1973): 207-222.
[5] Haber, Ralph Norman. "How we remember what we see." *Scientific American* 222, no. 5 (1970): 104-115.
[6] Levin, Joel R., and Alan M. Lesgold. "On pictures in prose." *ECTJ* 26, no. 3 (1978): 233-243.
[7] Simpson, Cynthia Lane. A comparative study of teachers' perceptions of traditional teaching and teaching with technology: Pre-technology era and post-technology era. University of Alabama, 2013.
[8] Chambers, Bette, Alan CK Cheung, Nancy A. Madden, Robert E. Slavin, and Richard Gifford. "Achievement effects of embedded multimedia in a success for all reading program." *Journal of Educational Psychology* 98, no. 1 (2006): 232.
[9] Asyhar, Rayandra. "Kreatif mengembangkan media pembelajaran." (2021).
[10] Mayer, Richard E. "Cognitive theory and the design of multimedia instruction: an example of the two-way street between cognition and instruction." *New Directions for Teaching and Learning* 2002, no. 89 (2002): 55-71.
[11] Zou W, Li Y, Shan X, Wu X. Application of Data Fusion and Image Video Teaching Mode in Physical Education Course Teaching and Evaluation of Teaching Effect. *Security and Communication Networks*. 2022 Mar 21;2022.
[12] Zhao M. Effect of Interactive Multimedia PE Teaching Based on the Simulated Annealing Algorithm. *Journal of Information Processing Systems*. 2022 Aug 1;18(4):562-74.
[13] Chen H, Yang Y, Xie S. Topic Search Algorithm for Network Multimedia Tennis Teaching Resources Using 5G-Enabled Internet of Things Technology. *Wireless Communications and Mobile Computing*. 2022 May 9;2022.
[14] Liu G, Zhuang H. Evaluation model of multimedia-aided teaching effect of physical education course based on random forest algorithm. *Journal of Intelligent Systems* 2022 Jan 1;31(1):555-67.
[15] Zhao M. College Physical Education Flipped Classroom Teaching Based on Multimedia Network Data Fusion. *Wireless Communications and Mobile Computing*. 2022 Mar 7;2022.
[16] Lian S. Experimental Research on Badminton Teaching of Physical Education Major Based on Deep Learning in the Multimedia Environment. *Computational Intelligence and Neuroscience*. 2022 Mar 16;2022.
[17] Gu Y. Deep Integration of Physical Education and Multimedia Technology Using Internet of Things Technology. *Wireless Communications and Mobile Computing*. 2022 Jun 23, 2022.

[18] Hu X, Peng C, Li M. Multimedia Image in Physical Education. *Wireless Communications and Mobile Computing*. 2022 May 4;2022.

[19] Dan L. Study on the college physical education mode utilizing multimedia technology. In 2013 *Fourth International Conference on Intelligent Systems Design and Engineering Applications* 2013 Nov 6 (pp. 601-604). IEEE.

[20] Tan Z, Li S. Multimedia technology in physical education. In *2009 International Symposium on Computer Network and Multimedia Technology* 2009 Jan 18 (pp. 1-4). IEEE.

[21] Xin Y. Analyzing the quality of business English teaching using multimedia data mining. *Mobile Information Systems*. 2021 May 17;2021.

[22] Cheng X, Liu K. Application of multimedia networks in business English teaching in vocational college. *Journal of Healthcare Engineering*. 2021 Apr 29;2021.

[23] Xing Y. Application of Multimedia Technology in Business English Interactive Teaching. In *Journal of Physics: Conference Series* 2019 Oct 1 (Vol. 1314, No. 1, p. 012166). IOP Publishing.

[24] Karpova O. The implementation of the multimedia approach to teaching business English. *Advanced Education*. 2017 Dec 27:10-5.

[25] Zhang B. Research on the Construction and Development Prospect of Aided Business English Teaching System Based on Computer Multimedia Technology. *Mobile Information Systems*. 2022 Jul 31;2022.

[26] Kumar T, Malabar S, Benyo A, Amal BK. Analyzing multimedia tools and language teaching. *Linguistics and Culture Review*. 2021 Aug 6;5(S1):331-41.

10

Assessment of Adjusted and Normalized Mutual Information Variants for Band Selection in Hyperspectral Imagery

Bhagyashree Chopade, Vikas Gupta and Divyesh Varade*

Technocrats Institute of Technology, Bhopal, India and Indian Institute of Technology Jammu, Jammu, India

Abstract

Similarity measures from information theory are widely used in feature selection, particularly based on mutual information. Although several methods exist for feature selection in hyperspectral data utilizing information theory-based approaches, seldom are all aspects of information utilized in the developed techniques. Various normalization, adjustment and weighing schemes have been proposed in the literature for mutual information. However, a detailed investigation of these schemes for feature selection is lacking. In this study, we investigate the normalization scheme for different variants of mutual information for unsupervised feature selection in hyperspectral data. We also examine the potential of adjusted mutual information for the selection of best bands in hyperspectral data. We define a novel scheme for the computation of the expectation of mutual information based on the concept that the mutual information between the mean filtered hyperspectral bands at different neighbourhood sizes yield different mutual information with respect to a reference image. Using this concept to determine the expectation of mutual information satisfies the constant baseline criteria used in the adjusted mutual information. The first principal component is used for the reference image. Further, we propose a novel scheme to utilize weighted normalized mutual information for computing the adjusted mutual information. The weights for the mutual information normalization are computed based on the sharpness factor of the images that is determined by subtracting a median filtered image from itself. The potential of the different normalized and adjusted mutual information

**Corresponding author*: varadedm@gmail.com

Suman Kumar Swarnkar, J P Patra, Sapna Singh Kshatri, Yogesh Kumar Rathore and Tien Anh Tran (eds.) Supervised and Unsupervised Data Engineering for Multimedia Data, (217–246) © 2024 Scrivener Publishing LLC

for feature selection is identified by performing a supervised classification of the selected bands using the Random Forest classifier. The investigations are conducted using four state-of- the-art hyperspectral datasets including the Indian Pines, Salinas, Pavia University and Dhundi datasets. We performed experiments following a two-case strategy where in the first case, the training samples were fixed at 20% and in the second case, the number of selected bands were fixed at 20. The experimental results revealed that for the first case, the weighted normalized and weighted adjusted sum variants of mutual information were observed to show better performance for feature selection. For the second case, the sum variants of normalized and adjusted sum variants of mutual information are observed to perform better for feature selection. In general, it can be noted that the normalization by sum of individual entropies can be preferred for development of feature selection methods incorporating mutual information.

Keywords: Mutual information, normalized mutual information, adjusted mutual information, feature selection, band selection, hyperspectral

Introduction

With the advances in electronic chip manufacturing and sensor technology, hyperspectral imaging has seen a rapid development and significant application as an emerging scientific tool. Hyperspectral imaging derives its essence by enabling direct identification of surfaces by imaging [1]. Hyperspectral imaging sensors have been utilized in various applications, including material characterization to Earth observation [2]. In a study, hyperspectral data was used for the identification of different tree species corresponding to various forest and vegetation classes [3]. Hyperspectral imaging has also essentially developed as an imaging modality in medical sciences for surgical operations and diagnosis [4].

Hyperspectral imaging techniques have also been utilized in recent studies for investigations of the quality of agricultural produce such as fruits and vegetables [5]. Hyperspectral data combined with various processing techniques have also been used for investigating plant biodiversity and mapping specific invasive species [6, 7]. Other studies have shown the capability of hyperspectral signatures in the investigations of faunal biodiversity of fisheries [8]. Varade *et al.* [9] utilized hyperspectral data for the retrieval of various spectral indices for identification of vegetation and snow. With a plethora of techniques based on hyperspectral data, there have been significant developments in Earth observation, particularly focused on vegetation, agriculture, soil, geology, urban, land use land cover

(LULC), water resources and disasters [10]. However, in several of these applications, the issues related to the higher dimensionality in striking a tradeoff between the requisite precision, resource, and computational efficiency have to be dealt with [11–13].

Issues of Higher Dimensionality

Typically, a hyperspectral sensor provides spectral imaging in hundreds of narrow continuously spaced bands over a wide range of the electromagnetic spectrum covering the visible and short-wave infrared regions [14]. Understandably, having a larger number of bands of narrow spectral width is advantageous in classification of complex scenarios such as in LULC applications [14]. However, the availability of a higher number of narrow hyperspectral bands demands the requirement of an exponentially increased number of training samples to ensure statistical confidence in the classification results [13].

For example, consider a scenario for identification of 10 classes based on a hyperspectral dataset comprising 100s of narrow bands and a coverage of 1000x1000 pixels. The classification process will require an extremely large training sample set for each of the classes to ensure high classification accuracy. In essence, broadband multispectral images can be classified in a much simpler manner using fewer training samples for each class. However, the higher dimensionality of hyperspectral data allows not only identification of a greater number of classes but possibilities for identifying micro-level classes also. For establishing sufficient classification accuracy, classifier training is often challenging considering the large volume of samples required for training. The classifier training may thus often be an issue during the lack of sufficient training samples with a higher dimensionality of the data [14, 15]. Hence, the benefits of hyperspectral imaging are curbed by the issues of dimensionality often associated with what is known as the Hughes Phenomenon or the curse of dimensionality [15].

Dimensionality Reduction

Dimensionality reduction is simply the process of obtaining a set of principal variables from a number of random variables. In the case of hyperspectral imagery, this corresponds to the extraction of most informative bands or features accomplished through two well-defined processes, i.e., feature extraction and feature selection. Dimensionality reduction introduces the benefits of increased computational efficiency and performance, and decreased constraints on model training time. Additional advantages of dimensionality reduction have been known to be removal of noise in the hyperspectral data, avoidance of model overfitting issue, ease in data visualization, and data compression.

Feature Extraction

Feature extraction aims to reduce the hyperspectral data by generating smaller partitions of the initial set of observations that can be used for model training and analysis. The general traits of feature extraction algorithms include selection, integration, or assimilation of different variables into features that represent efficiently the full scope of the large volume data to be analysed or processed. Simultaneously, the higher performance or efficiency of the retrieved information needs to be ensured in feature extraction [14, 16, 17]. Feature extraction methods in hyperspectral dimensionality reduction based on statistical component analysis transforms have been widely known to be efficient [16]. However, feature extraction algorithms are used in applications that require label prediction and avoided in applications requiring analysis based on the reflectance spectra since these algorithms alter the source reflectance characteristics of the data [18].

Feature Selection

The narrowband imaging, meaning very low separation between adjacent wavelengths in hyperspectral remote sensing, introduces two issues. Firstly, a significant level of redundance in the information retrieval from the adjacent bands of the same broad wavelength spectrum, and secondly, the poor signal-to- noise ratio in some of the bands, typically the shortwave infrared bands which exhibit relatively lower target reflectance. Subsequently, most of the meaningful information can be represented by a smaller subset of the source hyperspectral feature set. The process of determination of this smaller subset is typically referred to as feature selection or in the case of hyperspectral data as band selection [16]. The methods for feature selection are broadly categorized into wrapper, filter, embedded and hybrid approach [19].

The univariate statistics such as the correlation coefficient that defines the intrinsic properties of bands are used in the filter methods. Typically, such methods are parametric in a sense that a parameter such as the correlation coefficient has to be derived for each combination of bands for their ranking. However, advances in such approaches include methods which derive similarity of each of the bands with respect to a reference [20], and are focused on in this study. Wrappers search the full dimensionality of the source data for bands, and utilizing classifier learning with band sets to ascertain their quality. Usually, these are supervised methods and are relatively computationally exhaustive. Embedded methods combine the advantages of wrappers and filters iteratively in an optimization scheme based on specific application models such as classification, target detection, etc. Hybrid methods implement multiple hybrid schemes combining the wrapper and filter methods for selecting the most informative band set [19].

The General Architecture of Feature Selection Experiments

In the previous section, we observed that feature extraction and feature/band selection techniques are widely used for the dimensionality reduction of hyperspectral data. In general, it is known that before the deployment of any technique, it must be validated with respect to a reference. The common strategy for the evaluation of the band selection methods is shown in Figure 10.1. Due to the high dimensionality (100s of bands in hyperspectral data), it is not possible to manually organize the bands with respect to their level of information to match the best bands determined by the selection technique. However, it is possible to ascertain the potential of the selected band set with respect to the reference data or ground truth. This is possible by employing supervised classification techniques and observing the accuracy statistics. However, two problems persist with conventional feature selection methods, (1) determination of the number of bands to be selected which is often a user-supplied parameter, (2) loss of information when an inappropriate band is a selection. The latter is easily identified from the reduced classification accuracy with respect to the reference.

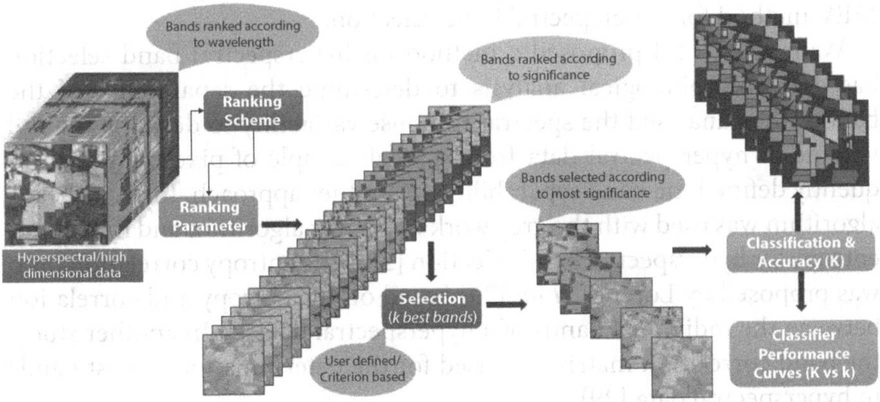

Figure 10.1 Evaluation strategy for band selection methods used for dimensionality reduction of hyperspectral data.

The general approach as shown in Figure 10.1 follows a ranking scheme for the hyperspectral bands based on ranking parameters such as the correlation coefficient or mutual information, and subsequently the bands are ranked in descending order of their significance. A user-defined or criterion-based number of bands k are then selected from the ranked list of bands. The most informative band subset is then passed to a classifier to assess the accuracy. In order to assess the appropriateness of the selected band set a performance curve representing the comparison of Kappa coefficient and the number of bands is generated to evaluate the band selection method.

Developments in Feature Selection Methods

Edge-preserved filtering for improving the classification results was used for identification of best bands in hyperspectral data in a wrapper method by [21]. In a study, a multigraph determinantal point process (MDPP) model based on the structure between various bands of hyperspectral data was developed for band selection [22]. Nagasubramanian *et al.* [23] proposed an approach combining support vector machines with genetic algorithms for hyperspectral band selection in an effort to detect early detection of diseases in Soybeans. Cao *et al.* [24] developed a spectral-spatial approach in a semi-supervised framework for improving hyperspectral band selection with a lower volume of training samples. They proposed two algorithms, the first was based on utilizing the classification map to derive statistical characteristics for predicting the sample quality, and the second was based on Markov random field (MRF) model. The maximum ellipsoid volume (MEV) was used for hyperspectral band selection in [25]. [26] combined a sequential forward search algorithm with the MEV method for hyperspectral band selection.

Wang *et al.* [27] proposed a method for hyperspectral band selection based on morphological analysis to determine the separability of the bands. They analysed the spectral response variability to describe the full volume of hyperspectral data from a small sample of pixels, and subsequently defined the band separability. In another approach, fuzzy c-means algorithm was used with the grey work optimizer algorithm and maximum entropy for hyperspectral band selection [28]. The entropy correlation ratio was proposed by Lorencs *et al.* [29] based on the entropy and correlation between the individual bands of a hyperspectral dataset. In another study, the band correlation matrix was used for the determination of best bands in hyperspectral data [29].

Habermann *et al.* [30] proposed a supervised approach for band selection utilizing a binary single layer neural network for discriminating each class from the other for generating weights for each of the classes in an effort to select best bands. Luo *et al.* [31] developed an approach for band selection based on the active gradient reference (AGR) index derived iteratively from a reference gradient map. Several approaches have also existed based on application of deep learning and machine learning techniques for hyperspectral band selection [32]. In Jiang *et al.* [33], a two-step strategy is utilized where first the bands are grouped and each group is selected to ensure that the linear reconstruction error between the selected bands from the consecutive groups is minimized. Varade *et al.* [20] developed an approach for band selection based on the denoising error response of the individual bands. For each band of the dataset, the denoising error was compared with a reference for ranking the bands using different matching parameters.

Varade *et al.* [34] proposed pre-clustering of bands for the computation of mutual information for band selection. Varade *et al.* [35] proposed an advancement of the mutual information-based approach for band selection utilizing pre-clustering of bands for computation of weighted mutual information with respect to the first principal component as a reference best band. They proposed two methods for computing the weights. The first technique utilized the inter-cluster to intra-cluster distance ratio for using weighted entropies in the computation of the normalized mutual information. The second techniques utilized the fuzzy c-means cluster centroids for the weights for the entropies of the fuzzy cluster memberships in the computation of the normalized mutual information. Both these techniques utilize only the cluster properties of the bands and the reference and were found to be influenced by the presence of noise in the hyperspectral data. Chowdhury *et al.* [36] developed an approach for band selection based on entropy and mutual information utilizing a fuzzy rule-based system incorporating ant colony optimization. Pan *et al.* [37] proposed the partition optimal band selection (POBS) method for band selection based on a weight calculation formula incorporating the standard deviation, information entropy and the correlation coefficient.

Although the literature provides several methods for band selection in hyperspectral data, seldom are all aspects of information utilized in the developed techniques. A common issue with methods based on the normalized mutual information is related to the type of normalization. In the literature, investigations remain virtually unobserved to identify the optimal normalization scheme [38] for the selection of best bands in the hyperspectral data. An alternative to normalization to account for the uncertainties in the mutual information owing to the discrepancies in the individual and joint entropy is to use weighted mutual information.

Moreover, the various normalization schemes, particularly the adjusted mutual information, need to be explored from the perspective of hyperspectral band selection. Subsequently, the objective of this study is to analyse the applicability of the different normalization schemes for mutual information for hyperspectral band selection.

Test Datasets

The experiments to evaluate the potential of various MI variants were conducted using four hyperspectral datasets that includes the Indian Pines dataset, Dhundi dataset, Pavia University dataset and the Salinas dataset summarized in Table 10.1.

Table 10.1 Summary of the test datasets including the Indian Pines, Salinas, Dhundi and the Pavia University.

Indian Pines		**Salinas**	
Class	Samples	Class	Samples
Alfalfa	46	Broccoli green weeds 1	2009
Corn notill	1428	Broccoli green weeds 2	3726
Corn mintill	830	Fallow	1976
Corn	237	Fallow rough plow	1394
Grass pasture	483	Fallow smooth	2678
Grass trees	730	Stubble	3959
Grass pasture mowed	28	Celery	3579
Hay windrowed	478	Grapes untrained	11271
Oats	20	Soil vinyard develop	6203
Soybean notill	972	Corn senesced green weeds	3278
Soybean mintill	2455	Lettuce romaine 4wk	1068
Soybean clean	593	Lettuce romaine 5wk	1927
Wheat	205	Lettuce romaine 6wk	916

(Continued)

Table 10.1 Summary of the test datasets including the Indian Pines, Salinas, Dhundi and the Pavia University. (*Continued*)

Indian Pines		**Salinas**	
Class	Samples	Class	Samples
Woods	1265	Lettuce romaine 7wk	1070
Buildings Grass Trees Drives	386	Vinyard untrained	7268
Stone Steel Towers	93	Vinyard vertical trellis	1807
Pavia University		Dhundi	
Class	Samples	Class	Samples
Asphalt	6631	Snow type 1	311
Meadows	18649	Snow type 2	2211
Gravel	2099	Bare soil/land	4288
Trees	3064	Forest	127
Painted metal sheets	1345	Shadow	4097
Bare Soil	5029	Cloud	729
Bitumen	1330		
Self-blocking bricks	3682		
Shadows	947		

The Indian Pines dataset corresponds to a scene captured by the Airborne Visible/Infrared Imaging Spectrometer (AVIRIS) sensor with a spatial extent of 145x145 pixels. The scene was acquired over the Indian Pines test site in Indiana with 200 bands between 400-2500 nm wavelengths [39]. This dataset includes micro classes in vegetation and urban structure. The Dhundi dataset corresponds to a subset derived from the Hyperion imagery over the Manali region in Himachal Pradesh, India, comprising 200x200 pixels with 196 spectral bands including the primary classes attributed to snow covered Himalayas [34]. The Salinas dataset comprises a scene acquired over the Salinas valley in California comprising 204 AVIRIS bands at a spatial extent of 512x217 pixels [40] and includes primarily agricultural micro classes. The Pavia University dataset [41] covers semi-urban classes of the Pavia University area from the Reflective Optics System Imaging Spectrometer (ROSIS-3) airborne sensor. The spectral range of ROSIS-3 is between 430 to 860 nm with 115 bands. However, the Pavia University dataset comprises 103 bands as 12 noisy bands were removed. The spatial resolution of this dataset is about 1.3m, and the dimensions per band are 610x340.

Methodology

Background

The mutual information of two random variables is defined using the individual entropies of the random variables and their joint entropy. Consider a discrete random variable *A* such that *A* comprises a set of values {a1, a2, a3...., an} with a probability distribution of *P*(*A*), then the entropy of *A* is given as follows.

$$H(A) = \sum_{j=1}^{n} p(a)\, ln(p(a)) \tag{10.1}$$

Now, we may consider another discrete random variable *B*, defined by the probability distribution of *P*(*B*) taking on values {b1, b2, b3...., bn}. If the variables *A* and *B* are jointly distributed, their joint probability distribution will be defined as *P* (*A*, *B*) and the joint entropy will be defined as follows.

$$H(A,B) = \sum_{j=1}^{n} p(a,b)\, ln(p(a,b)) \tag{10.2}$$

The information similarity or the independence of the variables *A* and *B* can be measured by evaluating the MI between these variables as follows.

$$\left.\begin{aligned} I(A,B) &= \sum_{j=1}^{n} p(a,b)\, ln\left(\frac{p(a,b)}{p(a)p(b)}\right) \\ &= H(A) + H(B) - H(A,B) \end{aligned}\right\} \tag{10.3}$$

where I indicate the MI between the two random variables A and B. For any two random variables that are statistically dependent, MI > 0 and when they are statistically independent, the MI=0. However, MI is not by itself a suitable measure of statistical dependency or independency between two random variables. For example, MI can be low when either A and B present a weak relation, or their entropies are small. Thus, normalization of mutual information is widely used [42, 43].

Normalization and Adjustment Schemes for Mutual Information

The normalization of a similarity metric or distance metric is carried out to restrict its range within a fixed interval, typically [0, 1]. There are different normalization schemes possible to constrain the range of MI, such that 1 represents the strongest relationship between the two random variables, and 0 represents their independency. Additionally, the metrics should exhibit the constant baseline property such that its expected values at random samples should remain constant. Typically, the baseline value should remain zero. However, seldom do any metrics follow the constant baseline property. Thus, an adjustment scheme was proposed by Vinh *et al.* [44] to account for this issue. The various schemes for normalized MI (NMI) and corresponding adjustment MI (AMI) are shown in Table 10.2 [44].

Computation of the Mutual Information Variants

As evident from the previous background, the proposed strategy for investigating the various normalization and adjustment schemes for hyperspectral band selection first requires the determination of the individual and the joint entropies. Varade *et al.* [34] indicated an alternative approach to the forward search strategy for band selection by utilizing the global mutual information computed between each of the hyperspectral bands and a reference that is the ground truth for the supervised selection and the first principal component in the case of unsupervised selection. Further, in Varade *et al.* [35], the first principal component was shown to produce relatively better classification results as compared to the best band of hyperspectral datasets. In the proposed approach, as shown in Figure 10.1, we follow a similar strategy. Thus, the individual entropy for a particular band (X) amongst the N bands of hyperspectral data (X) and the joint entropy of X with the first principal component PC1 which is selected as reference R. Then the mutual information between the band X and the reference R is shown in equation 10.4.

Table 10.2 The different types of NMI and corresponding AMI variants according to Vinh *et al.* [44].

Variant	Normalization scheme	Relation
Normalized Mutual Information	Joint entropy	$NMI_{jt} = \frac{I(A,B)}{H(A,B)}$
	Maximum of individual entropies	$NMI \frac{I(A,B)}{\max\{H(A),H(B)\}}_{max}$
	Sum of individual entropies	$NMI_{sum} = \frac{2I(A,B)}{H(A)+H(B)}$
	Square root of the product of individual entropies	$NMI_{sqrt} = \frac{I(A,B)}{\sqrt{H(A)H(B)}}$
	Minimum of individual entropies	$NMI \frac{I(A,B)}{\min\{H(A),H(B)\}}_{min}$
Adjusted Mutual Information	Maximum of individual entropies	$AMI \frac{I(A,B)-E\{I(A,B)\}}{\max\{H(A),H(B)\}-E\{I(A,B)\}}_{max}$
	Sum of individual entropies	$AMI_{sum} = \frac{I(A,B)-E\{I(A,B)\}}{\frac{1}{2}[H(A)+H(B)]-E\{I(A,B)\}}$
	Square root of the product of individual entropies	$AMI_{sqrt} = \frac{I(A,B)-E\{I(A,B)\}}{\sqrt{H(A)H(B)}-E\{I(A,B)\}}$
	Minimum of individual entropies	$AMI \frac{I(A,B)-E\{I(A,B)\}}{\min\{H(A),H(B)\}-E\{I(A,B)\}}_{min}$

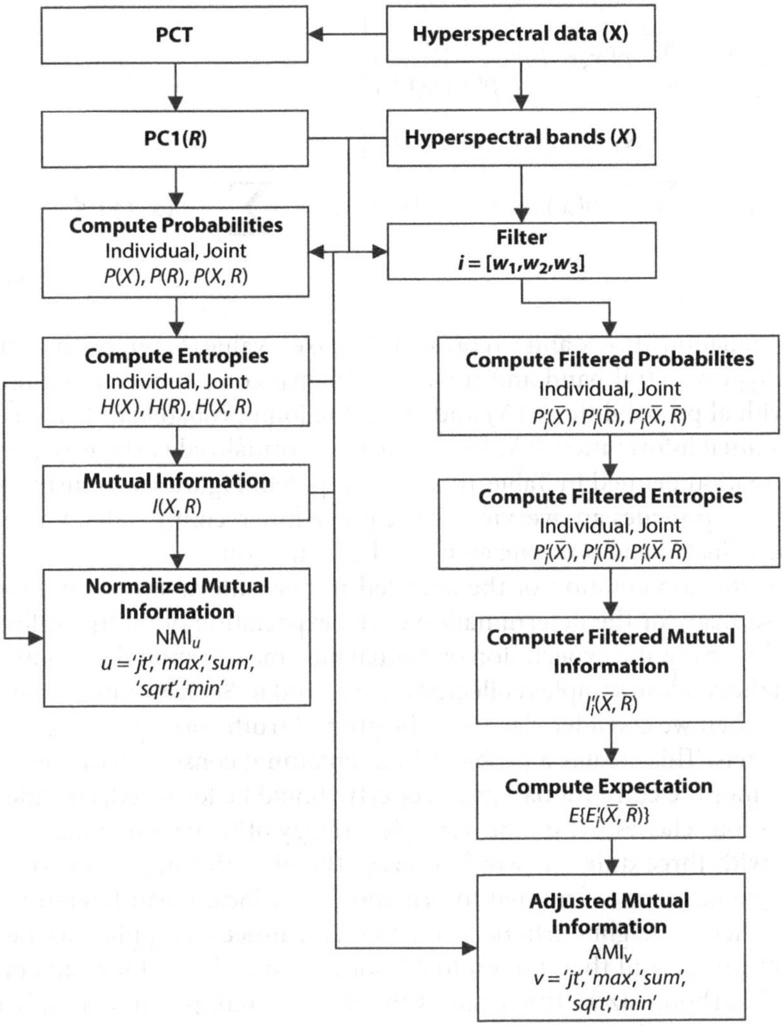

Figure 10.2 Workflow delineating the proposed approach for the computation of the normalized mutual information and the adjusted mutual information.

$$\left.\begin{aligned} I(X,R) &= \sum_{j=1}^{N} p(x,r)\, ln\left(\frac{p(x,r)}{p(x)p(r)}\right) \\ &= H(X)+H(R)-H(X,R) \end{aligned}\right\};$$

$$H(X) = -\sum_{j=1}^{N} p(x)\, ln(p(x)), H(X,R) = -\sum_{j=1}^{N} p(x,r)\, ln(p(x,r)) \tag{10.4}$$

In equation 10.4, x and r represent the pixels values taken by the particular hyperspectral band and the first principal component. Based on the individual probabilities $H(X)$ and $H(R)$, the joint probability $H(X, R)$, and the mutual information $I(X, R)$, the various normalized variants of mutual information defined in Table 10.2 are computed. Figure 10.2 illustrate the workflow provides an overview of the procedure recommended for calculating adjusted and normalized mutual information.

For the computation of the adjusted mutual information, we define a new strategy for the determination of the expectation of mutual information. Typically, the expectation of mutual information should be computed from the random samples collected from X, and R. Such a strategy does not work when we consider classes in the ground truth corresponding to very few pixels. This creates a problem in maintaining constant baseline property. Since the constant baseline property should be localized, considering the various classes, we define a simple strategy utilizing a moving average filter with three different window sizes. The objective here is to compute multiple instances of mutual information for a local mean filtered image with different neighbourhood sizes. The same process is applied to the reference image, and then the mutual information is derived for each of the neighbourhood sizes. The mean of the derived multiple mutual information is used as the expectation of mutual information. For simplicity and lower run time, we restrict the number of filter iterations to 3 with neighbourhood sizes 3, 5 and 7 corresponding to w1, w2 and w3.

Weighted Adjusted Mutual Information for Hyperspectral Band Selection
The concept of weighted mutual information is not new and has been explored widely in the literature. However, it has not gained popularity due to its limited applications. There are several ways in which weights can be utilized for the computation of the mutual information, the most popular being weighing the individual entropies, since devising weights for the joint distribution of the two random variables, say A and B as mentioned

before, is a complicated process. Hence, in the proposed method, we also utilize the weighted individual entropies for the computation of the normalized mutual information. The weighted mutual information, in this case, is shown in equation 10.5.

$$I^w(X, R) = w_X H(X) + w_R H(R) - H(X, R) \tag{10.5}$$

where w_X and w_R are the weights for the hyperspectral band and the reference first principal component, respectively and I^w is the weighted mutual information. The normalized weighted information, for example, for the case of normalization by the sum of the individual entropies, i.e., NMI^w_{sum} is shown as shown in equation 10.6.

$$WNMI_{sum} = NMI^w_{sum} = \frac{I^w(X,R)}{w_X H(X) + w_R H(R)} \tag{10.6}$$

$$WAMI_{sum} = AMI^w_{sum} = \frac{I^w(X,R) - E\{I^w(X,R)\}}{\{w_X H(X) + w_R H(R)\} - E\{I^w(X,R)\}} \tag{10.7}$$

Similarly, following the previous scheme in section 4.3, the adjusted mutual information from equation 10.6 can be computed as shown in equation 10.7. In equations 10.5, 10.6 and 10.7, we need the strategy to determine the weights. We know that the difference of the median filtered image from the image itself is a good indicator of the sharpness of the images. This is an example of a typical high pass filter that enhances the class edges providing spatial information regarding the structure of the classes. We refer to this difference as the sharpness factor in the present study. The sharpness factor is used in the proposed approach for the computation of the weights for the hyperspectral bands and the reference first principal component, rendering the proposed approach to be a spectral-spatial method for hyperspectral band selection. Let us say that the sharpness factors be dX and the dR for the hyperspectral band and the reference first principal components, then the corresponding weights w_Xand w_Rare determined as shown in equation 10.8. The expectation of the weighted mutual information is computed similarly, as explained in the previous section but now based on the weighted mutual information.

$$w_X = \frac{dX}{dX + dR}, w_R = \frac{dR}{dX + dR} \tag{10.8}$$

Statistical Accuracy Investigations

To evaluate the potential of the proposed method for hyperspectral band selection, we analyze the supervised classification accuracy of the selected bands. The supervised classification is performed using the Random Forest classifier with 100 trees. The analysis is performed based on two strategies; (1) Analysis of the classification accuracy corresponding to the percentage of training samples, (2) analysis of the classification accuracy corresponding to the number of bands selected. The potential of the mutual information variants and the proposed method is assessed based on the mean classification accuracy for the two cases mentioned above. The classification accuracy is determined using the error matrix or the confusion matrix and the overall accuracy and the Kappa coefficient derived from it.

Confusion Matrix

The pairwise comparison of the individual classes in the classification map with respect to the ground truth in an error matrix or the confusion matrix is a widely approached method for evaluating the classification accuracy. The left diagonal comparison in the confusion matrix represents the direct match of the class labels observed in the classification result and the reference. In other terms, the left diagonal elements of the confusion matrix represent the true predictions and the right diagonal represents the false predictions for a class. Several statistical inferences can be further derived from the confusion matrix which reveal the performance of the classifier.

Table 10.3 Confusion matrix.

i **= Rows (Predicted)**	***j*** **= Columns (Ground truth)**				**Rows total (n_{i+})**
	Class	**1**	**2**	**k**	
	1	n_{11}	n_{12}	n_{1k}	n_{1+}
	2	n_{21}	n_{22}	n_{2k}	n_{2+}
	k	n_{31}	n_{32}	n_{3k}	n_{k+}
Column Total (n_{+j})		n_{+1}	n_{+2}	n_{+k}	n

A sample confusion matrix based on Congalton and Green [45] is shown in Table 10.3, where, k represents the number of classes, n_{ij} represents the total samples classified into i^{th} class but actually in the jth class in ground truth data, n_{i+} is number of samples classified in i^{th} class by the classifier and n_{+j} is number of samples in j^{th} class in ground reference data.

Overall Accuracy and the Kappa Coefficient

The overall accuracy (OA) represents the fraction of correctly predicted labels accounting for all the classes considered in the confusion matrix. This is simply the sum of the left diagonal elements of the confusion matrix divided by the total number of samples (n). The OA as shown in equation 10.9 is often identified as a fraction between 0 to 1, or given in percentages by multiplying the fraction with 100.

$$OA = \frac{\sum_{i=1}^{k} n_{ii}}{n} \tag{10.9}$$

The overall accuracy is often misleading and can remain high even when a significant misclassification is observed for an individual class or several classes. Hence, OA is often regarded as a naïve measure.

A better metric to evaluate the classification accuracy is the Kappa coefficient that is generated as a statistical test to evaluate the accuracy of classification. The Kappa coefficient evaluates how well the classifier assigned pixels to the classes as compared to the random assigning of pixels. The Kappa coefficient may hold values -1(worse than random), 0 (random) and 1 (significantly better than random). Kappa coefficient is computed from the confusion matrix, as shown below.

$$\text{K} = \frac{\frac{1}{n}\sum_{i=1}^{k} n_{ij} - \frac{1}{n^2}\sum_{i=1}^{k} n_{i+}n_{+j}}{1 - \frac{1}{n^2}\sum_{i=1}^{k} n_{i+}n_{+j}} \tag{10.10}$$

Evaluation Strategy

The potential candidate bands for selection are derived using sorted NMI and AMI based on the expressions defined in Table 10.2. Additionally, weighted NMI and weighted AMI derived using equations 10.6 and 10.7 were sorted for the determination of potential bands for selection. The local maxima of the descending values of the MI variants and the proposed weighted NMI and AMI variants are used to determine the best bands and amongst these the user-defined number of bands are selected, following the approach defined by Varade *et al.* [20].

The strategy by Varade *et al.* [35] is utilized where the reference best band for the computation of the mutual information variants was considered as the first principal component. The Kappa coefficient is used for the assessment of classification accuracy determined using the error matrix or the confusion matrix. To evaluate the potential of the proposed method for hyperspectral band selection, we analyse the supervised classification accuracy of the selected band set. The supervised classification is performed using the Random Forest classifier with 100 trees. The analysis is performed based on two strategies: (1) analysis of the classification accuracy corresponding to the percentage of training samples, (2) analysis of the classification accuracy corresponding to the number of bands selected. A comparison for each of the case is carried out by evaluating the classification accuracy determined by the Kappa coefficient for two cases.

Results and Discussion

Evaluation of MI Variants with Respect to Fixed Training Samples

As mentioned earlier, we evaluate the various MI variants discussed in Table 10.2 based on the Kappa coefficient derived from the confusion matrix from the classification results and the reference data. In this case, the training percentage of the Random Forest classifier was fixed to 20% samples extracted randomly from the reference data. For each MI variant the selected bands were stacked into different multi-band images comprising 10, 20, 30, 40, 50, and 60 bands, similar to Varade *et al.* [35]. These multi-band images were each classified with the aforementioned settings using a Random Forest classifier.

Figure 10.3 shows the variation of Kappa coefficient for each of the band sets for the different hyperspectral datasets used for evaluation of the various MI variants. Figure 10.4 shows the mean classification Kappa for the different number of bands when 20% training samples are used for classifier training. The red-ended and the orange-ended bars indicate the best performing variants amongst the AMI and the NMI variants, respectively. In general, we observe that the Kappa coefficient increases with an increase in the selected bands used for classification.

For the Indian Pines dataset (Figure 10.3a), some inconsistency is observed for 10 and 20 selected bands for the variants AMIsum, NMIsqrt, and NMImax.

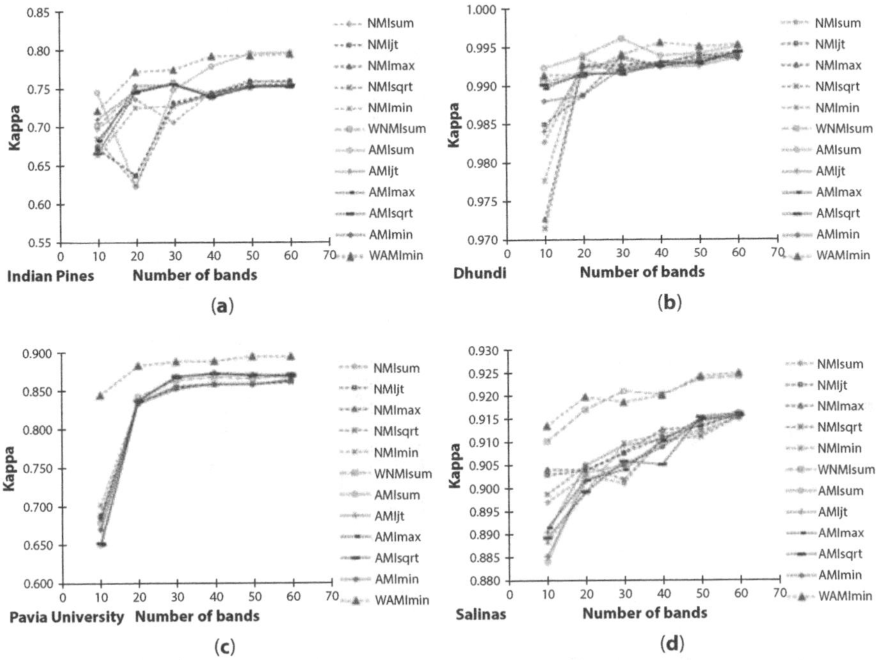

Figure 10.3 Classification accuracy (Kappa coefficient) for the different variants of mutual information with respect to the different number of bands for the (a) Indian Pines dataset, (b) Dhundi dataset, (c) Pavia University dataset, (d) Salinas dataset, for 20% random training samples using the Random Forest classifier.

For this dataset, the best and worst overall performance is exhibited by WAMIsum and NMIsqrt, respectively, as shown in Figure 10.4a. For the Dhundi dataset (Figure 10.3b), the NMIsqrt, NMImax, and the NMImin variants show significantly poor classification accuracy at 10 bands. For this dataset, the WAMIsum and the AMIsum variants show very good classifier performance as compared to the NMIsqrt variant that shows relatively poor classifier performance, as observed from Figure 10.4b. In the case of the Pavia University dataset (Figure 10.3c), for the best 10 selected bands, except WAMIsum, the other variants show significantly reduced classification accuracy (Figure 10.4c). The WAMIsum by far outperforms the other variants for this dataset compared to the least performing NMIsqrt variant. In Figure 10.3d for the Salinas dataset, we observe a cluster of variants, where the weighted MI variants show much better classification accuracies compared to the other variants. The average performance of the other variants determined by the mean Kappa coefficient is fairly similar as observed in Figure 10.4d.

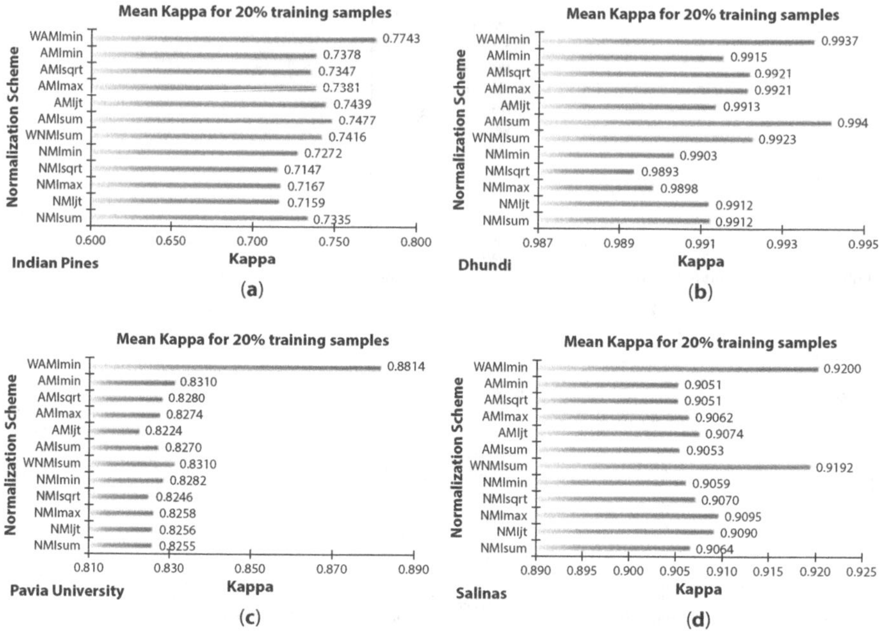

Figure 10.4 Mean Kappa Coefficient for the different variants of mutual information for the different number of bands for the (a) Indian Pines dataset, (b) Dhundi dataset, (c) Pavia University dataset, (d) Salinas dataset.

Evaluation of MI Variants with Respect to Fixed Number of Bands

Following a similar approach, we evaluated the various MI variants with respect to the varying volume of training samples. The number of bands in this case are fixed to 20, where typically peak accuracies have been observed in the previous studies on hyperspectral band selection [19]. The volume of training samples for the training the classifier was varied at intervals of 15 from 15 to 90%. The best selected 20 bands from each of the MI variants were stacked to develop multi-band images which were used for the assessment based on the classification accuracy. To maintain consistency, the classifier settings were ensured to remain the same.

Figure 10.5 shows the classification accuracies (Kappa coefficients) for the various volumes of the training data. In contrast to the previous case, here no single variant has been observed to show consistently higher accuracy. Subsequently, the mean values of the Kappa coefficient (from Figure 10.5) were assessed as shown in Figure 10.6 following a similar strategy as in Figure 10.4. In Figure 10.5a for the Indian Pines dataset, two cluster of variants are observed, where in general we observe the AMI variants to show better classifier performance than the NMI variants.

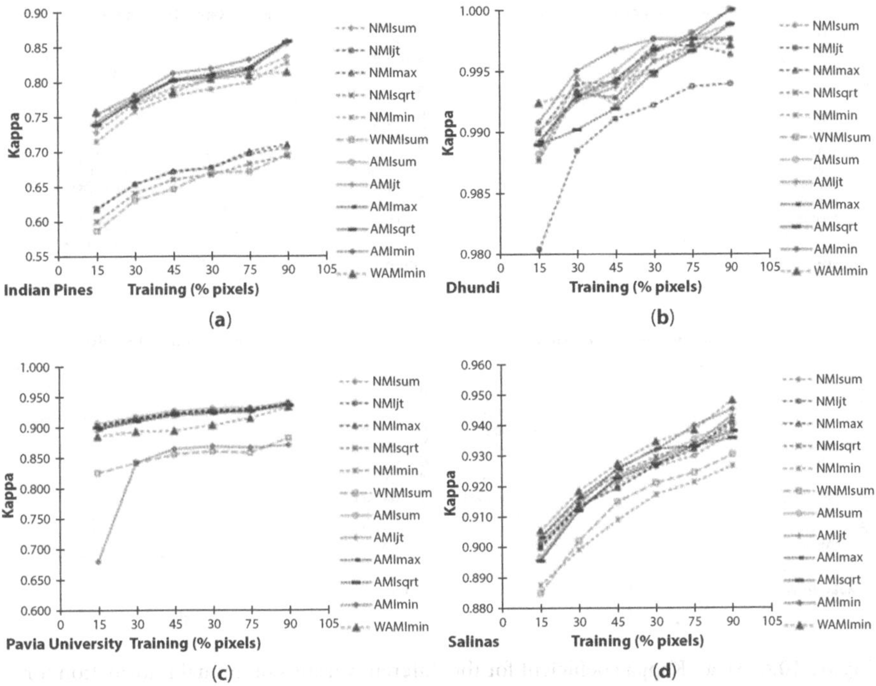

Figure 10.5 Classification accuracy (Kappa coefficient) for the different variants of mutual information with respect to the different volume of training samples for the (a) Indian Pines dataset, (b) Dhundi dataset, (c) Pavia University dataset, (d) Salinas dataset, for 20 selected best bands based on the Random Forest classifier.

The NMImin variant which can be observed in the topmost cluster showed much better performance amongst the other NMI variants. On average, the best and the worst performing variants are observed to be AMImin and WNMIsum, respectively, as seen in Figure 10.6a.

For the Indian Pines and the Dhundi datasets, the AMImin variant showed better overall Kappa coefficient amongst all the variants. For the Pavia University and the Salinas datasets, the AMIsum and WAMIsum variants exhibited better performance as determined by mean Kappa values. For these datasets, the NMIsqrt variant showed better performance amongst other normalized MI variants. A similar observation can be made for the Dhundi dataset in Figure 10.5b, where the AMI variants excluding AMIsqrt show better classification accuracies. The NMIjt variant is observed to show significantly poor classification performance, especially at 15% training volume compared to all other variants, as observed in both Figure 10.5b and 10.6b. The best performing variant for the Dhundi

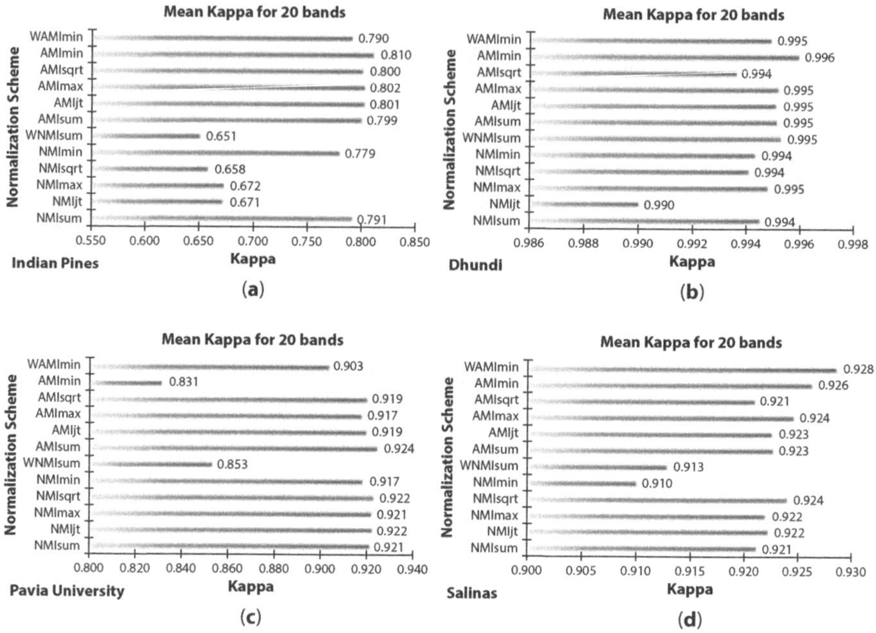

Figure 10.6 Mean Kappa coefficient for the different variants of mutual information for the different volume of training data for the (a) Indian Pines dataset, (b) Dhundi dataset, (c) Pavia University dataset, (d) Salinas dataset.

dataset is observed to be AMImin (Figure 10.6b). Similar to the Indian Pines dataset, we observe two cluster of variants in Figure 10.5c, where the AMImin and WNMIsum variants show significantly poor classification accuracies. For 15% training samples, the AMImin variant significantly underperforms as compared to the WNMIsum variant in the same cluster. Figure 10.6c shows that the performance of the other NMI variants is very similar. The AMIsum and the AMImin variants are the best and worst performing in terms of the mean Kappa values. In the Salinas dataset, as shown in Figure 10.5d, excluding the NMImin and the WNMImin variants the performance of the other variants is relatively similar with best classification accuracies observed for the WAMIsum variant and the AMImin variant, as shown in Figure 10.6d.

Overall Evaluation Based on Test Datasets

In general, it is observed that the AMI-based variants result in significantly better classification accuracy as compared to the NMI variants, as shown in Figure 10.6a. It is observed that the mean Kappa coefficient for 10, 20,

30, 40, 50 and 60 bands at 20% training is the highest for the WAMIsum followed by WNMIsum which is 0.8924 and 0.8710, respectively. For the case of 20 bands with training sample volumes varying between 15, 30, 45, 60, 75 and 90, the mean Kappa coefficient of 0.9102 for the AMIsum is marginally better. Overall, it is observed that the WAMIsum shows the best accuracy over the mean of the two cases, as mentioned above, as shown in Table 10.2 and Figure 10.7. From the analysis, it was observed that the normalization by the sum of the individual entropies showed relatively higher performance for band selection both in the case of weighted NMI and weighted AMI for 20% training samples at varying number of selected bands, as observed in Figure 10.7. The observed optimal "sum" normalization scheme is observed to be in agreement with the normalization scheme used for band selection in Uso *et al.* [42] and Varade *et al.* [20, 35].

The main ideas of the content up to this point have been what sign language is and why American sign language was chosen above other sign languages. What compelled us even more to research this topic? Now the question is, how are we going to accomplish such a task? To answer that, we must be able to comprehend the idea that this research is trying to portray as well as the procedures or strategies that will be employed to carry out this research sequentially.

In the case of the proposed methods based on weighted mutual information, it is observed that at 20% random training samples, these methods significantly outperform the other MI variants. For the other case of 20 bands, the mean Kappa is significantly influenced by the much lower Kappa values observed in the case of the Indian Pines and the Pavia University dataset for both WNMIsum and WAMIsum and particularly WNMIsum. An illustration of the workflow that outlines the suggested method for the computation of the normalized mutual information and the adjusted mutual information is shown in Figure 10.2.

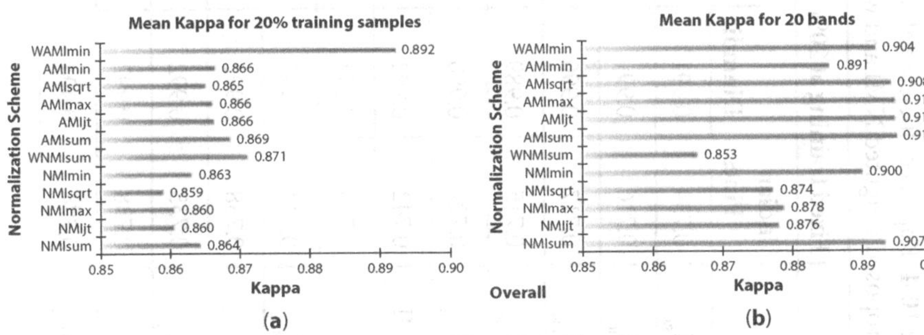

Figure 10.7 Mean classification accuracy for fixed training at 20% samples and 20 selected bands over the four test datasets for each of the MI variants in (a) and (b).

Table 10.4 Kappa coefficient values for the two cases used in strategic evaluation of the potential of the NMI/AMI variants and the proposed weighted NMI and weighted AMI for hyperspectral band selection.

	Fixed training at 20%					**Fixed bands 20**				
	Indian Pines	**Dhundi**	**Pavia University**	**Salinas**	**AVG**	**Indian Pines**	**Dhundi**	**Pavia University**	**Salinas**	**AVG**
NMI_{sum}	0.734	0.991	0.826	0.906	0.864	0.791	0.994	0.921	0.921	0.907
NMI_{jt}	0.716	0.991	0.826	0.909	0.860	0.671	0.990	0.922	0.922	0.876
NMI_{max}	0.717	0.990	0.826	0.910	0.860	0.672	0.995	0.921	0.922	0.878
NMI_{sqrt}	0.715	0.989	0.825	0.907	0.859	0.658	0.994	0.922	0.924	0.875
NMI_{min}	0.727	0.990	0.828	0.906	0.863	0.779	0.994	0.918	0.910	0.900
$WNMI_{sum}$	0.742	0.992	0.831	0.919	0.871	0.651	0.995	0.853	0.913	0.853
AMI_{sum}	0.748	0.994	0.827	0.905	0.869	0.799	0.995	0.924	0.923	0.910
AMI_{jt}	0.744	0.991	0.822	0.907	0.866	0.801	0.995	0.919	0.923	0.910
AMI_{max}	0.738	0.992	0.827	0.906	0.866	0.802	0.995	0.917	0.925	0.910
AMI_{sqrt}	0.735	0.992	0.828	0.905	0.865	0.800	0.994	0.919	0.921	0.908
AMI_{min}	0.738	0.992	0.831	0.905	0.866	0.810	0.996	0.831	0.926	0.891
$WAMI_{sum}$	0.774	0.994	0.881	0.920	0.892	0.790	0.995	0.903	0.929	0.904

Excluding the Indian Pines Dataset

Figure 10.8 shows the mean Kappa values for the two cases and the mean for these two cases for the various MI variants, including the proposed weighted ones excluding the Indian Pines dataset. It is observed that in this case, the proposed method WAMIsum significantly outperforms the other MI variants. In this case, for the first case with fixed training percentage of 20% random samples selected from the ground truth, the proposed

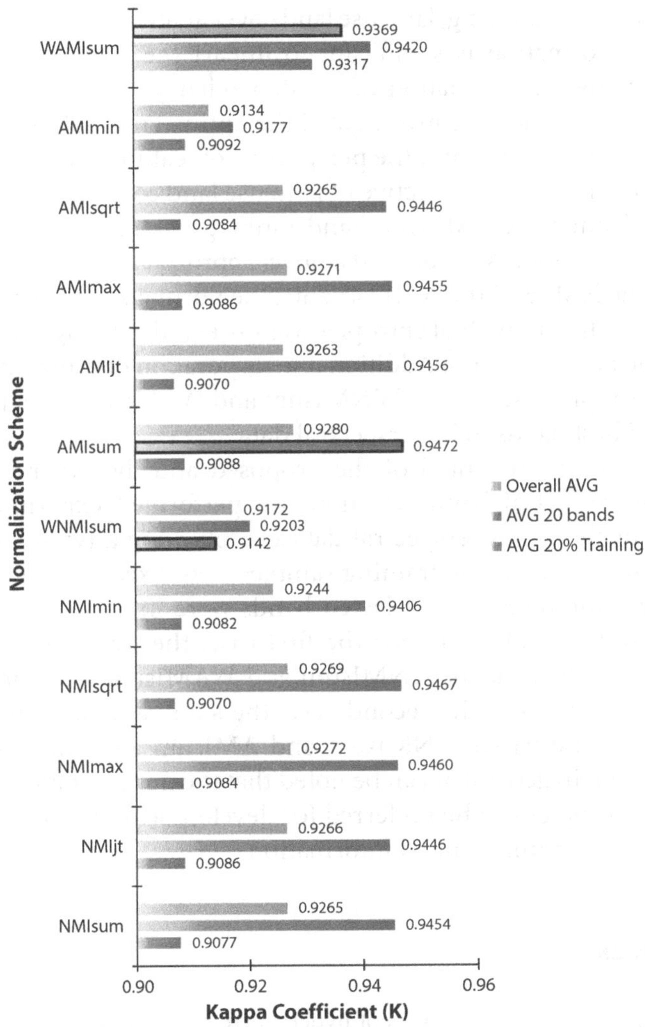

Figure 10.8 Mean Kappa coefficient for the two cases and their average excluding the Indian Pines dataset.

WNMIsum significantly outperformed the other MI variants. For the second case, with 20 selected bands, the mean Kappa values for most MI variants are relatively similar, excluding WNMIsum and AMImin.

Conclusion

Mutual information and techniques based on mutual information have been widely used in the literature for feature selection in numerous areas, including medical imaging, land use land cover analysis, etc. Normalization of mutual information is significant to impart the essential qualities of a metric for the determination of the dependency between two random variables. In this study, we investigated the optimal normalization scheme for mutual information from the perspective of feature selection in hyperspectral data from the perspective of land use land cover classification. We further examined the AMI as a band ranking parameter for hyperspectral feature selection. We proposed a novel approach for deriving the AMI. Amongst the NMI and the AMI variants, the normalization scheme based on the sum of the individual entropies was observed to be significantly better than the other schemes. Additional incorporation of utilizing weighted entropies was proposed as the WNMIsum and WAMIsum variants for the selection of best bands in hyperspectral data.

To examine the potential of the proposed and the other variants of MI for hyperspectral band selection, we performed experiments with four state-of-the-art hyperspectral datasets following a two-case strategy where in the first case, the training samples were fixed at 20% and in the second case, the number of selected bands were fixed at 20. The experimental results revealed that for the first case, the weighted normalized and adjusted sum variants WNMIsum and WAMIsum are more suitable for band selection. For the second case, the sum variants of normalized and adjusted sum variants NMIsum and AMIsum are more suitable for band selection. In general, it can be noted that the normalization by sum of individual entropies can be preferred for development of feature selection methods incorporating mutual information.

References

[1] Goetz, A. F.H., Three decades of hyperspectral remote sensing of the Earth: A personal view. *Remote Sensing of Environment*, 113, D13, S5-S16, 2009.

[2] Mateen, M., Wen, J., Nasrullah, and Azeem, M., The Role of Hyperspectral Imaging: A Literature Review. *ijacsa*, 9, 8, 2018.

[3] Doktor, D., Lausch, A., Spengler, D., and Thurner, M., Extraction of Plant Physiological Status from Hyperspectral Signatures Using Machine Learning Methods. *Remote Sensing*, 6, 12, pp. 12247–12274, 2014.

[4] Lu, G. and Fei, B., Medical hyperspectral imaging: A review. *Journal of Biomedical Optics*, 19, 1, p. 10901, 2014.

[5] Li, X., Li, R., Wang, M., Liu, Y., Zhang, B., and Zhou, J., Hyperspectral Imaging and Their Applications in the Nondestructive Quality Assessment of Fruits and Vegetables. in *Hyperspectral Imaging in Agriculture, Food and Environment*, A. I. L. Maldonado, H. R. Fuentes, and J. A. V. Contreras (eds.), InTech, 2018.

[6] Underwood, E., Mapping nonnative plants using hyperspectral imagery. *Remote Sensing of Environment*, 86, 2, pp. 150–161, 2003.

[7] Dominiak-Swigon, M., Olejniczak, P., Nowak, M., and Lembicz, M., Hyperspectral imaging in assessing the condition of plants: Strengths and weaknesses. *Biodiversity Research and Conservation*, 55, 1, pp. 25–30, 2019.

[8] Kolmann, M. A. *et al.*, Hyperspectral data as a biodiversity screening tool can differentiate among diverse Neotropical fishes. *Scientific Reports*, 11, 1, p. 16157, 2021.

[9] Varade, D., Maurya, A. K., and Dikshit, O., Development of spectral indexes in hyperspectral imagery for land cover assessment. *IETE Technical Review*, pp. 1–9, 2018.

[10] Transon, J., d'Andrimont, R., Maugnard, A., and Defourny, P., Survey of Hyperspectral Earth Observation Applications from Space in the Sentinel-2 Context. *Remote Sensing*, 10, 3, p. 157, 2018.

[11] Datta, D., Mallick, P. K., Bhoi, A. K., Ijaz, M. F., Shafi, J., and Choi, J., Hyperspectral Image Classification: Potentials, Challenges, and Future Directions. *Computational Intelligence and Neuroscience*, 2022, p. 3854635, 2022.

[12] Mianji, F. A., Zhang, Y., Sulehria, H. K., Babakhani, A., and Kardan, M. R., Super-Resolution Challenges in Hyperspectral Imagery. *Information Technology J.*, 7, 7, pp. 1030–1036, 2008.

[13] Nasrabadi, N. M., Hyperspectral Target Detection: An Overview of Current and Future Challenges. *IEEE Signal Process. Mag.*, 31, 1, pp. 34–44, 2014.

[14] Varshney, P. K. and Arora, M. K., *Advanced image processing techniques for remotely sensed hyperspectral data*. Berlin, Heidelberg, Springer, 2010.

[15] Hughes, G., On the mean accuracy of statistical pattern recognizers. *IEEE Trans. Inform. Theory*, 14, 1, pp. 55–63, 1968.

[16] Chang, C.-I. *Hyperspectral data processing: Algorithm design and analysis*, Hoboken, NJ, Wiley-Interscience, 2013.

[17] Wang, L. and Zhao, C., *Hyperspectral image processing*. Heidelberg, Springer, 2016.

[18] Amigo, J. M. e., *Hyperspectral imaging*. Amsterdam, Elsevier, 2019.

[19] Sun, W. and Du, Q., Hyperspectral Band Selection: A Review. *IEEE Geosci. Remote Sens. Mag.*, 7, 2, pp. 118–139, 2019.

[20] Varade, D., Maurya, A. K., and Dikshit, O., Unsupervised hyperspectral band selection using ranking based on a denoising error matching approach. *International Journal of Remote Sensing*, 70, 2, pp. 1–23, 2019.

[21] Cao, X., Wei, C., Han, J., and Jiao, L., Hyperspectral Band Selection Using Improved Classification Map. *IEEE Geosci. Remote Sensing Lett.*, 14, 11, pp. 2147–2151, 2017.

[22] Yuan, Y., Zheng, X., and Lu, X., Discovering Diverse Subset for Unsupervised Hyperspectral Band Selection. *IEEE Transactions on Image Processing: A Publication of the IEEE Signal Processing Society*, 26, 1, pp. 51–64, 2017.

[23] Nagasubramanian, K., Jones, S., Sarkar, S., Singh, A. K., Singh, A., and Ganapathysubramanian, B., Hyperspectral band selection using genetic algorithm and support vector machines for early identification of charcoal rot disease in soybean stems. *Plant Methods*, 14, p. 86, 2018.

[24] Cao, X. *et al.*, A semi-supervised spatially aware wrapper method for hyperspectral band selection. *International Journal of Remote Sensing*, 39, 12, pp. 4020–4039, 2018.

[25] Geng, X., Sun, K., Ji, L., and Zhao, Y., A Fast Volume-Gradient-Based Band Selection Method for Hyperspectral Image. *IEEE Trans. Geosci. Remote Sensing*, 52, 11, pp. 7111–7119, 2014.

[26] Zhang, W., Li, X., Dou, Y., and Zhao, L., A geometry-based band selection approach for hyperspectral image analysis. *IEEE Transactions on Geoscience and Remote Sensing*, 56, 8, pp. 4318–4333, 2018.

[27] Wang, J., Wang, X., Zhang, K., Madani, K., and Sabourin, C., Morphological band selection for hyperspectral imagery. *IEEE Geoscience and Remote Sensing Letters*, 15, 8, pp. 1259–1263, 2018.

[28] Xie, F., Lei, C., Li, F., Huang, D., and Yang, J., Unsupervised hyperspectral feature selection based on fuzzy c -means and grey wolf optimizer. *International Journal of Remote Sensing*, 40, 9, pp. 3344–3367, 2018.

[29] Lorencs, A., Mednieks, I., and Sinica-Sinavskis, J., Selection of informative hyperspectral band subsets based on entropy and correlation. *International Journal of Remote Sensing*, pp. 1–18, 2018.

[30] Habermann, M., Fremont, V., and Shiguemori, E. H., Supervised band selection in hyperspectral images using single-layer neural networks. *International Journal of Remote Sensing*, 40, 10, pp. 3900–3926, 2019.

[31] Luo, X., Shen, Z., Xue, R., and Wan, H., Unsupervised Band Selection Method Based on Importance-Assisted Column Subset Selection. *IEEE Access*, 7, pp. 517–527, 2019.

[32] Sawant, S. S., Manoharan, P., and Loganathan, A., Band selection strategies for hyperspectral image classification based on machine learning and artificial intelligent techniques – Survey. *Arab J Geosci*, 14, 7, a5, 2021.

[33] Jiang, X., Lin, J., Liu, J., Li, S., and Zhang, Y., A Coarse-to-Fine Optimization for Hyperspectral Band Selection. IEEE Geosci. *Remote Sensing Lett.*, 16, 4, pp. 638–642, 2019.

[34] Varade, D., Maurya, A. K., Sure, A., and Dikshit, O., Supervised classification of snow cover using hyperspectral imagery. in *International Conference on Emerging Trends in Computing and Communication Technologies, Dehradun, India*, pp. 1–7, IEEE, 2017.

[35] Varade, D., Maurya, A. K., and Dikshit, O., Unsupervised Band Selection of Hyperspectral Data Based on Mutual Information Derived from Weighted Cluster Entropy for Snow Classification. *Geocarto International*, 2019.

[36] Chowdhury, A. R., Hazra, J., Dasgupta, K., and Dutta, P., Fuzzy rule-based hyperspectral band selection algorithm with ant colony optimization. *Innovations Syst Softw Eng*, 37, 6, p. 2631, 2022.

[37] Pan, Y., Xing, S., and Liu, D., Partition Optimal Band Selection Method for Hyperspectral Image. *J. Phys.: Conf. Ser.*, 2005, 1, p. 12054, 2021.

[38] Amelio, A. and Pizzuti, C., Correction for Closeness: Adjusting Normalized Mutual Information Measure for Clustering Comparison. *Computational Intelligence*, 33, 3, pp. 579–601, 2017.

[39] Baumgardner, M., Biehl, L., and Landgrebe, D., 220 Band AVIRIS hyperspectral image data set: June 12, 1992 Indian Pine Test Site 3, Purdue University Research Repository.

[40] Plaza, A., Martinez, P., Plaza, J., and Perez, R., Dimensionality reduction and classification of hyperspectral image data using sequences of extended morphological transformations. *IEEE Trans. Geosci. Remote Sensing*, 43, 3, pp. 466–479, 2005.

[41] Graña, M., Veganzons,, M. A., and Ayerdi, B., Hyperspectral Remote Sensing Scenes, 2021. https://www.ehu.eus/ccwintco/index.php/Hyperspectral_Remote_Sensing_Scenes#Pavia_Centre_and_University

[42] Uso, A. M., Pla, F., Sotoca, J. M., and García-Sevilla, P., Clustering-based hyperspectral band selection using information measures. *IEEE Transactions on Geoscience and Remote Sensing*, 45, 12, pp. 4158–4171, 2007.

[43] Cover, T. M. and Thomas, J. A., *Elements of Information Theory*, 2nd ed. Hoboken, N.J., Wiley and Chichester: John Wiley, 2006. http://www.loc.gov/catdir/enhancements/fy0624/2005047799-d.html

[44] Vinh, N. X., Epps, J., and Bailey, J., Information Theoretic Measures for Clusterings Comparison: Variants, Properties, Normalization and Correction for Chance. *Journal of Machine Learning Research*, 11, 95, pp. 2837–2854, 2010. http://jmlr.org/papers/v11/vinh10a.html

[45] Congalton, R. G. and Green, K., *Assessing the Accuracy of Remotely Sensed Data: Principles and Practices*, 3rd ed. Boca Raton, London, New York, CRC Press, Taylor & Francis Group, 2019.

11

A Python-Based Machine Learning Classification Approach for Healthcare Applications

Vishal Sharma

Birla Institute of Technology and Science, Pilani, India

Abstract
Machine learning (ML) approaches have been an important technique in various applications. To know a possible future illness by deploying particular health data has represented a vibrant area for these applications. This chapter investigates the important patterns of different ML classification techniques, and its ability and application in discovering future illness. In addition, this chapter aims to perform an effective ML classification method that can effectively tell the symptoms of illness of a person, based on the received symptoms from the model under development. Let us go through in detail how we can develop such a machine learning model.

***Keywords*:** Machine learning, healthcare, classification, Gaussian Naive Bayes, support vector machine (SVM)

Introduction

Machine learning algorithms deploy numerous mathematical techniques to train from previous available data and find out meaningful insights from enormous, unstructured and complex data sets [1]. These ML techniques have various applications, covering text categorization [2], anomaly detection [3], e-mail filtration [4], credit card fraud prevention [5], detection of

Email: bits.vishal11@gmail.com

Suman Kumar Swarnkar, J P Patra, Sapna Singh Kshatri, Yogesh Kumar Rathore and Tien Anh Tran (eds.) Supervised and Unsupervised Data Engineering for Multimedia Data, (247–262) © 2024 Scrivener Publishing LLC

the customer purchase behavior [6], manufacturing optimization process [7] and modelling for a particular illness [8]. Many of these use cases have been performed using supervised learning [4, 5, 8] of the ML techniques instead of unsupervised. In the supervised approach, a prediction model is constructed by training a data set where the class is already familiar and then the output of unlabeled illustrations can be said [9]. This chapter analyses the performance of the various ML classification approaches. Illness prediction and medical data analytic and informatics have achieved important attention from the machine learning research community. This is basically due to the wide acceptance of digitization into the healthcare field in various forms (e.g., e-health records and other related administrative data) and the presence of big health databases for researchers. Further, these e-data are deployed in a different field of health-related research fields, for example, the examining of healthcare usefulness [10], computing the feasibility of a hospital network [11], finding patterns and price [12], constructing illness risk forecasting machine learning model [13, 14], any chronic illness monitoring [15], and comparison of illness prevalence and drug outcomes [16]. In this chapter we are considering various classification algorithms [8, 17, 18].

Methodology

We generally follow the following basic steps for the illness classification.
First Step - Data collection: This is the first step for any ML problem statement. Here, we are taking data into consideration from the Kaggle website, which has two different CSV data files. The first is a training data set, the other a testing data set. In the deployed dataset, we have 133 columns; 132 columns are for illness symptoms, and one end column denotes prediction.

Second Step - Data Cleaning: This step is also known as data pre-processing and is one of the important steps in machine learning model development. The accuracy of the finally developed ML method depends on the accuracy of the data deployed for model development; it is therefore necessary to refine the data before applying actual machine learning model. Once data cleaning is achieved, we use that data further for training and testing. All these processes are considered as exploratory data analysis (EDA). Further analyzing our data set, we came to know that all the columns in the dataset are numerical. In addition to these, our target variable, prognosis, is a kind of string data type which is encoded into the numerical form by the help of a label encoder. Here in this chapter, all these processes are implemented in Python.

Third Step - Model Development: At this stage of model development, our data is now ready to use for training in the desired machine learning model. Here, we are interested in a Python-based implementation of various classification algorithms such as Naive Bayes, Random Forest, and Support Vector machine. All these algorithms will be trained by this pre-processed data, and further we test the quality of the developed machine learning model with the use of confusion matrix. We will study in detail about the confusion matrix. Till this point, we have trained all the three classification algorithms.

Fourth Step - Inference: Here, we can use the already trained algorithms in the previous step for predicting the symptoms of a particular illness. The input symptoms can be fed as an input into these trained models. In addition to this, we can combine the predictions generated from all these three models to confirm that the final prediction is as per the expectations that is more accurate and robust.

After all these important steps, we write a user defined function which considers symptoms as input which are separated by commas. Further, these trained models predict the illness based on these inputs, and finally returns into a JSON file.

Python-Based Implementation Steps

Figure 11.1 describes each and every step of the models used for classification. For better understanding of the algorithm implementation part, just make sure that you have uploaded the data sets (for training and testing in csv format). For Python-based implementation, one can use either a separate Jupiter notebook or a Google Colaboratory (Google Colab). It's a product from Google Research and a free GPU, TPU is available over the cloud.

Reading the Required Data

The required data set is loaded from the already saved folders using the rich library set of Python i.e., Pandas library. In the data reading process, we drop the null values. In this clean data set we have all the feature with binary values 0's and 1's. In all the classification algorithms while implementing we check for the balanced values achieved for the target variable. For validating this we deploy bar plot technique to confirm the data set is balanced or imbalanced. We write the Python code to read the dataset under consideration

Python-Based Implementation Steps

By close observation from the below plot, it is now clear that each illness has 120 samples which indicates that the data set is now a balanced

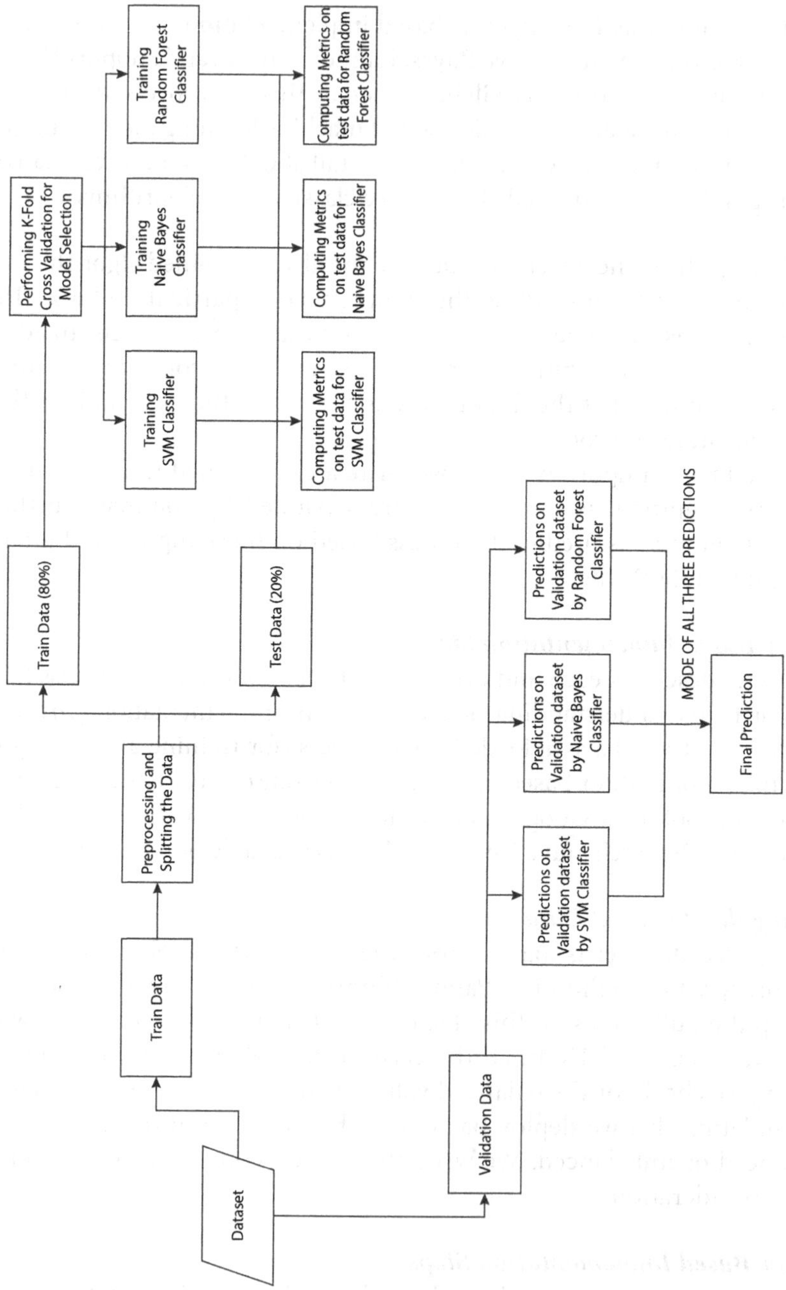

Figure 11.1 An overview of all the three classifiers.

dataset. At this stage we confirm that further there is no balancing exercise required. Here we observe that the target column (prognosis column) is an object datatype, which is not desirable for training a machine learning model. At this stage, first we need to convert this object datatype into a numerical datatype. For this conversion, we take help of a label encoder. In this process, label encoder assigns a different index to each label. This indexing is achieved in such a way that if n is the total number of labels, then each label is numbered from 0 to (n - 1).

Splitting the Data Set in Training and Testing

After cleaning data set, null values are eliminated, and numerical format of different labels are achieved. Now we split the deployed data set into training and testing and then we develop the model. For this we split the data set in the ratio of 80:20. This ratio indicates that 80% of the data set is deployed for training and the remaining 20% data set is deployed for the testing the model under development. In other words we can say that 20% of the data set is deployed for investigating the performance of the developed model.

Based on Python implementation, we get the following results Train which showed in Figure 11.2: (3936, 132), (3936)

Test: (984, 132), (984)

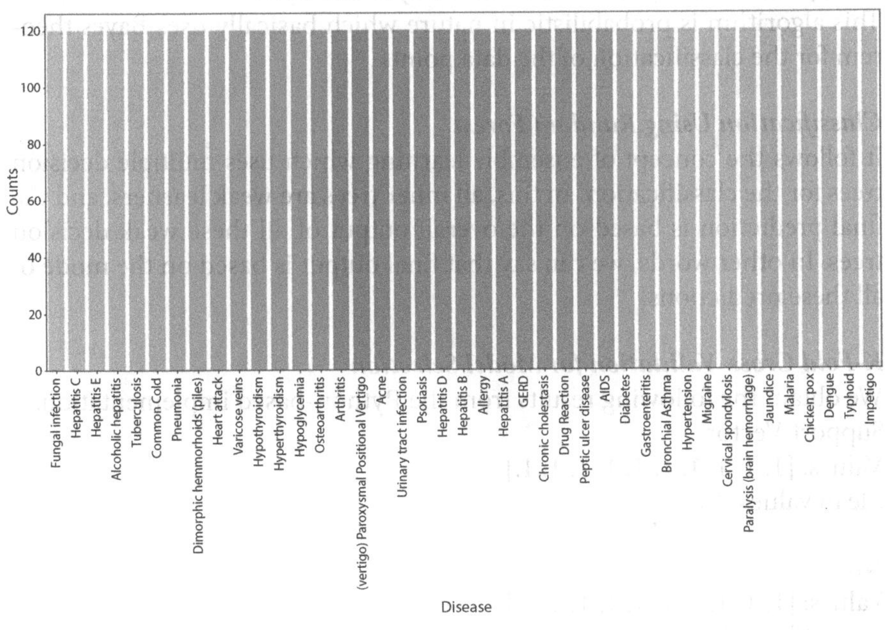

Figure 11.2 Output of the Python implementation.

Machine Learning Model Development

At this stage we develop the model. For evaluation of the model, we consider K-Fold cross-validation. Further, in the current chapter, we study the following classification algorithms and perform a Python-based implementation. The classification algorithms for the current study are Random Forest (RF), Support Vector machine (SVM), and Gaussian Naive Bayes (NB). To check the performance of all these classification algorithms, we use K-Fold cross-validation. At this point, let's first be familiar with the various classification algorithms and their performance evaluator, i.e., K-Fold cross-validation.

K-Fold Cross-Validation Method

Here, the complete data set is first split into k subsets, called as folds, and then the training part is accomplished on the (k 1) subsets. Finally, the model performance evaluation is achieved by deploying the remaining one subset.

Classification Using Support Vector Classifier

This type of classifier is also known as discriminative classifier. It means when we feed a labeled training data, an optimum hyperplane is computed by the algorithm which distinguishes the dataset accurately in distinct classes in that hyperspace under consideration.

Classification Using Gaussian Naive Bayes Classifier

This algorithm is probabilistic in nature which basically uses Bayes theorem for the classification of the data points.

Classification Using Random Forest

It follows the concept of ensemble learning which uses multiple decision trees for the classification. In this, all inner trees are weak learners, and the final prediction is based on the overall output of all these weak decision trees. In other words, we can say that final output is based on the mode of all these predictions.

K-Fold Cross-Validation for Model Selection

We obtain the following results from the Python-based implementation.
Support Vector
Values: [1. 1. 1. 1. 1. 1. 1. 1. 1. 1.]
Mean values: 1.0

NB
Values: [1. 1. 1. 1. 1. 1. 1. 1. 1. 1.]
Mean Value: 1.0

RF
Values: [1. 1. 1. 1. 1. 1. 1. 1. 1. 1.]
Mean Value: 1.0

From these values, we can observe the results obtained after applying K-Fold cross-validation. The mean scores in such a case are very high. To make it more accurate and robust, let's combine all these models and calculate the mode of forecasting of these three models, so that if one model predicts a wrong result, at least we can get correct predictions from the remaining two models. This type of strategy helps us to predict accurately the unseen data sets. Here we are implementing in Python where at the end we are taking into account all the three models.

Confusion Matrix (CM)

In machine learning, a confusion matrix is a table used to assess the performance of a classification algorithm. Figures 11.3, 11.4 and 11.5 show how the findings are divided into four categories. It is an investigation tool for various classification algorithms used in the machine learning. It is in the form of a table which reflects the classification performance which is basically based on the test data set for that the true values are already familiar.

A CM is a tabular summary of the various right and wrong forecasts generated by a classification algorithm. We can use it to investigate the realization of a classification system. It can be deployed to compute the realization of a particular classification system through the computation of the various realization metrics.

Before taking into consideration the confusion matrix, we must go through the terms used to analyze and understand the results from these matrices.

The CM tabular data is deployed to find out the efficiency of the classification algorithm by the comparison between predicted and actual classes.

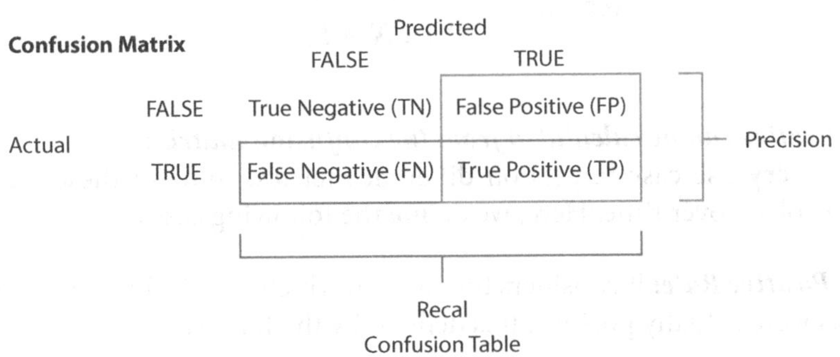

Figure 11.3 Confusion table.

n = 165	Predicted: NO	Predicted: YES
Actual: NO	50	10
Actual: YES	5	100

Figure 11.4 Example for the confusion matrix.

n = 165	Predicted: NO	Predicted: YES	
Actual: NO	TN = 50	FP = 10	60
Actual: YES	FN = 5	TP = 100	105
	55	110	

Figure 11.5 Example for the confusion matrix.

Here we can observe that in general the binary confusion matrix can be represented by square cells.

Following is the important terminology to understand the concept of a confusion matrix.

The accuracy test is calculated from the given confusion matrix tabular data. The following ratio is used to calculate the accuracy test:

$$Accuracy = \frac{\boldsymbol{TP + TN}}{\boldsymbol{P + TN + FP + FN}}$$

What ratios can be calculated from the confusion matrix?

Since every use case targets on different metrics, some of these metrics have evolved over time. Here, we define the following cases:

True Positive Rate: It considers the cases in which positively classified data points were actually positive. It is defined by the following ratio:

$$\frac{TP}{TP+FN}$$

True Negative Rate: It considers all those cases in which negatively classified data points were actually negative. It is expressed by the following ratio:

$$\frac{TN}{TN+FP}$$

Precision: This metric indicates the correctness of the positive label. It computes how likely outcome of the (+ive) class is accurate. Precision is defined as the relative frequency of correctly, positively classified subjects. Further it can be written as

$$\frac{TP}{TP+FP}$$

Sensitivity: It calculates the fraction of positive classes accurately found out. It provides how well the model is to identify positive class.

$$\text{Recall} = \frac{TP}{TP+FN}$$

What can we Understand from the Above Confusion Matrix?

If you were forecasting about the illness, "yes" indicates having an illness, and "no" means not having that illness.

ML classification generates a total of 165 forecast (For example, 165 sufferers were being tested for that illness).

From 165 cases, the machine learning classifier predicted "yes" 110 times, and predicted "no" 55 times.

In actual case, 105 sufferers in that sample have the illness, and 60 sufferers do not.

Accuracy: It reflects the number of times the ML classifier is right

$$\frac{(TP+TN)}{SUM} = \frac{(100+50)}{165} = 0.91$$

Misclassification Rate: Totally, how many times is it incorrect?

$$\frac{\boldsymbol{(FP+FN)}}{\boldsymbol{Total}}=\frac{\mathbf{(10+5)}}{\mathbf{165}}=0.09$$

True Positive Rate: When it's yes, how many times does it forecast yes?

$$\frac{\boldsymbol{True\ Positive}}{\boldsymbol{Actual\ Yes}}=\frac{\mathbf{100}}{\mathbf{105}}=0.95$$

False Positive Rate: When it's actually no, how many times does it forecast yes?

$$\frac{\boldsymbol{False\ Positive}}{\boldsymbol{Actual\ No}}=\frac{\mathbf{10}}{\mathbf{60}}=0.17$$

True Negative Rate: When it's actually no, how many times does it forecast no?

$$\frac{\boldsymbol{False\ Negative}}{\boldsymbol{Actual\ No}}=\frac{\mathbf{50}}{\mathbf{60}}=0.83$$

Precision: When it forecasts yes, how many times is it right?

$$\frac{\boldsymbol{TP}}{\boldsymbol{AForecasted\ Yes}}=\frac{\mathbf{100}}{\mathbf{110}}=0.91$$

Prevalence: How many times does the yes condition actually happened in the sample?

$$\frac{\boldsymbol{Actual\ Yes}}{\boldsymbol{Sum}}=\frac{\mathbf{105}}{\mathbf{165}}=0.64$$

***Combining all the three models**
Output of the support vector classifier (as shown in Figure 11.6) is as follows:
Efficiency on train data by SV Classifier: 100.0
Test data efficiency by SV Classifier: 100.0

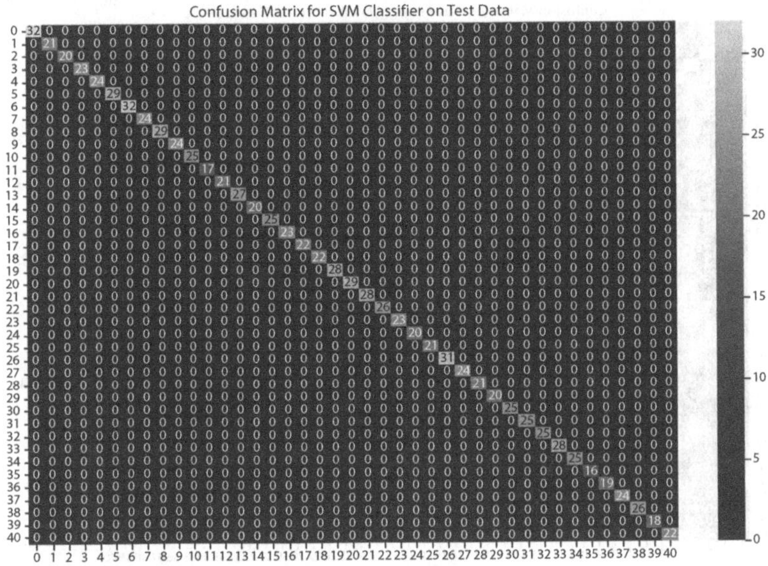

Figure 11.6 Confusion matrix.

Output of the Naive Bayes Classifier (as shown in Figure 11.7) is as follows:
Train data accuracy by NB Classifier: 100.0 Test data accuracy by NB Classifier: 100.0

Output of the Random Forest (as shown in Figure 11.8) is as follows:
Train data accuracy by RF Classifier: 100.0 Test data accuracy by RF Classifier: 100.0

At this stage, observing all these matrices, we conclude that the systems are giving good results on new values. Here, one can train a system on complete train value available in data set which was earlier downloaded and then finally we perform testing operation on the available test data set.

Model Fitting on the Whole Data set and Test Data set Validation
Output of the Python Implementation (as shown in Figure 11.9) is as follows:
Test data accuracy by the combined model: 100.0

At this stage we conclude all the data set is classified accurately by the used combined model. Now finally we create a user-defined function which accepts symptoms as input and predicts the output as illness. For accomplishing this, we consider all the models all together.

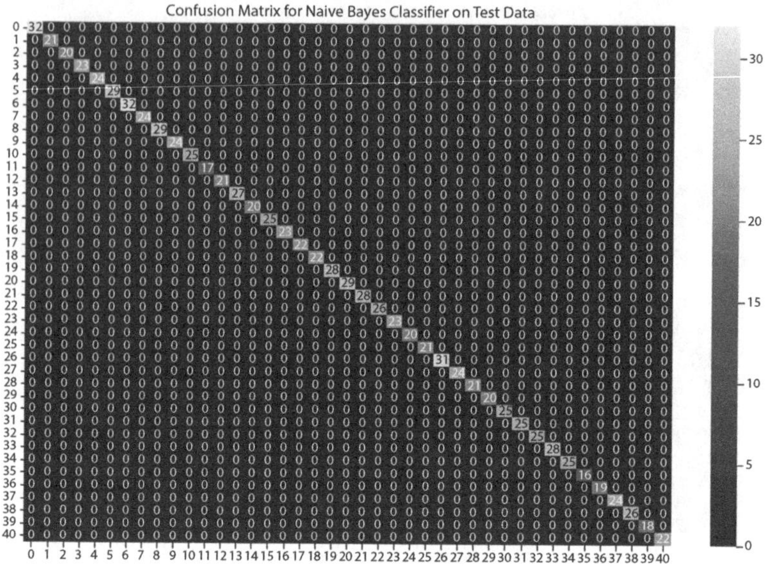

Figure 11.7 Confusion matrix.

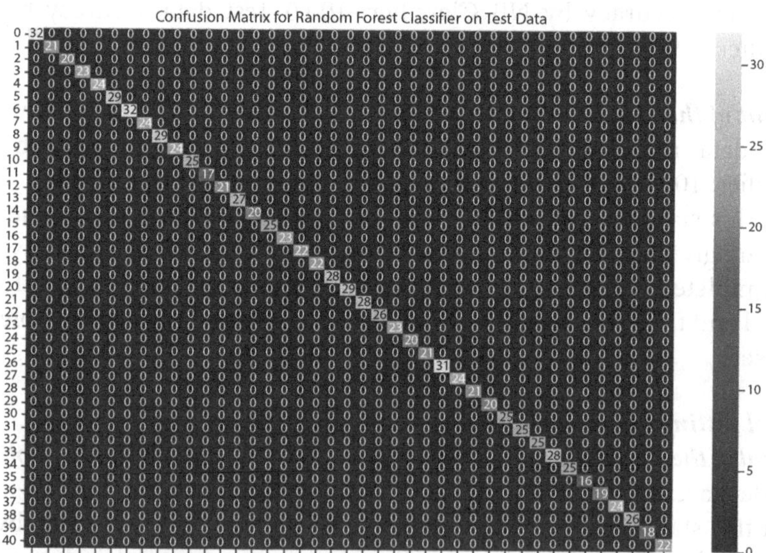

Figure 11.8 Confusion matrix.

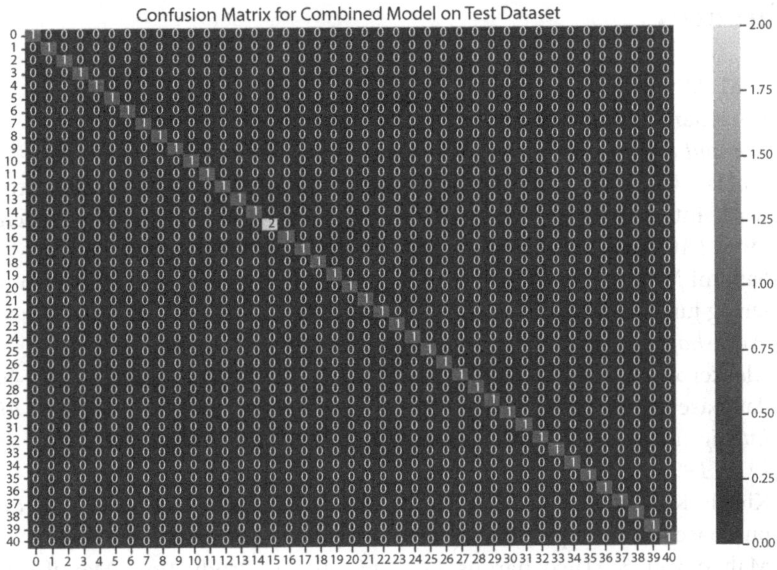

Figure 11.9 Confusion matrix.

Creation of a User-Defined Function Which Accepts Input Symptoms and Forecasts About the Possible Illness

Output of the Python Implementation is as follows:
'RF forecast': 'Fungal infection', 'NB forecast': 'Fungal infection', 'SVM forecast': 'Fungal infection', 'Final forecast': 'Fungal infection'

Here it is necessary that whatever symptoms we are providing to the user defined function as an input they should be among the 132 symptoms available in the data set.

Discussion

We analyzed ML classification techniques for the forecasting of symptoms for a particular type of illness. Because the medical data and its research changes at a large extent between such illness prediction use cases, a comparative analysis can be made when a general benchmark on data set and its existence is maintained. Hence, we only selected studies that performed various ML approaches on similar data set and illness forecasting for their comparison. Despite changes on repetition and their merits, produced outcomes indicate the immense power of those categories of classification techniques in the illness forecasting.

References

[1] T. M. Mitchell, *Machine Learning*. McGraw-Hill Boston, MA: 1997.

[2] Sebastiani F. Machine learning in automated text categorization. *ACM Comput Surveys (CSUR)*. 2002;34(1):1–47.

[3] Sinclair C, Pierce L, Matzner S. An application of machine learning to network intrusion detection. In: *Computer Security Applications Conference, 1999. (ACSAC'99) Proceedings. 15th Annual; 1999*. pp. 371–7. IEEE.

[4] Sahami M, Dumais S, Heckerman D, Horvitz E. A Bayesian approach to filtering junk e-mail. In: *Learning for Text Categorization: Papers from the 1998 Workshop*, vol. 62; 1998. pp. 98–105. Madison, Wisconsin.

[5] Aleskerov E, Freisleben B, Rao B. Cardwatch: A neural network-based database mining system for credit card fraud detection. In: *Computational Intelligence for Financial Engineering (CIFEr)*, 1997, *Proceedings of the IEEE/IAFE 1997*; 1997. pp. 220–6. IEEE.

[6] Kim E, Kim W, Lee Y. Combination of multiple classifiers for the customer's purchase behavior prediction. *Decis Support Syst*. 2003;34(2):167–75.

[7] Mahadevan S, Theocharous G. "Optimizing Production Manufacturing Using Reinforcement Learning," in *FLAIRS Conference*; 1998. pp. 372–7.

[8] Yao D, Yang J, Zhan X. A novel method for disease prediction: hybrid of random forest and multivariate adaptive regression splines. *J Comput*. 2013; 8(1):170–7.

[9] R. S. Michalski, J. G. Carbonell, and T. M. Mitchell, *Machine Learning: an Artificial Intelligence Approach*. Springer Science & Business Media, 2013.

[10] Culler SD, Parchman ML, Przybylski M. Factors related to potentially preventable hospitalizations among the elderly. *Med Care*. 1998; 1:804–17.

[11] Uddin MS, Hossain L. Social networks enabled coordination model for cost Management of Patient Hospital Admissions. *J Healthc Qual*. 2011;33(5):37–48.

[12] Lee PP, *et al.* Cost of patients with primary open-angle glaucoma: a retrospective study of commercial insurance claims data. *Ophthalmology*. 2007;114(7):1241–7.

[13] Davis DA, Chawla NV, Christakis NA, Barabási A-L. Time to CARE: a collaborative engine for practical disease prediction. *Data Min Knowl Disc*. 2010;20(3):388–415.

[14] McCormick T, Rudin C, Madigan D. A hierarchical model for association rule mining of sequential events: an approach to automated medical symptom prediction; 2011.

[15] Yiannakoulias N, Schopflocher D, Svenson L. Using administrative data to understand the geography of case ascertainment. *Chron Dis Can*. 2009; 30(1):20–8.

[16] Fisher ES, Malenka DJ, Wennberg JE, Roos NP. Technology assessment using insurance claims: example of prostatectomy. *Int J Technol Assess Health Care*. 1990;6(02):194–202.

[17] Farran B, Channanath AM, Behbehani K, Thanaraj TA. Predictive models to assess risk of type 2 diabetes, hypertension and comorbidity: machine-learning algorithms and validation using national health data from Kuwait-a cohort study. *BMJ Open*. 2013;3(5):e002457.
[18] Ahmad LG, Eshlaghy A, Poorebrahimi A, Ebrahimi M, Razavi A. Using three machine learning techniques for predicting breast cancer recurrence. *J Health Med Inform*. 2013;4(124):3.

12

Supervised and Unsupervised Learning Techniques for Biometric Systems

Pallavi Pandey*, Yogita Yashveer Raghav, Sarita Gulia, Sagar Aggarwal and Nitin Kumar

Department of Computer Science and Engineering, School of Engineering and Technology, KR Mangalam University, Gurugram, India

Abstract

In the domain of biometric systems, where individual identities are confirmed through distinctive traits like fingerprints, facial geometry, and gait patterns, the application of supervised and unsupervised machine learning techniques plays a pivotal role. This chapter provides a comprehensive examination of these approaches within the context of biometric systems. Supervised learning, which relies on labeled data to train models for predicting outcomes, has proven effective in various biometric applications, employing algorithms such as Convolutional Neural Networks, Support Vector Machines, logistic regression, and Decision trees. Unsupervised learning, in contrast, excels in automatic feature extraction, data analysis, and learning strategy creation. While it may not be the primary choice for identification, it contributes significantly to improved feature fusion and data analysis. This chapter offers a detailed exploration of these machine learning techniques, assessing their suitability for both identification and verification processes. Furthermore, it addresses the persistent challenges faced in biometric system development, ranging from handling numerous identities and security concerns to extracting relevant data from noisy inputs. Privacy, data breaches, and the evolving nature of biometric attributes are also discussed. With biometrics increasingly integrated into everyday devices like smartphones, this chapter underscores the balance required between security and usability, exploring the motivations driving enhancements in biometric recognition methods to meet the growing demands for performance, usability, and security. Additionally, the chapter provides a comprehensive overview of various biometric techniques, highlighting their respective advantages and challenges,

**Corresponding author*: jipallavi@gmail.com

Suman Kumar Swarnkar, J P Patra, Sapna Singh Kshatri, Yogesh Kumar Rathore and Tien Anh Tran (eds.) Supervised and Unsupervised Data Engineering for Multimedia Data, (263–300) © 2024 Scrivener Publishing LLC

thereby offering insights into their uniqueness and application suitability. In summary, this chapter serves as an invaluable resource for those involved in the dynamic and ever-evolving field of biometrics.

***Keywords*:** Biometrics, supervised learning, unsupervised learning, identification, verification, challenges, techniques, machine learning

Introduction

It is well known that the biometric system refers to a real-time system that uses an individual's distinctive traits, including fingerprints and facial geometric patterns, to confirm their identity. In addition to fingerprints and facial data, there are other biometric traits like gait pattern, periocular region, sclera, ears and iris data. Gait patterns are the patterns which are created during walking. That is, when a person walks, he or she creates a pattern called gait pattern. The two methods of machine learning generally used for developing a biometric system are supervised learning and unsupervised learning. Although there is one more method called reinforcement learning, in this chapter, only supervised and unsupervised methods used in the multimedia data related to biometric system have been explored. The machine learns while being watched over in supervised learning as the name suggests supervised. It has a model that can forecast outcomes using labelled data. A dataset with tags indicates that the intended result is already known. With unsupervised learning, a computer uses unlabeled data to learn on its own. In order to produce results or make predictions based on the inputted data, machine learning makes extensive use of structured data. These data include images, videos and sounds and are also called multimedia data.

Supervised learning has benefited various biometric applications using several existing techniques. Convolution-based neutral networks, Support Vector Machines, logistic regression, and Decision trees are a few of the algorithms. Biometrics that use unsupervised machine learning ensure good learning processes, better classification, and precise location of biometric features. It is possible to fully extract the automatic finger pattern using unsupervised methods. But it could be applied in the preliminary stage for improved feature fusion, data analysis, and learning strategy creation.

This chapter deals with the various machine learning techniques that fall under supervised or unsupervised methods used in the literature for biometric systems. Moreover, the comparison between these two learning methods will also be done to find out which one should be better for biometric identification and verification. Biometric identification is a matching process that matches the current test data to the available N data stored in the system, whereas biometric verification involves one to one matching regarding whether this person is Mr. X or not. The chapter covers both the biometric systems, that is, identification and verification. There can be works that can use a combination of both the learning methods as a fusion approach can be a good approach for developing a biometric system so these types of works will also be elaborated in the chapter.

In recent years, machine learning tasks involving computer vision, natural language processing, and speech processing have seen impressive progress. Biometrics largely makes use of supervised learning and unsupervised learning approaches because it is concerned with using attributes to identify individuals. Biometrics is the field of identification that uses a person's physical/behavioral traits. Physical traits including a person's face, fingerprints, and iris are used in physiological biometrics. Behavior-based biometrics are highly influenced by various socioenvironmental elements and are dependent on an individual's actions. In order to be successful in practical applications, biometric systems must overcome some related difficulties [1].

Challenges in developing a biometric system

Numerous identities: Biometric recognition requires identifying possibly millions of people, each with subtle unique characteristics. To identify people on this scale, extremely complicated models are needed.

Invasion of biometric systems: There are several different ways that biometric systems can be attacked. Such attacks must be recognized as a part of the recognition system.

Intrapersonal variations: To fully capture variations in attributes, typically numerous samples of an individual are needed. Sometimes, these intraperson variations may be greater than differences between individuals.

Biometric data extraction: Extraction of pertinent biometric data from noisy input data necessitates extensive preprocessing (like extraction of a person's face from a crowded background or a person's speech signal from a noisy background).

Persistence: Biometric attributes may not be constant because they are dependent on human characteristics. While behavioral biometrics also depend on socio-environmental factors, physiological biometrics gradually change over time.

Distinctiveness: It's unknown whether a person may be identified exclusively by a single biometric characteristic. Particularly, the majority of behavioral biometrics are only utilized for verification because they are ineffective for identification.

Privacy as well as data breach: Biometrics is an access control method that is secure because biological traits are distinctive and nearly impossible to duplicate. On the other hand, because people maintain their passwords, passwords can be exchanged and readily obtained by hackers. Since the world can see the essential components of recognition, biometrics present a challenge to privacy. For instance, someone else may capture speech, use a photo for facial recognition without permission, or even duplicate fingerprints from a surface anyone can have touched.

Biometric information may be stolen or leaked by hackers if identity management systems are compromised. Because biometric data cannot be replaced, malevolent individuals can continue their illicit acts as long as they have access to it.

There are other challenges also which are related separately with modalities-based biometric systems, like in speech-based system, the voice of a human has been impacted by weather in everyday life. Also, if a person has a cough or a fever, it is quite challenging to recognize their voice. The frequency range between the caller and the receiver changes often. The performance of the microphone is once more impacted by the telephone frequency encoding and decoding procedure. Moreover, vocabulary and speech style are also a challenge to create a voice-based biometric system. Similarly, with palm print, it goes well with offline recognition [2, 3], but it does not work with an offline system [4]. Other challenges related to separate modalities are mentioned in section 2.

Motivations

On smartphones, tablets, laptops, and desktops, authentication is the primary method for establishing a user's identity and preventing illegal access. The use of biometrics on mobile devices is increasing since the majority of current smartphone models have at least one built-in biometric verification method, most typically face or fingerprint recognition. These might serve as a secure and useful alternative to PINs or passwords. However, there are still flaws in biometric systems, such as the ability to fake biometrics or be attacked directly by the devices and systems. Organizations can use this advice to weigh the advantages of implementing biometrics in devices against potential security issues. Studies' interest in boosting the effectiveness of biometric recognition methods is motivated by a variety of factors.

Devices that use biometric authentication may benefit greatly. The majority of consumers are already quite comfortable with using biometric authentication to unlock a device; therefore the system's simplicity will probably lead to a high uptake rate. Additionally, biometrics can offer a secure alternative to passwords and are typically much more practical than passwords, especially on the majority of modern cell phones. As a backup, smartphones still need the device passcode. However, because passcodes will be input much less frequently, organizations can impose passcodes that are more complicated without significantly reducing usability.

Various Biometric Techniques

Automated biometric authentication systems use a variety of physiological and behavioural characteristics. Every biometric attribute has benefits and drawbacks, and the choice of biometric technique depends on the application. No single biometric characteristic is expected to completely meet the requirements of all applications. The suitability of a specific biometric authentication technique for a specific application depends on both the manner in which the application is utilised and the features of the biometric feature. Brief descriptions of each currently used or being developed biometric feature are provided below.

Fingerprints

Fingerprint-based authentication has been shown to be the most dependable, efficient, and popular technique for human identity and verification. Every finger of a single person has a unique print. The first seven months of foetal development determine how a fingerprint, a pattern of ridges and valleys on the surface of a fingertip, will grow. The only elements that distinguish a fingerprint are the local ridge characteristics and how they interact. The ridges and valleys in a fingerprint alternate and move in a localised, predictable direction. The two most obvious local ridge characteristics are ridge bifurcation and ridge termination. Ridge termination refers to the point when a ridge abruptly ends. A ridge bifurcation occurs when a ridge divides into branch ridges. All of these details are referred to as minutiae. The bulk of fingerprint matching systems are built on four main fingerprint representation schemes: grayscale picture, phase image, skeleton image, and minutiae. Because it is distinct, condensed, and compatible with characteristics utilised by experts in the field of human fingerprints, minutiae-based representation has become the most widely used fingerprint representation system [5].

Benefits

- These systems are typically easy to install and utilise.
- It takes low-cost equipment with typically minimal power requirements.

- A fingerprint pattern is made up of components that are unique to each individual and that remain constant over time.
- Fingerprints are essentially global. Only 2% of the population of humans cannot utilise fingerprints because of skin injury or genetic issues.
- The most popular biometric is fingerprints.
- Passwords shouldn't need to be remembered; just swipe your finger across the scanner to complete the transaction.
- The technique is very secure since biometric fingerprint scanners offer a way to record an identifying point that is very difficult to forge.
- It is simple to use and has a fast and accurate verification process.

Challenges

- A fingerprint scanner may be inaccurate since it only scans a portion of the finger. Many scanning systems have the potential to be hacked by exhibiting fake fingers or someone else's finger.
- People who work in the chemical industries typically have their fingerprints altered.
- Cuts and markings change fingerprints, which frequently affects performance.
- Fingerprints are not confidential. Everywhere we go, we all leave our fingerprints. Once the fingerprints are taken, they are permanently taken! It's possible that you never return to a secure position.

Signature

A biometric signature is a type of biometric authentication that uses an individual's signature as the basis for identity verification. This typically involves capturing a digital image of an individual's signature and comparing it to reference signatures stored in a database. The system then uses pattern recognition and other techniques to determine if the two signatures match and if the individual should be granted access. Biometric signatures are commonly used in financial transactions and other high-security environments. It can provide a high level of accuracy and security but is difficult to implement and may not be suitable for all types of applications.

Benefits

- Signature biometrics are non-intrusive and easily integrated into existing processes.

- Signature biometrics can provide a high degree of security by making it difficult for someone to forge someone else's signature.
- Signature biometrics may be easier to use than other types of biometrics. This includes fingerprint or iris scans that may be considered invasive or intimidating.
- Biometric signatures can be used in a variety of applications, including financial transactions, government services, and other high-security environments.
- Signature biometrics are more reliable than other types of authentication, such as passwords or PIN, which are easily forgotten or stolen. Signature biometrics can provide an audit trail that allows organizations to track and verify the authenticity of transactions [5-7].

Challenges

- Signature biometrics can be vulnerable to forgery, especially if the reference signature does not adequately represent an individual's natural signature.
- Signature biometrics can be difficult to implement and may require specialized hardware such as signature pads to acquire and process the signature data.
- Signature biometrics may not be as accurate as other types of biometrics such as fingerprints or iris scans and can provide a higher level of uniqueness and individuality.
- Signature biometrics can be affected by changes in an individual's physical condition, such as aging or injury, which can change the signature's appearance over time. Signature biometrics can be less secure than other biometric methods in certain situations. For example, when a person signs a document in the presence of another person, who else can see the signature?

Gait

Gait biometrics, also known as gait analysis or gait recognition, is a form of biometrics that uses an individual's unique walking patterns to verify their identity. This typically involves capturing an image or video of a person walking and using computer vision and machine learning algorithms to analyze the person's movements and identify the unique characteristics of their gait. Ambulatory biometric systems can be used in a variety of applications, including security systems and surveillance, healthcare and sports performance analysis. Potential benefits of ambulatory biometrics include high accuracy, contactless measurement, and the ability to work remotely. However, this technology also has limitations and challenges: It requires special hardware and has potential for false positives or false negatives.

Benefits

- Gait biometrics can provide high accuracy because human gait is unique and difficult to imitate.
- Ambulatory biometrics can be unobtrusive because the person does not need to perform any special actions or touch the device.
- Ambulatory biometrics can be captured by cameras and other sensors without direct human involvement, so they can be used remotely.
- Gait biometrics can be robust against certain types of spoofing attacks, such as using a photo or video of a person to imitate walking.
- Gait biometrics can provide additional information that may be useful for other applications, such as speed, stride length, and a person's posture. Ambulatory biometrics can be used in a variety of settings, including security systems, surveillance, healthcare, and sports performance analysis [5,6].

Challenges

- Ambulatory biometrics can be affected by changes in a person's physical condition, such as injury, illness, or weight change that may alter gait.
- Gait biometrics are difficult to implement and can require specialized hardware such as cameras and motion sensors to capture and process the gait data.
- Ambulatory biometrics can be less accurate than other types of biometrics that offer a higher level of uniqueness and individuality, such as fingerprints and iris scans.
- Ambulatory biometrics may not be suitable for people with certain disabilities, such as movement disorders that affect the ability to walk.
- Gait biometrics can be vulnerable to impersonation attacks such as mimicking human gait using prosthetics or robotic

devices. Ambulatory biometrics may not be suitable for all types of applications, such as situations where a person is sitting or stationary.

Palm print

A palm print is a type of biometric identification that uses the unique patterns on the palm of a person's hand to identify them. This type of identification is often used in security systems because the palm of the hand is difficult to replicate and is unique to each individual. To create a palm print for biometric identification, a person typically places their hand on a scanner that captures the image of their palm. This image is then processed by a computer algorithm that extracts the unique features of the palm, such as the lines and ridges, and creates a template that can be used for identification. This template is stored in a database and can be compared to other palm print images to verify a person's identity.

Advantages

There are several advantages to using palm prints for biometric identification, including:

- **High level of accuracy**: Palm prints are unique to each individual and are difficult to replicate, making them a reliable method of identification.
- **Non-intrusive**: Unlike other biometric methods, such as fingerprints, palm prints can be captured without the person having to touch a scanner or provide any physical contact. This makes the process more convenient and hygienic.
- **Fast and efficient**: Palm print scanners are fast and can capture a high-quality image of a person's palm in a matter of seconds. This makes the identification process quick and efficient.
- **Versatility**: Palm print scanners can be used in a variety of settings, such as airports, government buildings, and office buildings, to provide secure access control.
- **Cost-effective**: Palm print technology is relatively inexpensive compared to other methods, like iris or facial-based authentication. This makes it a cost-effective option for organizations looking to implement biometric identification systems.

Challenges

There are a few challenges to using palm prints for biometric identification, including:

- **Poor image quality**: In some cases, the quality of the palm print image may be poor, making it difficult for the computer algorithm to accurately extract the unique features of the palm. This can lead to a high rate of false rejections or false acceptances, which can compromise the security of the system.
- **Limited data**: Unlike fingerprints, which are commonly used for biometric identification, there is not as much data available on palm prints. This can make it difficult for the computer algorithm to accurately identify individuals based on their palm prints.
- **User cooperation**: In order for a palm print to be captured accurately, the user must cooperate and place their hand on the scanner in the correct position. If the user does not cooperate, the quality of the palm print image may be poor, leading to inaccurate identification.
- **Limited use cases**: Palm print technology is not as versatile as other biometric methods, such as fingerprints or facial recognition. This means that it may not be suitable for all biometric identification applications.
- **Privacy concerns**: As with any biometric identification method, there are concerns about the potential for palm print data to be misused or accessed without the user's consent. This can raise privacy concerns and may deter some people from using palm print technology [7].

Hand geometry

Hand geometry is a type of biometric identification that uses the shape and size of a person's hand to identify them. This method is often used in security systems because the shape and size of the hand is difficult to replicate and is unique to each individual. To create a hand geometry biometric, a person typically places their hand on a scanner that captures the dimensions of their hand, such as the length and width of the fingers, the palm, and the overall hand shape. This information is then processed by a computer algorithm that creates a template that can be used for identification. This template is stored in a database and can be compared to other hand geometry biometrics to verify a person's identity.

Benefits

There are several benefits to using hand geometry for biometric identification, including:

- **High level of accuracy**: Hand geometry is a reliable method of identification because the shape and size of a person's hand is unique and difficult to replicate.
- **Non-intrusive**: Unlike other biometric methods, such as fingerprints or palm prints, hand geometry does not require the person to make any physical contact with a scanner. This makes the process more convenient and hygienic.
- **Fast and efficient**: Hand geometry scanners are fast and can capture the dimensions of a person's hand in a matter of seconds. This makes the identification process quick and efficient.
- **Versatility**: Hand geometry scanners can be used in a variety of settings, such as airports, government buildings, and office buildings, to provide secure access control.
- **Cost-effective**: Hand geometry technology is relatively inexpensive compared to other biometric methods, such as iris or facial recognition. This makes it a cost-effective option for organizations looking to implement biometric identification systems.

Challenges

There are a few challenges to using hand geometry for biometric identification, including:

- **Poor image quality:** In some cases, the dimensions of the hand may not be captured accurately, leading to a high rate of false rejections or false acceptances. This can compromise the security of the system.
- **Limited data:** Unlike fingerprints, which are commonly used for biometric identification, there is not as much data available on hand geometry. This can make it difficult for the computer algorithm to accurately identify individuals based on their hand geometry.
- **User cooperation:** In order for hand geometry to be captured accurately, the user must cooperate and place their hand on the scanner in the correct position. If the user does

not cooperate, the dimensions of the hand may not be captured accurately, leading to inaccurate identification.

- **Limited use cases:** Hand geometry technology is not as versatile as other biometric methods, such as fingerprints or facial recognition. This means that it may not be suitable for all biometric identification applications.
- **Privacy concerns:** As with any biometric identification method, there are concerns about the potential for hand geometry data to be misused or accessed without the user's consent. This can raise privacy concerns and may deter some people from using hand geometry technology.

Voice

Voice biometrics, also known as voice recognition or voice authentication, is a type of biometrics that uses a person's unique voice characteristics to verify their identity. This usually involves recording a person's voice and analysing the voiceprint using a computer algorithm. This is the set of unique features of the human voice. Voice biometric authentication systems can be used in a variety of applications, including security systems, customer service, and voice control devices. Potential advantages of voice biometrics include high accuracy, convenience, and the ability to work remotely. However, this technology also has limitations and challenges: the need for high-quality audio recordings and the potential for false positives or false negatives [8].

Benefits

- the human voice is unique and difficult to imitate, so voiceprint recognition can provide high accuracy.
- Voice biometrics are convenient and easy to use because they do not require the person to take any special actions or touch the device.
- Voice biometrics can be captured using microphones and other sensors without direct human involvement, so they can be used remotely.
- Voice biometrics can be robust against certain types of spoofing attacks, such as recordings of a person's voice to mimic voiceprints.

- Voice biometric authentication can provide additional information such as: It may also be useful for other applications, such as a person's emotional state, accent, and speaking speed. Voice biometric authentication can be used in a variety of environments, including security systems, customer service, and voice-enabled devices.

Challenges

- Voice biometrics can be affected by changes in a person's physical condition, such as a cold or sore throat that can change your voice.
- Voice biometrics can be difficult to implement and may require special hardware such as microphones and noise-cancelling technology to capture and process voice data.
- Voice biometrics can be less accurate than other types of biometrics such as fingerprints and iris scans, providing a higher level of uniqueness and individuality.
- Voice biometrics may not be suitable for people with certain disabilities, such as a language disorder affecting speech ability.

Voice biometric authentication can be vulnerable to spoofing attacks such as using recordings of a person's voice to mimic voiceprints. Voice biometrics may not be suitable for all types of applications, such as in a noisy environment where people's voices are difficult to hear.

Iris

Iris recognition is a sort of biometric identification that recognizes people by their eyes' distinctive iris patterns. This method is often used in security systems because the iris is unique to each individual and is difficult to replicate. To create an iris biometric, a person typically looks into a scanner that captures an image of their iris. This image is then processed by a computer algorithm that extracts the unique features of the iris, such as the patterns and colors, and creates a template that can be used for identification. This template is stored in a database and can be compared to other iris biometrics to verify a person's identity.

Benefits

There are several benefits to using iris recognition for biometric identification, including:

- **High level of accuracy**: Iris recognition is a highly accurate method of identification because the iris is unique to each individual and is difficult to replicate.
- **Non-intrusive**: Unlike other biometric methods, such as fingerprints or palm prints, iris recognition does not require the person to make any physical contact with a scanner. This makes the process more convenient and hygienic.
- **Fast and efficient**: Iris recognition scanners are fast and can capture an image of a person's iris in a matter of seconds. This makes the identification process quick and efficient.
- **Versatility**: Iris recognition scanners can be used in a variety of settings, such as airports, government buildings, and office buildings, to provide secure access control.
- **Cost-effective**: Iris recognition technology is relatively inexpensive compared to other biometric methods, such as facial recognition. This makes it a cost-effective option for organizations looking to implement biometric identification systems.

Challenges

There are a few challenges to using iris recognition for biometric identification, including:

- **Poor image quality**: In some cases, the quality of the iris image may be poor, making it difficult for the computer algorithm to accurately extract the unique features of the iris. This can lead to a high rate of false rejections or false acceptances, which can compromise the security of the system.
- **Limited data**: Unlike fingerprints, which are commonly used for biometric identification, there is not as much data available on iris recognition. This can make it difficult for the computer algorithm to accurately identify individuals based on their iris.
- **User cooperation**: In order for an iris biometric to be captured accurately, the user must cooperate and look into the scanner in the correct position. If the user does not cooperate, the quality of the iris image may be poor, leading to inaccurate identification.

- **Limited use cases**: Iris recognition technology is not as versatile as other biometric methods, such as fingerprints or facial recognition. This means that it may not be suitable for all biometric identification applications.
- **Privacy concerns**: As with any biometric identification method, there are concerns about the potential for iris biometric data to be misused or accessed without the user's consent. This can raise privacy concerns and may deter some people from using iris recognition technology.

Retina

Iris recognition is a sort of biometric identification that uses the distinctive patterns of an individual's eyes to identify them. This method is often used in security systems because the retina is unique to each individual and is difficult to replicate. To create a retina biometric, a person typically looks into a scanner that captures an image of their retina. This image is then processed by a computer algorithm that extracts the unique features of the retina, such as the blood vessels and the nerve fibers, and creates a template that can be used for identification. This template is stored in a database and can be compared to other retina biometrics to verify a person's identity [9].

There are several advantages to using retina recognition for biometric identification, including:

- **High level of accuracy**: Retina recognition is a highly accurate method of identification because the retina is unique to each individual and is difficult to replicate.
- **Non-intrusive**: Unlike other biometric methods, such as fingerprints or palm prints, retina recognition does not require the person to make any physical contact with a scanner. This makes the process more convenient and hygienic.
- **Fast and efficient**: Retina recognition scanners are fast and can capture an image of a person's retina in a matter of seconds. This makes the identification process quick and efficient.
- **Versatility**: Retina recognition scanners can be used in a variety of settings, such as airports, government buildings, and office buildings, to provide secure access control.
- **Cost-effective**: Retina recognition technology is relatively inexpensive compared to other biometric methods, such as facial recognition. This makes it a cost-effective option for organizations looking to implement biometric identification systems.

Infrared thermogram

An infrared thermogram is a type of biometric identification that uses the heat signatures of a person's face to identify them. This method is often used in security systems because the heat patterns on a person's face are unique and difficult to replicate. To create an infrared thermogram biometric, a person typically looks into a scanner that captures an image of their face using infrared light. This image is then processed by a computer algorithm that extracts the unique heat signatures of the face and creates a template that can be used for identification. This template is stored in a database and can be compared to other infrared thermogram biometrics to verify a person's identity.

Benefits

- **High level of accuracy**: Infrared thermograms are a reliable method of identification because the heat patterns on a person's face are unique and difficult to replicate.
- **Non-intrusive**: Unlike other biometric methods, such as fingerprints or palm prints, infrared thermograms do not require the person to make any physical contact with a scanner. This makes the process more convenient and hygienic.
- **Fast and efficient**: Infrared thermogram scanners are fast and can capture an image of a person's face in a matter of seconds. This makes the identification process quick and efficient.
- **Versatility**: Infrared thermogram scanners can be used in a variety of settings, such as airports, government buildings, and office buildings, to provide secure access control.
- **Cost-effective**: Infrared thermogram technology is relatively inexpensive compared to other biometric methods, such as facial recognition. This makes it a cost-effective option for organizations looking to implement biometric identification systems [9].

Face

A form of biometric identification known as facial recognition uses the distinctive features of a person's face to identify them. This method is often used in security systems because the face is unique to each individual and is difficult to replicate. To create a facial recognition biometric, a person typically looks into a scanner that captures an image of their face. This image is then processed by a computer algorithm that extracts the unique features of the face, such as the shape of the eyes, nose, and mouth, and creates a template that can be used for identification. This template is stored in a database and can be compared to other facial recognition biometrics to verify a person's identity.

Challenges

To keep your personal information secure, it is crucial to weigh the risks and drawbacks of facial recognition technology despite its many advantages.

- **Individual and social privacy may be violated.**
  The potential risk to personal privacy presented by facial recognition technology is a severe negative. People object to having photos of their faces collected and stored in databases for a potential future use.
- **Data vulnerabilities are produced.**
  There is a chance that facial recognition data stored in databases will be compromised. Hackers have gained access to databases that house facial scans that have been gathered and used by banks, police forces, and defence companies.
- **It presents chances for fraud and other criminal activity.**
  Criminals may utilise facial recognition technology to target helpless victims when committing their crimes. They can obtain sensitive information about people, such as photos and videos taken via facial scans and stored in databases, in order to commit identity fraud. A thief might use this information to open credit cards or bank accounts in the victim's name, or even steal the victim's identity to perpetrate crimes.
- **Technology is fallible.**
  A number of other factors, such as camera angles, illumination, and image or video quality, could influence the technology's ability to recognise faces. Facial recognition software can potentially be tricked by wearing disguises or slightly changing one's look.

DNA

DNA biometric identification is a method that uses the unique genetic code of an individual to identify them. This method is often used in forensic science and law enforcement because DNA is unique to each individual and is difficult to replicate. To create a DNA biometric, a sample of a person's DNA, such as a saliva or blood sample, is collected and processed by a computer algorithm that extracts the unique genetic code of the individual and creates a template that can be used for identification. This template is stored in a database and can be compared to other DNA biometrics to verify a person's identity [9].

Benefits

- **It is a minimally invasive testing method.**
  For matching and comparison, a DNA sample is necessary. Material retrieval is a quick and painless technique because DNA may be discovered in various bodily fluids and tissues. Many collectors take saliva from the mouth for testing using a cotton swab. It is also possible to use hair follicles. This lowers the cost of collection and does away with the inconvenience of using needles to take blood.
- **It can be used for criminal justice purposes.**
  Although the criminal justice system may employ DNA fingerprinting to build genetic profiles for suspects, this technology is capable of much more. People can learn more about their heritage with the use of products like 23andMe and AncestryDNA. DNA comparisons can be used to determine which family members are related.
- **It can be used to identify inherited diseases.**
  DNA fingerprinting is commonly used to identify specific genetic illnesses, some of which could be fatal if not properly recognised.

Challenges

- **It creates issues with privacy.**
  An immortal database can hold a DNA sample that has been collected and analysed using modern technology. If this information is accessed, privacy issues can be raised, especially if the DNA was obtained illegally.
- **Hacking becomes a significant problem.**
  Databases containing DNA information may possibly be accessed due to security weaknesses. This might lead to a new kind of identity theft because it would make it possible for outside parties to get DNA fingerprinting data.

Major Biometric-Based Problems from a Security Perspective

There are a few researches that focus on machine learning and biometric identification from the standpoint of security. Because the most often utilized recognition method is biometry, the approach for our investigation was carried out utilizing the procedures below. These are:

- The WOS database studies from 2010 to 2016 were used for this investigation.
- While scanning research, the terms machine learning, security, and biometric recognition are searched for.
- It was observed that machine learning methods are employed not only for the biometric recognition and authentication process but also to limit user-caused vulnerabilities and to create a safe platform for biometric applications. Due to these factors, the biometric identification process has been examined in terms of biometric application vulnerabilities, user convenience, and usage contexts. Appropriate studies have also been chosen for these criteria.
- The findings of this analysis have been used to identify and assess common approaches and methodologies. The observed results demonstrate machine learning techniques for security viewpoint.
- The literature search using the keywords "biometric application" and "security" has shown four primary issues. These include recording user session information, retaining characteristic data, exploiting institutional or organisational weaknesses when employing biometric applications, and leveraging biometric data for financial gain. According to these four objectives, studies were created. Machine learning algorithms, and their success rates, application domains, and datasets were all examined from a security standpoint.

During the biometric recognition process, machine learning methods are used for a variety of objectives in addition to characterizing traits. Among these varied goals are increasing speed and reliability through developed biometric methods, liveness recognition of biometric features, classifying biometric data sets to analyse and conduct the classification procedure in order to improve the statistical method used in the biometric authentication process, and so on [12], [13-15], [16-18], [19-30]. The preservation of the biometric traits, the security of the biometric traits' attributes, and issues that arise while employing biometric applications are viewed as the major shortcomings of the process [3]. Therefore, in this chapter, the biometric identification process has been examined in light of user-friendliness, programmed vulnerabilities, and utilization areas.

Thanks to the security measures and protocols we've already mentioned, a trustworthy biometric system can be installed on the platforms. Despite all safeguards, a number of circumstances may impair data availability, confidentiality, and integrity. The violation of this law constitutes an outright violation of the person's privacy and personal information. Depending on who took the photo, there are several options for what to do if someone's biometric data is hacked. To demonstrate the potential misuse of people, systems, factors, methodologies, techniques, and technology during biometric authentication, we can suggest and explain a number of situations.

- Case I: Information about such a user's session may be recorded. An attacker can have the same permissions as the user due to the biometric feature used for login. It is common knowledge that someone's private information, including their first and last names, address, phone number, email address, passwords, and in some situations even their credit card number, may be compromised. With the usage of the private information, people may potentially unintentionally become involved in crimes.
- Case II: Any assault has the potential to compromise the private data. These data could be distributed or sold for commercial or other gain.
- Case III: Biometric characteristics may be gathered from organisational or institutional weaknesses. For instance, national ID numbers from Brazil, the United States, Turkey, and other countries have lately been posted online.
- Case IV: Biometric data may be gathered from outside sources and utilised to create other biometric data, such as personality data derived from facial traits [10], [11].
- Case V: It is risky to use biometric characteristics for passwords or other similar applications. That is due to the restriction of having unique values. For instance, when a biometric characteristic is recorded, a person's password is acquired. As a result, it immediately breaches integrity and secrecy.

As can be observed from the aforementioned situations, biometric systems have certain flaws and some crucial components that need to be safeguarded in order to provide data confidentiality, integrity, and availability using the methods and technology at hand.

There are a few researches that focus on machine learning and biometric identification from the standpoint of security. Because the most often utilised recognition method is biometry, the WOS database studies from 2010 to 2016 were used for this investigation. When "Security" and "biometric recognition" are searched for, the keywords "PCA, LDA, KNN, Naive Bayes, SVM, GMM, ANN, HMM, LBP" are also queried. The findings of this scan have been used to identify and assess common approaches and methodologies.

Biometrics machine learning solutions from a security point of view
In these situations, these two essential factors must be taken into account while creating a secured biometric identification platform:

- The data that was gathered throughout the application process can be safely preserved.
- Application security flaws that could be discovered during the implementation phase of the project should be kept to a minimum.

In this part, the research has been assessed using the five examples previously mentioned in terms of the application, user, and usage areas. Additionally, machine learning approaches that are used to increase the security of built apps have been examined and given in Table 12.1.

Supervised Learning Methods for Biometric System

In comparison to iris recognition, the retinal imaging biometric is dependent on each individual's retina's distinctive patterns. It predates iris scanning, another procedure that makes use of the ocular region. In the inside of the eye, it makes up 65% of the inner wall of the eyeball; there are distinctive blood vessels that are recognized by pattern. The innermost layer of that eye has a thin tissue called the retina that is composed of neural cells. Even identical twins have unique optic patterns that stay unchanged throughout life. The retina cannot be duplicated, it is destroyed so rapidly after death, it can only be examined on a living person. The standard size

Table 12.1 Security perspective, properties, data sets, and success criteria comparison of used machine learning techniques.

Ref.	Features	Security perspective	Developed/ used/ proposed methods	Success rate	Data set	Case
[12]	Face/Palmprint	Make a new cancelable biometric template generation technique utilising one-way modulus hashing and Gaussian random vectors.	Gaussian Random Vector/PCA/ LDA	Average EER for PCA was 0.05%; average EER for LDA was 0.03%; average EER for LDA was 0.2%; and average palm EER was 0.05%.	ORL/Yale/Indian Face/ PolyU/Casia	I, II, V
[13]	Face	Describe a novel method for protecting facial biometrics during recognition that makes use of so-called cancellable biometrics.	2DPCA	Up to 3% more accurate than the original data	ORL	I, II, V
[14]	Face	Create safe facial biometric templates using a revolutionary biometric protection technique to be utilised with statistical recognition algorithms.	2DPCA	3% and 4.5% more accurate recognition than the original and other altered data	ORL	I, II, V

(*Continued*)

Table 12.1 Security perspective, properties, data sets, and success criteria comparison of used machine learning techniques. (*Continued*)

Ref.	Features	Security perspective	Developed/ used/ proposed methods	Success rate	Data set	Case
[15]	Fingerprint	Present a novel binary length-fixed fingerprint feature generating approach.	BCH/Reed–Solomon/ LDPC	4.58% zeroFAR	FVC2002 DB2	I, V
[17]	Fingerprint	Concentrate on implementing and evaluating a biometric cryptosystem using a variety of fingerprint texture descriptors.	Gabor Filter/ LBP	EER of the fingerprint texture descriptors for Finger Code 10.96%, LBP8-22.79%, LBP16-19.54%, LBP24-24.6%, LBPu2 -22.88% LBPri-29.56%, and LDP 15.95%	FVC2000 DB2a	I, II, III, IV, V
[19]	Iris	Identify printed-iris attacks/ Resist attacks based on high-quality printing	SVM, LBP Linear Kernel, Gabor Sobel Filter	FGR 2.25/FFR 0.25/ HTER 1.25	Miche Database/ Mobio-fake Database	I, V

(*Continued*)

Table 12.1 Security perspective, properties, data sets, and success criteria comparison of used machine learning techniques. (*Continued*)

Ref.	Features	Security perspective	Developed/ used/ proposed methods	Success rate	Data set	Case
[20]	Mouse Dynamics	Examine biometric authentication systems using a variety of analytical methods, and compare static and dynamic trust models.	SVM, ANN, Multi Classifier Fusion (MCF), LibSVM	FMR 0.37%/FNMR 1.12%	Their approach, which is based on data from 28 users and focuses on various mouse occurrences	I
[21]	Face	Biometrics research is now active as a result of growing privacy and security concerns as well as the requirement to accurately determine an individual's identification.	SVM with AD, EM algorithm with NB	-	VidTIMIT dataset/ MBGC dataset	I, II
[22]	Face/ Fingerprint/ Iris	The proposed approach uses online learning to update the selection process continually.	SVM, Fusion algorithms	FAR 0.01%	WVU/LEA	I, II, III, V

(*Continued*)

Table 12.1 Security perspective, properties, data sets, and success criteria comparison of used machine learning techniques. (*Continued*)

Ref.	Features	Security perspective	Developed/ used/ proposed methods	Success rate	Data set	Case
[23]	Face	Present a computational method for identifying people that integrates soft biometrics relating to the face and body.	SVM, Gaussian kernel, SUM, Bayesian, Fuzzy Logic	identification rate of 88%	ORLAT&T/Yale/ MUCT	IV
[24]	Iris	Leave the detection and feature extraction issues in the background and concentrate on recognition	ANN,SVM	FRR average value of 19.80%	CASIA-Iris V1 database	I, II, III, IV, V

(*Continued*)

Table 12.1 Security perspective, properties, data sets, and success criteria comparison of used machine learning techniques. (*Continued*)

Ref.	Features	Security perspective	Developed/ used/ proposed methods	Success rate	Data set	Case
[25]	Fingerprint	Biometric technologies inability to meet the demands for reliability and high accuracy In ideal settings, biometric verification systems are trustworthy, but they might be extremely sensitive to actual environmental variables.	SVM, RSVM	EER 0.13%	FVC2006 datasets	I, V
[26]	Teeth	Enhance recognition precision while reducing computational complexity	PCA/LDA/ EHMM	FDR and FRR error rate of 8.85%	Database Consisting of Teeth Images	I, V

of the retina templates is 40–96 bytes. It has a 1 in 10,000,000 failure rate. Going to invade and slowly, enrolling and retinal scanning. Banking, the military, and governments all use retinal biometrics [31].

Since the retina cannot be seen directly, blood vessels are lit by a low-intensity ray of infrared, or the processed retinal patterns are then photographed using visible light that is then traced over the retina. Retinal pattern variances are turned into digital code kept in databases. A person receiving retinal imaging is supposed to fixate on a separate place for nearly 15 seconds and keep their eyes focused on the scanner and remain still. The blood vessels are found by the coupler [2]. Although the retina scan has already been employed in jail, military sites, nuclear reactors, and other extremely secure locations as well as in medical applications, it is not suitable in many applications just because it requires user cooperation. It is not yet readily available on the market and is presently in the prototype development stage. Retinal image acquisition is challenging and calls for a particular technology and software [32][34].

Researchers pertaining to biometrics determined that a person's hand, especially the palm, possesses specific characteristics that might be applied for authentication purposes. These parameters, which include the palm's thickness and the width regarding the number of fingers, among others, are not special. In later life, the structure of the hand becomes stable. For verification, only the characteristics of the hand are insufficient. However, after the dimensions of the hand and fingers are paired with different ordinary person attributes, they are reliable for identifying purposes. Due to disease, aging, or weight changes, the shape of the hand may change, and this is a time-sensitive issue [31]. Every person has a unique hand shape, and this probably won't change quickly in the future. Hand geometry biometrics, developed in the 1970s, is more ancient than palm print biometrics. It uses straightforward processing methods and is a widely established technology. The study of novel acquisition, preprocessing, and verification techniques starts with hand geometry. The various hand geometry measures are shown in Figure 12.1 below.

The two different forms of hand geometry systems are contact-based and contactless. With the use of five pins, the claimant's hand is put and adjusted in contact-based technology so that it is properly positioned for the camera. The hand image is immediately acquired in contactless. There are two categories of optical scanners. Using a black and white camera and light, the first category a hand in white and black on a bit map is produced. Only 2D aspects of the hand are present in the bitmap image that the computer software is processing. The other category makes advantage of all 3D elements of the hand and detects using two sensors the hand's shape both

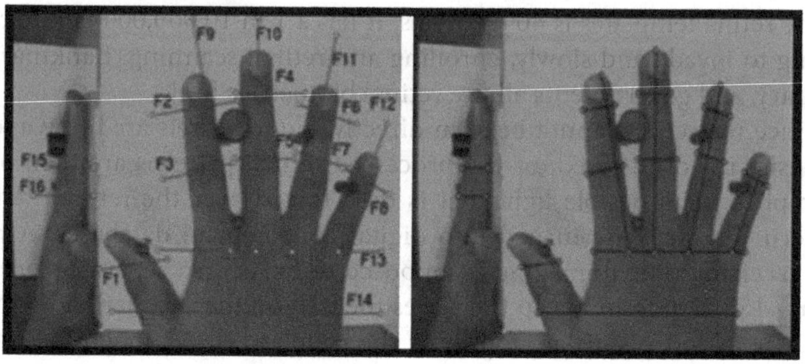

Figure 12.1 Hand geometry [35].

vertically and horizontally. Some scanners only produce the visual signal of the hand shape. To obtain the desired image of the hand, these image signals are digitally processed in the computer [35].

The palm and sides of the hand can be captured in two orthogonal 2D images using an optical camera. Up to 90 dimensions are often measured for the hand geometry, including the finger's height, length, and width, the distance between joints, and the morphologies of knuckles. Systems for recognizing hands solely on their shape rather than their fingerprints. The reader can read even unclean hands. Following the reading, a hand template is created using the hand's geometrical traits, and it is then saved for use in comparing various using hands. When the user touches the scanner with their hand, it typically creates a 3D representation of their hand and measures the size and shape of their wrists and fingers. It simply takes a few seconds for the complete process for the device to compare it with previous database patterns that have been saved. Many offices and factories, as well as laboratories and other business organizations, utilize hand scanners today.

The skin has multiple layers, each of which has unique morphologies and visual characteristics. It has two layers: an outer layer called the epidermis and an interior one called the dermis. Luminism proved that individual differences in the skin's absorption spectrum exist. The two characteristics of the skin that can be utilized [31] to identify a person are its electrical and light properties. Different light wavelengths are sent into the skin via a variety of LEDs, where they are scattered and read by photodiodes for analysis and verification. When light reflects from the skin, there are typically two distinct reflection components: a surface-based specular or interface reflection component that occurs with a diffuse or body reflection component, only in one direction that is formed when some of the sporadic light returns to the skin's surface and emerges through it in various ways. Both individuals' distinctive biological "spectral signature" and information about their skin is tone makeup. The researchers examine the skin with infrared light.

Safie *et al.* [36] have used ECG to create a biometric system. They have used a new feature extraction method called PAR (Pulse Active Ratio) to create a biometric authentication system. In this work, new ECG feature vectors are created using PAR. The proposed approach is tested on 112 participants with 9800 ECG comparisons, yielding a 10% accuracy improvement over other traditional temporal and amplitude feature extraction techniques.

The ECG captures the numerous electrical potentials the heart creates on the surface of the body and is typically taken using electrodes attached to the skin. These electrodes record voltage changes brought on by the heart cells undergoing depolarization and repolarization, causing the heart muscle to contract and relax [37]. The recent increase in the number of accessible portable ECG sensors available for use in innovative applications like fitness monitoring and wearable biometric identification devices has enabled the ubiquitous collection of ECG data.

Sidek *et al.* [38] examine the reliability of electrocardiogram (ECG) signal-based biometric identification in a mobile setting. We put our suggested biometric sample extraction method into practice to evaluate its applicability to various classifiers. The dependability and stability of the subject recognition techniques were validated using subjects from the MIT-BIH Normal Sinus Rhythm Database (NSRDB). Discriminatory features that were extracted from the experiments were then applied to various classifiers to measure performance based on the complexity of our proposed sample extraction method when compared to other related algorithms, the total execution time (TET) applied on various classifiers in various mobile devices, and the classification accuracy when applied to various classification techniques. The results of the experiments demonstrated that their solution reduces the computational complexity of the biometric identification process when compared to other relevant methods. This was demonstrated by the fact that TET values on mobile devices were much lower than those on non-mobile devices while still retaining high accuracy rates in the range of 98.30% to 99.07% across several classifiers. These results therefore validate the applicability of ECG-based biometric identification in a mobile setting.

Benouis *et al.* [39] suggested the use of an improved 1D local binary pattern to derive the most important elements for ECG-based human recognition. ECG signal characteristics typically provide some significant issues due to their inherent sensitivity to noise, artefacts, emotional and behavioral disorders, and other variable factors. In order to address this crucial problem, we employ a one-dimensional local difference pattern (1D-LDP) operator to extract the statistical features that can be used to differentiate between different ECG recordings by comparing the differences between successive neighboring samples. This method captures information about both the micro- and macro-patterns in the heartbeat activity while minimizing the local and global variation that occurs in ECG over time. K-nearest neighbors (KNN), linear support vector machines (SVM), and neural networks were used as the classifier to test its resilience. Results obtained demonstrate that using the MIT-BIH Normal Sinus Rhythm and ECG-ID database, the 1D-LDP operator significantly outperforms the already available 1D-LBP variations.

Uwaechia *et al.* [40], [41] have presented various biometric authentication-based studies using ECG. They have given an overview and discussion of ECG signal preprocessing, feature extraction, feature selection, and feature modification. In order to assess and compare the acquisition procedure, acquisition hardware, and acquisition resolution (bits) for ECG-based biometric systems, they also gave a study of the available ECG databases. Thirdly, they provided a survey on several approaches, including deep learning methods for ECG signal classification, including deep supervised learning, deep semi-supervised learning, and deep unsupervised learning. Finally, they have discussed cutting-edge methods for information fusion in multimodal biometric systems.

Unsupervised Learning Methods for Biometric System

Unsupervised learning involves an architecture receiving inputs x1, x2, x3,... and creating models of the input that may be used for making decisions, predicting inputs in the future, effectively conveying inputs to another machine, etc. Unsupervised learning can be described as the method by which the data shows patterns that go beyond what would be considered unstructured noise. In this sense, the major objectives of unsupervised learning are tasks including dimensionality reduction and grouping.

Several methods have been created to accomplish this, but most strategies are founded on:

- k-means
- Algorithm of expectation-maximization

- Hebbian learning methodology
- CNN
- Gaussian Mixture Models

Unsupervised algorithms for biometric applications are primarily concerned with securing personal data by performing tasks such as behavior pattern recognition, feature level fusion, and meaning extraction from biometric data in an encrypted manner. Additionally, the installation of biometric systems through the use of unsupervised learning proves the precise positioning of biometric characteristics, ensuring improved registration and the creation of learning policies, leading to better categorization. One successful speaker verification system developed by MIT Lincoln Laboratories, for instance, used a global background model with 2048 Gaussian components with diagonal covariance [32]. In addition, Vlachos and Dermatas propose a novel clustering method called the nearest neighbor clustering algorithm (NNCA), which is unsupervised and has been used successfully for retinal vessel segmentation. The Tardos fingerprint recognition code was also improved with an iterative Expectation-Maximization technique for collusion strategy adaptation. Because it is unsupervised, it may be used for highly automated finger vein pattern extraction.

In conclusion, it can be said that unsupervised learning is an effective technique for identifying biometric patterns. However, in most cases, it just serves as a preliminary stage for data analysis, the creation of stronger learning policies, feature fusion (clustering tasks), etc. It may be seen as an early data issue solution method to more accurately categorize labours.

Fifty individuals (female and male) were photographed with a mobile phone (8 megapixels, 3264 x 2448) in [33]. Five photos total were obtained throughout each of the two sessions, with three days remaining to record the second session. There were 500 photos in all. Since rotations around the x and y axes might distort the shape information, they tried to keep all of the photos with a small amount of rotation around the z-axis, between -45 and 45 degrees, of the hand upright. The hands appear horizontal in shots because the photo was taken using a mobile phone. To make hand segmentation easier, all hand photos were placed against a dark background in the foreground. Knowing that the shape is unaffected by image scaling, they have reduced all of the images in VSHI to 0.125 of their original size in order to speed up the authentication process. Their typical hand shape biometric system is shown in Figure 12.2.

Biometric recognition of gait enables the authentication of people based on how they walk. Due to the particular amplitude, frequency, and

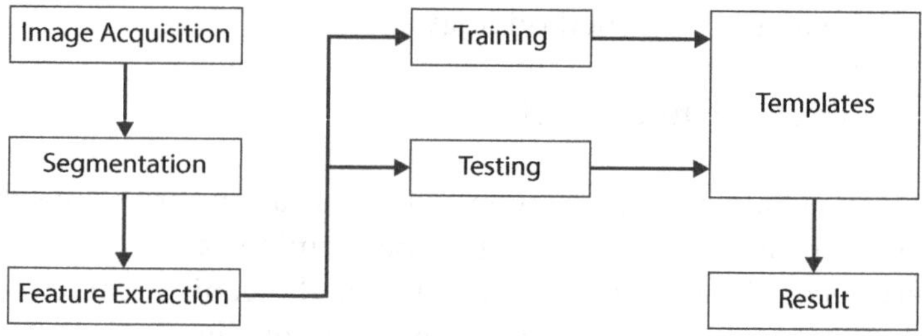

Figure 12.2 A typical hand-shape biometric system.

length of an arm swing, it is a distinctive trait among people. There are various simple techniques to identify this trait. One of them allows for gait biometrics authentication via mobile devices and comes from Inertial Measurement Units (IMU), which include a gyroscope and an accelerometer. In Mantyjarvi *et al.*, a case study of this was given. The accelerometer's gait biometrics data were employed in a framework of template matching and cross-correlation to achieve a combined error rate of 7%. (EER). Many researchers adopted this strategy, suggesting fresh research in the literature as per the analysis of Sprager and Juric [37].

Due to their ability to extract more robust and discriminative features, Deep Learning (DL) techniques have taken the lead in the gait detection field in recent years. One of the first CNN-based DL-based systems was created by Gadaleta and Rossi in Gadaleta and Rossi [37]. The authors outperformed earlier techniques using pre-defined and frequently arbitrary characteristics by using Gait biometrics feature extractors that are universal detection of high rates of misclassification of all features.

RNNs are also among the most effective DL methods for temporal sequences. The OU-ISIR dataset was utilized in a novel strategy that Ackerson *et al.* developed [34]. RNNs with long short-term memories (LSTM), were one of the earliest algorithms created by the authors, and it resulted in an EER of 7.55%.

Zou *et al.* offered an exciting new plan of action [42]. For more robust characteristics, a hybrid DL model incorporating CNNs and LSTM was developed. The suggested model combined the improvements of CNNs and RNNs by removing discriminative features from convolutional maps (processing features as temporal sequences). With 118 participants and data taken from the gyroscope and accelerometer of mobile devices used in the wild, an accuracy of 93.7% was obtained.

Face recognition is a technique that is still in its infancy but is constantly evolving. Researchers in the domains of pattern recognition, image processing, computer vision, neural networks, optics, security, and psychology have all shown an interest in face recognition. The most important use is visual analysis and comprehension, which was created not just by engineers but also by neuroscientists [31].

A common and unobtrusive technique is face recognition. Face recognition is based on the proportions, measurements, and other physiological characteristics of the face. Humans can recognize and distinguish depending on the size of faces, placement, shape, and spatial connections of facial features such as the nose, mouth, eyes, chin, and jaw.

To recognize and find a face in a picture, the face detection process is the first action. The extraction procedure for features from the face is known as feature extraction. This stage is crucial in identifying facial expressions, which confirms the face's individuality and ability to distinguish between two people. Face recognition is the third and last step, and it incorporates the tasks of identification and authentication. The act of comparison between the face picture and the face image template and determining whether the given identification is true or fake is known as either verification or authentication.

The method of identification involves comparing two images of faces to many other face photographs in a database to determine the face's identification with some possibilities and to provide the most likely identification. The workflow of these processes on an input image is shown in Figure 12.3(b).

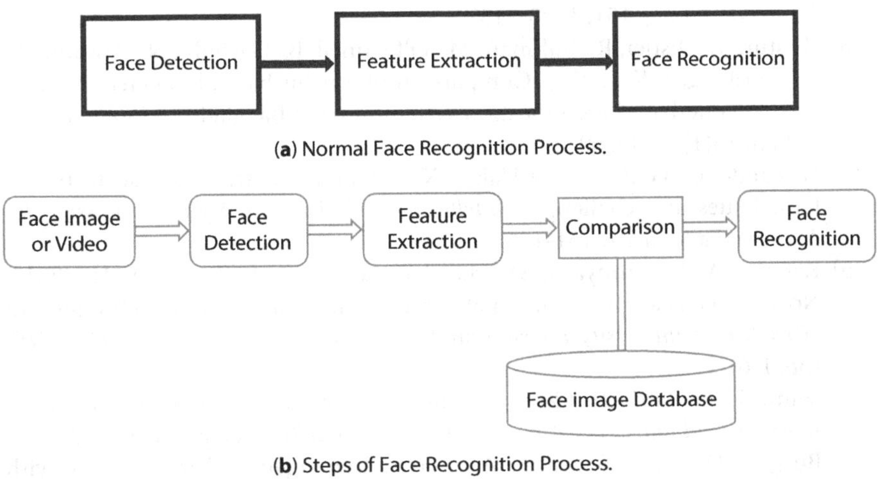

Figure 12.3 (a) standard face recognition procedure, (b) the process of face recognition.

In face recognition, there are three fundamental methods [1]. In the feature-based method, the local characteristics of the face, such as the eyes, mouth, and nose, are employed to segment the face and act as the input for face detection.

In a holistic approach, the full face is employed as an input for both face detection and face recognition. Feature-based and holistic techniques are used in a hybrid approach. The Template-Based Approach, another popular technique, determines the relationship between an input image and a typical face pattern by using all of the facial features [1].

Conclusion

This chapter includes various traits to be used as biometric techniques, their benefits as biometric techniques and the challenges that are involved using these traits to create a authentication system. Several studies have used supervised and unsupervised learning techniques to overcome those challenges that occurred in traditional biometric system.

References

[1] Sundararajan, K., & Woodard, D. L. (2018). Deep learning for biometrics: A survey. *ACM Computing Surveys (CSUR)*, 51(3), 1-34.

[2] Nigam, A., & Gupta, P. (2015). Designing an accurate hand biometric based authentication system fusing finger knuckleprint and palmprint. *Neurocomputing*, 151, 1120-1132.

[3] Khatun, F., Distler, R., Rahman, M., O'Donnell, B., Gachuhi, N., Alwani, M., ... & Friberg, I. K. (2022). Comparison of a palm-based biometric solution with a name-based identification system in rural Bangladesh. *Global Health Action*, 15(1), 2045769.

[4] Gawande, U., Golhar, Y., & Hajari, K. (2017). Biometric-based security system: Issues and challenges. *Intelligent Techniques in Signal Processing for Multimedia Security*, 151-176.

[5] Kataria, A. N., Adhyaru, D. M., Sharma, A. K., & Zaveri, T. H. (2013, November). A survey of automated biometric authentication techniques. In *2013 Nirma university international conference on engineering (NUiCONE)* (pp. 1-6). IEEE.

[6] Saini, R., & Rana, N. (2014). Comparison of various biometric methods. *International Journal of Advances in Science and Technology*, 2(1), 24-30.

[7] Burgan, D. A., & Baker, L. A. (2009). Investigating Self-Assembly with Macaroni. *Journal of Chemical Education*, 86(6), 704A.

[8] Bouridane, A. (2009). Introduction and Preliminaries on Biometrics and Forensics Systems. In *Imaging for Forensics and Security* (pp. 1-10). Springer, Boston, MA.
[9] Sharif, M., Raza, M., Shah, J. H., Yasmin, M., & Fernandes, S. L. (2019). An overview of biometrics methods. *Handbook of Multimedia Information Security: Techniques and Applications*, 15-35.
[10] Galbally, J., Fierrez, J., Ortega-Garcia, J. (2007). Vulnerabilities in biometric systems: Attacks and recent advances in liveness detection. *Database*, 1(3), 4.
[11] Jain, A. K., Nandakumar, K., Nagar, A. (2008). Biometric template security. *EURASIP Journal on Advances in Signal Processing*, 2008, 113.
[12] H. Kaur, P. Khanna, Gaussian Random Projection Based Non-invertible Cancelable Biometric Templates, *Procedia Computer Science*, vol. 54, pp. 661–670, 2015.
[13] M.A. Dabbah, W.L. Woo, S.S. Dlay, Secure authentication for face recognition, in *IEEE Symposium on Computational Intelligence in Image and Signal Processing, CIISP 2007*. hskip 1em plus 0.5em minus 0.4em2007, pp. 121–126.
[14] M.A. Dabbah, W.L. Woo, S.S. Dlay, Appearance-Based Biometric Recognition: Secure Authentication and Cancellability, in *IEEE 15th International Conference on Digital Signal Processing*. hskip 1em plus 0.5em minus 0.4em2007, pp. 479–482.
[15] P. Li, X. Yang, H. Qiao, K. Cao, E. Liu, J. Tian, An effective biometric cryptosystem combining fingerprints with error correction codes, *Expert Systems with Applications*, vol. 39, no. 7, pp. 6562–6574,2012.
[16] Dong, X., Jin, Z., Zhao, L., Guo, Z., (2021). BioCanCrypto: An LDPC coded bio-cryptosystem on fingerprint cancellable template, in: *2021 IEEE International Joint Conference on Biometrics (IJCB)*, Shenzhen, China, pp. 1-8.
[17] Y. Imamverdiyev, A.B.J. Teoh, J. Kim, Biometric cryptosystem based on discretized fingerprint texture descriptors, *Expert Systems with Applications*, vol. 40, no. 5, pp. 1888–1901, 2013.
[18] C. Rathgeb, C. Busch, Cancelable multi-biometrics: Mixing iris-codes based on adaptive bloom filters, *Computers & Security*, vol. 42, pp. 1–12, 2014.
[19] Gragnaniello, D., Sansone, C., Verdoliva, L. (2015). Iris liveness detection for mobile devices based on local descriptors. *Pattern Recognition Letters*, 57, 81-87.
[20] Mondal, S., Bours, P. (2015. A computational approach to the continuous authentication biometric system. *Information Sciences*, 304, 28-53.
[21] Chakraborty, S., Balasubramanian, V., Panchanathan, S. (2013). Generalized batch mode active learning for face-based biometric recognition. *Pattern Recognition*, 46(2), 497-508.
[22] Bharadwaj, S., Bhatt, H. S., Singh, R., Vatsa, M., Noore, A. (2015). QFuse: Online learning framework for adaptive biometric system. *Pattern Recognition*, 48(11), 3428-3439.

[23] Arigbabu, O. A., Ahmad, S. M. S., Adnan, W. A. W., Yussof, S. (2015). Integration of multiple soft biometrics for human identification. *Pattern Recognition Letters*, 68, 278-287.
[24] De Marsico, M., Petrosino, A., Ricciardi, S. (2016). Iris Recognition through Machine Learning Techniques: a Survey. *Pattern Recognition Letters.*
[25] Nanni, L., Lumini, A., Ferrara, M., Cappelli, R. (2015). Combining biometric matchers by means of machine learning and statistical approaches. *Neurocomputing*, 149, 526-535.
[26] Kim, D. J., Shin, J. H., Hong, K. S. (2010). Teeth recognition based on multiple attempts in mobile device. *Journal of Network and Computer Applications*, 33(3), 283-292.
[27] Bouadjenek, N., Nemmour, H., Chibani, Y. (2015). Robust softbiometrics prediction from off-line handwriting analysis. *Applied Soft Computing.*
[28] Kim, D. J., Chung, K. W., Hong, K. S. (2010). Person authentication using face, teeth and voice modalities for mobile device security. IEEE.
[29] Transactions on Consumer Electronics, 56(4), 2678-2685.[31] Hazen, T. J., Weinstein, E., Park, A. (2003, November). Towards robust person recognition on handheld devices using face and speaker identification technologies. In *Proceedings of the 5th International Conference on Multimodal Interfaces* (pp. 289-292). ACM.
[30] Tresadern, P. A., McCool, C., Poh, N., Matejka, P., Hadid, A., Levy, C., Marcel, S. (2012). Mobile biometrics (mobio): Joint face and voice verification for a mobile platform. *IEEE Pervasive Computing*, 99.
[31] Sabhanayagam, T., Venkatesan, V. P., & Senthamaraikannan, K. (2018). A comprehensive survey on various biometric systems. *International Journal of Applied Engineering Research*, 13(5), 2276-2297.
[32] Ortiz, N., Hernández, R. D., Jimenez, R., Mauledeoux, M., & Avilés, O. (2018). Survey of biometric pattern recognition via machine learning techniques. *Contemporary Engineering Sciences*, 11(34), 1677-1694.
[33] Hassanat, A. B., Btoush, E., Abbadi, M. A., Al-Mahadeen, B. M., Al-Awadi, M., Mseidein, K. I., ... & Al-alem, F. A. (2017, April). Victory sign biometrie for terrorists identification: Preliminary results. In *2017 8th International Conference on Information and Communication Systems (ICICS)* (pp. 182-187). IEEE.
[34] Jain, A. K., & Li, S. Z. (2011). *Handbook of Face Recognition* (Vol. 1). New York: Springer.
[35] Srivastava, H. (2013). Personal identification using iris recognition system, a review. *International Journal of Engineering Research and Applications (IJERA)*, 3(3), 449-453.
[36] Safie, S. I., Soraghan, J. J., & Petropoulakis, L. (2011). Electrocardiogram (ECG) biometric authentication using pulse active ratio (PAR). *IEEE Transactions on Information Forensics and Security*, 6(4), 1315-1322.

[37] Sahli, H., Mouelhi, A., Ben Slama, A., Sayadi, M., & Rachdi, R. (2019). Supervised classification approach of biometric measures for automatic fetal defect screening in head ultrasound images. *Journal of Medical Engineering & Technology*, 43(5), 279-286.

[38] Sidek, K. A., Mai, V., & Khalil, I. (2014). Data mining in mobile ECG based biometric identification. *Journal of Network and Computer Applications*, 44, 83-91.

[39] Benouis, M., Mostefai, L., Costen, N., & Regouid, M. (2021). ECG based biometric identification using one-dimensional local difference pattern. *Biomedical Signal Processing and Control*, 64, 102226.

[40] Uwaechia, A. N., & Ramli, D. A. (2021). A comprehensive survey on ECG signals as new biometric modality for human authentication: Recent advances and future challenges. *IEEE Access*.

[41] Madduluri, S., Kumar, T. K., (2023).Feature selection models using 2D convolution neural network for ECG based biometric detection - A brief survey, in: *2023 4th International Conference on Electronics and Sustainable Communication Systems (ICESC)*, Coimbatore, India, pp. 1650-1654.

[42] Zhou, M., Tang, Y., Tian, Z., & Geng, X. (2017). Semi-supervised learning for indoor hybrid fingerprint database calibration with low effort. *IEEE Access*, 5, 4388-4400.

About the Editors

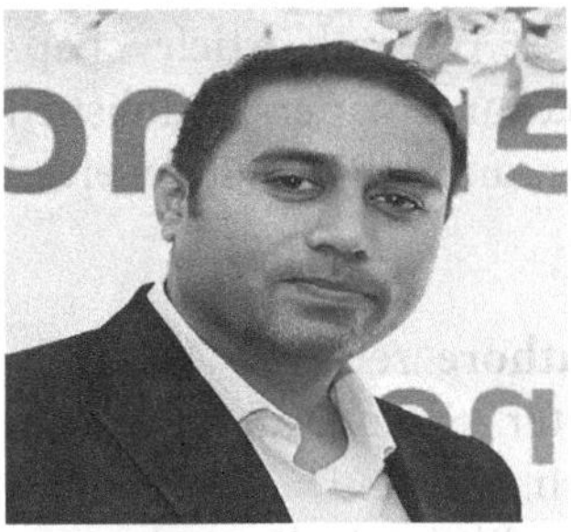

Dr. Suman Kumar Swanrkar received a Ph.D. (CSE) degree in 2021 from Kalinga University, Nayaraipur. He received M.Tech. (CSE) degree in 2015 from the Rajiv Gandhi Proudyogiki Vishwavidyalaya, Bhopal, India. He has 2+ year of experience in IT industry as Software Engineer and 8+ year of experience in Educational Institutes as Assistant Professor. Currently associated with Shri Shankaracharya Institute of Professional Management and Technology Raipur, Chhattisgarh, India as Assistant Professor in Computer Science & Engineering Department.

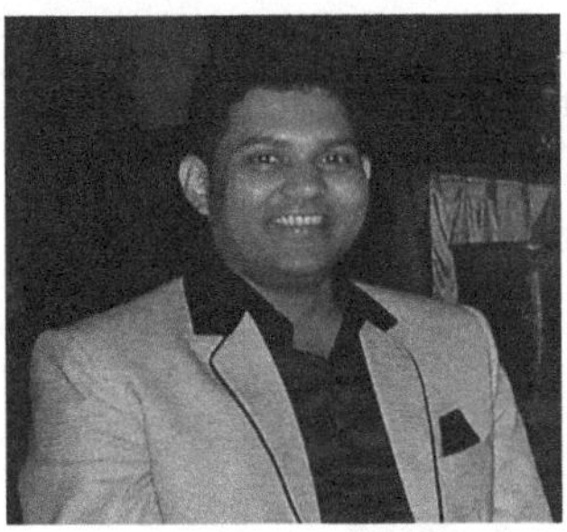

Dr. JP Patra is a Professor at Shri Shankaracharya Institute of Professional Management and Technology, Raipur under Chhattisgarh Swami Vivekanand Technical University, Bhilai, India. He holds more than 17 years of experience in research, teaching in these areas Artificial Intelligence, Analysis and Design of Algorithms, Cryptography and Network Security. He has Published and granted Indian/Australian patents. He has contributed to book chapters, published by Elsevier, Springer and IGI Global. He is associated with AICTE-IDEA LAB, IIT Bombay and IIT Kharagpur as a Coordinator.

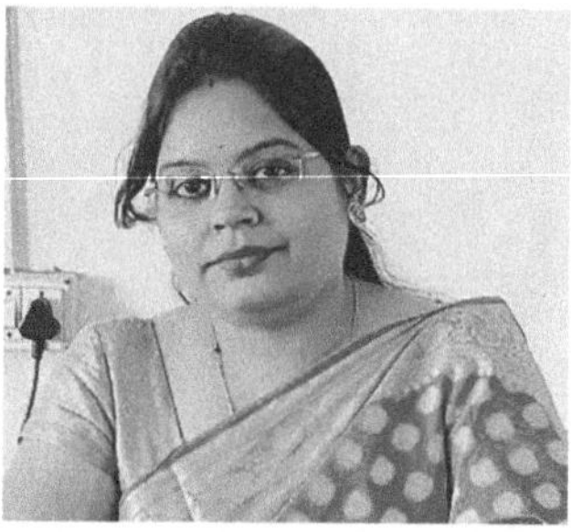

Dr. Sapna Singh Kshatri Received the Ph.D. degree from MATS University, Raipur. She has completed her M.C.A. from Rungta College of Eng. & Technology Bhilai, India. Recently She is working as Assistant Professor in Shri Shankaracharya Institute of Professional Management and Technology (SSIPMT), In Artificial Intelligence and Machine Learning Department. She has 6 years of teaching and academic experience over 15 research article, chapters, and national and international conference and papers, published international book in IGI global, wiley, Bentham and IIP. She is received Best Paper Awards in International Conferences.

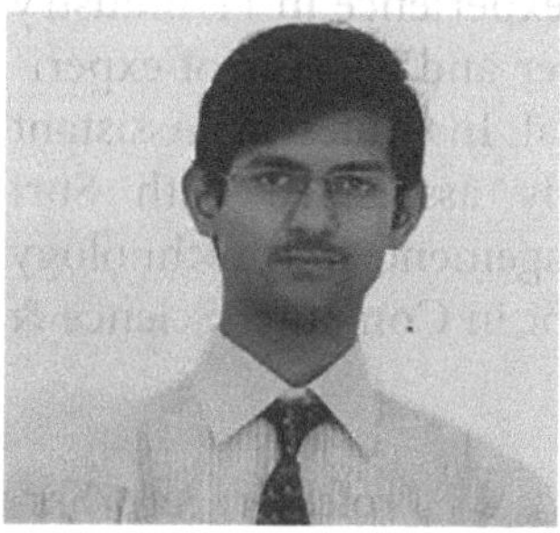

Yogesh Kumar Rathore received M. Tech. degree in Computer Science Engineering from Chhattisgarh Swami Vivekanand Technical University, Bhilai, India in the year 2010.He has 16 years experience of working, as an Assistant Professor (Department of Computer Science Engineering) at Shri Shankaracharya Institute of Professional Management and Technology, Raipur. Currently, he is also a Ph.D. scholar (part-time) at the Department of Information Technology, National Institute of Technology, Raipur. He has published more than 40 research papers in various conferences and journals including Scopus and SCI index.

Index

Also of Interest

Also in the Series, "Advances in Data Engineering and Machine Learning"

DATA ENGINEERING AND DATA SCIENCE: Concepts and Applications, Edited by Kukatlapalli Pradeep Kumar, Aynur Unal, Vinay Jha Pillai, Hari Murthy, and M. Niranjanamurthy, ISBN: 9781119841876. Written and edited by one of the most prolific and well-known experts in the field and his team, this exciting new volume is the "one stop shop" for the concepts and applications of data science and engineering for data scientists across many industries.

MEDICAL IMAGING, Edited by H. S. Sanjay, and M. Niranjanamurthy ISBN: 9781119785392. Written and edited by a team of experts in the field, this is the most comprehensive and up-to-date study of and reference for the practical applications of medical imaging for engineers, scientists, students, and medical professionals.

ADVANCES IN DATA SCIENCE AND ANALYTICS, Edited by M. Niranjanamurthy, Hemant Kumar Gianey, and Amir H. Gandomi, ISBN: 9781119791881. Presenting the concepts and advances of data science and analytics, this volume, written and edited by a global team of experts, also goes into the practical applications that can be utilized across multiple disciplines and industries, for both the engineer and the student, focusing on machining learning, big data, business intelligence, and analytics.

WIRELESS COMMUNICATION SECURITY: Mobile and Network Security Protocols, Edited by Manju Khari, Manisha Bharti, and M. Niranjanamurthy, ISBN: 9781119777144. Presenting the concepts and advances of wireless communication security, this volume, written and edited by a global team of experts, also goes into the practical applications for the engineer, student, and other industry professionals.

ARTIFICIAL INTELLIGENCE AND DATA MINING IN SECURITY FRAMEWORKS, Edited by Neeraj Bhargava, Ritu Bhargava, Pramod Singh Rathore, and Rashmi Agrawal, ISBN: 9781119760405. Written and edited by a team of experts in the field, this outstanding new volume offers solutions to the problems of security, outlining the concepts behind allowing computers to learn from experience and understand the world in terms of a hierarchy of concepts.

MACHINE LEARNING AND DATA SCIENCE: Fundamentals and Applications, Edited by Prateek Agrawal, Charu Gupta, Anand Sharma, Vishu Madaan, and Nisheeth Joshi, ISBN: 9781119775614. Written and edited by a team of experts in the field, this collection of papers reflects the most up-to-date and comprehensive current state of machine learning and data science for industry, government, and academia.

SECURITY ISSUES AND PRIVACY CONCERNS IN INDUSTRY 4.0 APPLICATIONS, Edited by Shibin David, R. S. Anand, V. Jeyakrishnan, and M. Niranjanamurthy, ISBN: 9781119775621. Written and edited by a team of international experts, this is the most comprehensive and up-to-date coverage of the security and privacy issues surrounding Industry 4.0 applications, a must-have for any library.

Check out these other related titles from Scrivener Publishing

MATHEMATICS AND COMPUTER SCIENCE VOLUME 2, Edited by Sharmistha Ghosh, M. Niranjanamurthy, Krishanu Deyasi, Biswadip Basu Mallik, and Santanu Das, ISBN: 9781119896326. This second volume in a new multi-volume set builds on the basic concepts and fundamentals laid out in the previous volume, presenting the reader with more advanced and cutting-edge topics being developed in this exciting field.

MATHEMATICS AND COMPUTER SCIENCE VOLUME 1: Concepts and Applications, Edited by Sharmistha Ghosh, M. Niranjanamurthy, Krishanu Deyasi, Biswadip Basu Mallik, and Santanu Das, ISBN: 9781119879671. This first volume in a new multi-volume set gives readers the basic concepts and applications for diverse ideas and innovations in the field of computing together with its growing interactions with mathematics.

DATA WRANGLING: Concepts, Applications, and Tools, Edited by M. Niranjanamurthy, Kavita Sheoran, Geetika Dhand, and Prabhjot Kaurk, ISBN: 9781119879688. Written and edited by some of the world's top experts in the field, this exciting new volume provides state-of-the-art research and latest technological breakthroughs in next-data wrangling, its theoretical concepts, practical applications, and tools for solving everyday problems.

CONVERGENCE OF DEEP LEARNING IN CYBER-IOT SYSTEMS AND SECURITY, Edited by Rajdeep Chakraborty, Anupam Ghosh, Jyotsna Kumar Mandal and S. Balamurugan, ISBN: 9781119857211. In-depth analysis of Deep Learning-based cyber-IoT systems and security which will be the industry leader for the next ten years.

MACHINE INTELLIGENCE, BIG DATA ANALYTICS, AND IOT IN IMAGE PROCESSING: Practical Applications, Edited by Ashok Kumar, Megha Bhushan, José A. Galindo, Lalit Garg and Yu-Chen Hu, ISBN: 9781119865049. Discusses both theoretical and practical aspects of how to harness advanced technologies to develop practical applications such as drone-based surveillance, smart transportation, healthcare, farming solutions, and robotics used in automation.

MACHINE LEARNING TECHNIQUES AND ANALYTICS FOR CLOUD SECURITY, Edited by Rajdeep Chakraborty, Anupam Ghosh and Jyotsna Kumar Mandal, ISBN: 9781119762256. This book covers new methods, surveys, case studies, and policy with almost all machine learning techniques and analytics for cloud security solutions.

Printed in the USA/Agawam, MA
September 16, 2026

910661.087